T0263303

Small Animal Orthopedic Medicine

Editors

FELIX DUERR
LINDSAY ELAM

VETERINARY CLINICS OF NORTH AMERICA: SMALL ANIMAL PRACTICE

www.vetsmall.theclinics.com

July 2022 • Volume 52 • Number 4

ELSEVIER

1600 John F. Kennedy Boulevard • Suite 1800 • Philadelphia, Pennsylvania, 19103-2899
http://www.vetsmall.theclinics.com

VETERINARY CLINICS OF NORTH AMERICA: SMALL ANIMAL PRACTICE Volume 52, Number 4 July 2022 ISSN 0195-5616, ISBN-13: 978-0-323-98795-0

Editor: Stacy Eastman
Developmental Editor: Axell Ivan Jade Purificacion

Veterinary Clinics of North America: Small Animal Practice (ISSN 0195-5616) is published bimonthly by Elsevier Inc., 360 Park Avenue South, New York, NY 10010-1710. Months of issue are January, March, May, July, September, and November. Business and Editorial Offices: 1600 John F. Kennedy Blvd., Ste. 1800, Philadelphia, PA 19103-2899. Customer Service Office: 3251 Riverport Lane, Maryland Heights, MO 63043. Periodicals postage paid at New York, NY and additional mailing offices. Subscription prices are $369.00 per year (domestic individuals), $980.00 per year (domestic institutions), $100.00 per year (domestic students/residents), $465.00 per year (Canadian individuals), $1029.00 per year (Canadian institutions), $503.00 per year (international individuals), $1029.00 per year (international institutions), $100.00 per year (Canadian students/residents), and $220.00 per year (international students/residents). To receive student/resident rate, orders must be accompanied by name of affiliated institution, date of term, and the *signature* of program/residency coordinator on institution letterhead. Orders will be billed at individual rate until proof of status is received. Foreign air speed delivery is included in all *Clinics* subscription prices. All prices are subject to change without notice. **POSTMASTER:** Send address changes to *Veterinary Clinics of North America: Small Animal Practice*, Elsevier Health Sciences Division, Subscription Customer Service, 3251 Riverport Lane, Maryland Heights, MO 63043. Customer Service (orders, claims, online, change of address): Elsevier Periodicals Customer Service, Elsevier Health Sciences Division Subscription **Customer Service 3251 Riverport Lane Maryland Heights, MO 63043. Tel: 1-800-654-2452 (U.S. and Canada); 314-447-8871 (outside U.S. and Canada). Fax: 314-447-8029. E-mail: journalscustomerservice-usa@elsevier.com (for print support); journalsonlinesupport-usa@elsevier.com (for online support).**

Reprints. For copies of 100 or more of articles in this publication, please contact the Commercial Reprints Department, Elsevier Inc., 360 Park Avenue South, New York, NY 10010-1710. Tel.: 212-633-3874; Fax: 212-633-3820; E-mail: reprints@elsevier.com.

Veterinary Clinics of North America: Small Animal Practice is also published in Japanese by Inter Zoo Publishing Co., Ltd., Aoyama Crystal-Bldg 5F, 3-5-12 Kitaaoyama, Minato-ku, Tokyo 107-0061, Japan.

Veterinary Clinics of North America: Small Animal Practice is covered in *Current Contents/Agriculture, Biology and Environmental Sciences, Science Citation Index, ASCA, MEDLINE/PubMed (Index Medicus), Excerpta Medica, and BIOSIS.*

Contributors

EDITORS

FELIX DUERR, Dr. med. vet., MS
Diplomate, American College of Veterinary Surgeons (Small Animal); Diplomate, European College of Veterinary Surgeons; Diplomate, American College of Veterinary Sports Medicine and Rehabilitation; Associate Professor, Small Animal Orthopedic Medicine and Mobility, Department of Clinical Sciences, Colorado State University Fort Collins, Colorado, USA

LINDSAY ELAM, DVM, MPH
Diplomate, American College of Veterinary Sports Medicine and Rehabilitation; Assistant Professor, Small Animal Orthopedic Medicine and Mobility, Department of Clinical Sciences, Colorado State University, Fort Collins, Colorado, USA

AUTHORS

LEILANI ALVAREZ, DVM, CVA, CCRT
Diplomate, American College of Veterinary Sports Medicine and Rehabilitation; Director, Integrative and Rehabilitative Medicine, Animal Medical Center, New York, New York, USA

JENNIFER BROWN, DVM
Diplomate, American College of Veterinary Sports Medicine and Rehabilitation; Florida Veterinary Rehabilitation and Sports Medicine, Tampa, Florida, USA

BRITTANY JEAN CARR, DVM, CCRT
Diplomate, American College of Veterinary Sports Medicine and Rehabilitation; The Veterinary Sports Medicine and Rehabilitation Center, South Carolina, USA

CHRIS W. FRYE, DVM
Diplomate, American College of Veterinary Sports Medicine and Rehabilitation; Assistant Clinical Professor and Section Chief of Sports Medicine, Department of Clinical Sciences, Cornell University College of Veterinary Medicine, Ithaca, New York, USA

LAURI-JO GAMBLE, DVM, CCRP, CVA
Diplomate, American College of Veterinary Sports Medicine and Rehabilitation; Sports Medicine and Rehabilitation Service, Ottawa Animal Emergency and Specialty Hospital, Ottawa, Ontario, Canada

JULIETTE HART, DVM, MS, CCRT, CVA
Diplomate, American College of Veterinary Sports Medicine and Rehabilitation; Diplomate, Sports Medicine and Rehabilitation – Small Animal; Specialty Advisory Board, Sports Medicine and Rehabilitation – NVA Compassion First Hospitals, Director, Sports Medicine and Rehabilitation Department, Medical Director, Animal Emergency and Specialty Center, Parker, Colorado, USA

NINA R. KIEVES, DVM
Diplomate, American College of Veterinary Surgeons (Small Animal); Diplomate American College of Veterinary Sports Medicine and Rehabilitation (Canine); Associate Professor, Small Animal Orthopedic Surgery, Director, Sports Medicine and Rehabilitation, The Ohio State University, Department of Veterinary Clinical Sciences, Columbus, Ohio, USA

DAVID LEVINE, PT, PhD, DPT, CCRP, FAPTA
Department of Health, Education and Professional Studies, The University of Tennessee, Department of Physical Therapy, The University of Tennessee at Chattanooga, Chattanooga, Tennessee, USA

PETER J. LOTSIKAS, DVM
Diplomate, American College of Veterinary Surgeons – Small Animal; Diplomate, American College of Veterinary Sports Medicine and Rehabilitation; Skylos Sports Medicine, Frederick, Maryland, USA

CAROLINA MEDINA, DVM, CVA, CVPP
Diplomate, American College of Veterinary Sports Medicine and Rehabilitation; Coral Springs Animal Hospital, Coral Springs, Florida, USA

ALLISON MILLER, DVM, CCRP
Lecturer, Department of Biomedical Sciences, Cornell University College of Veterinary Medicine, Ithaca, New York, USA

ERIN MISCIOSCIA, DVM, CVA
Diplomate, American College of Veterinary Sports Medicine and Rehabilitation; Clinical Assistant Professor, Department of Comparative, Diagnostic and Population Medicine, College of Veterinary Medicine, University of Florida, Gainesville, Florida, USA

CHRISTINA MONTALBANO, VMD, CCRP, CVA
NorthStar VETS, Robbinsville, New Jersey, USA

MEGAN NELSON, BS, CVT
Twin Cities Animal Rehabilitation and Sports Medicine Clinic, Burnsville, Minnesota, USA

CYNTHIA M. OTTO, DVM, PhD
Diplomate, American College of Veterinary Emergency and Critical Care; Diplomate, American College of Veterinary Sports Medicine and Rehabilitation; Penn Vet Working Dog Center, Clinical Sciences and Advanced Medicine, School of Veterinary Medicine, University of Pennsylvania, Philadelphia, Pennsylvania, USA

MEGHAN T. RAMOS, VMD
Penn Vet Working Dog Center, Clinical Sciences and Advanced Medicine, School of Veterinary Medicine, University of Pennsylvania, Philadelphia, Pennsylvania, USA

BARBARA ESTEVE RATSCH, PhD, DVM, CCRP
Department of Physical Medicine, Evidensia Sørlandet Animal Hospital, Hamresanden, Norway

JENNIFER REPAC, DVM, CVA, CCRT, CVCH, Certified Veterinary Chiropractic
Diplomate, American College of Veterinary Sports Medicine and Rehabilitation; Clinical Assistant Professor, Department of Comparative, Diagnostic and Population Medicine, College of Veterinary Medicine, University of Florida, Gainesville, Florida, USA

JULIA TOMLINSON, BVSC, MS, PhD
Diplomate, American College of Veterinary Surgeons; Diplomate, American College of Veterinary Sports Medicine and Rehabilitation; Twin Cities Animal Rehabilitation and Sports Medicine Clinic, Burnsville, Minnesota, USA

JOSEPH J. WAKSHLAG, DVM, PhD
Diplomate, American College of Veterinary Internal Medicine; Diplomate, American College of Veterinary Sports Medicine and Rehabilitation; Department of Clinical Sciences, Cornell University College of Veterinary Medicine, Ithaca, New York, USA

Contents

Preface: From Prevention to Injection: Exploring the Breadth of Orthopedic Medicine **xi**

Felix Duerr and Lindsay Elam

Canine Comprehensive Mobility Assessment **841**

Christina Montalbano

 Video content accompanies this article at http://www.vetsmall.theclinics.com.

A comprehensive mobility assessment goes beyond the orthopedic or neurologic examination for the localization of pathology. This assessment involves attention to the dog's posture and stance, a hands-on examination with special attention to soft tissue structures, and the performance of functional assessments. A comprehensive mobility assessment can guide advanced diagnostic testing as well as providing a foundation in the formulation of a successful treatment plan.

Objective Gait Analysis: Review and Clinical Applications **857**

Nina R. Kieves

Objective kinetic and kinematic data can be used as an objective measure of treatment intervention over time but can also be used to evaluate progress of clinical patients. Force plate and pressure sensitive walkway systems both offer the clinician the ability to obtain useful kinetic data, whereas additional equipment is required to obtain kinematic data. Which system is preferred depends on what specific data the researcher or clinician hopes to acquire; both are accurate and consistent, and each offers pros and cons compared with the other that must be considered.

Orthopedic Imaging: A Practical Clinical Guide **869**

Jennifer Brown

Many imaging options are available to the practitioner both in-house and on a referral basis to help make a definitive diagnosis for orthopedic injuries. To guide treatment, a complete understanding of the nature and extent of the injury is ideal. While a thorough orthopedic physical examination is the first step, a complete diagnostic work-up will include at least one and often more than one imaging modality. The goal of this article is to discuss the imaging options for some of the more common orthopedic issues encountered in dogs to help guide the practitioner through the selection of which should be considered to accomplish a diagnosis.

Canine Mobility Maintenance and Promotion of a Healthy Lifestyle **907**

Meghan T. Ramos and Cynthia M. Otto

This article highlights the recommendations and considerations for maintaining a healthy canine lifestyle. A key component of a healthy lifestyle is the enhancement and optimization of mobility. Mobility is essential in

maintaining a high quality of life and involves the interplay of a dog's structure, posture, body condition score, physical exercise, and a healthy human-animal bond throughout a dog's lifetime.

Evidence-Based Complementary and Alternative Canine Orthopedic Medicine **925**

Erin Miscioscia and Jennifer Repac

The use of complementary and alternative veterinary medicine (CAVM) continues to become more widespread, especially for the management of chronic pain conditions such as canine osteoarthritis. Many patients have comorbidities that preclude traditional medical options, have not adequately responded to conventional therapies, or have owners interested in pursuing a complementary approach. Evidence-based CAVM can serve as a safe and effective adjunct to manage chronic pain conditions. There is growing evidence in the veterinary literature for the use of acupuncture and some herbal supplements in the multimodal management of canine osteoarthritis. The majority of evidence supporting chiropractic is limited to equine and human literature.

Clinical Guide to Obesity and Nonherbal Nutraceuticals in Canine Orthopedic Conditions **939**

Barbara Esteve Ratsch, David Levine, and Joseph J. Wakshlag

The typical canine rehabilitation patient with orthopedic disease may differ in its nutritional needs, with the assumption that most patients will be on a complete and balanced commercial dog food that is not enriched with agents for ameliorating their condition. For a significant number of rehabilitation patients, obesity is a major issue where hypocaloric diet plans are often implemented and are covered extensively elsewhere (VCNA Small Animal Practice May 2021). The focus of this article will be implementation of physical activity or structured physical exercise protocols and how they might be used in combination with a typical hypocaloric diet plan, a diet low in calories. Considering the limited information regarding physical activity or structured exercise programs in dogs, a human comparative assessment of efficacy is fundamental as a baseline of information regarding typical interventions. In addition, many of these long-term rehabilitation cases typically exhibit osteoarthritis (OA) and as part of case management, there is a need to implement nutrient or nutraceutical intervention to either diminish the progression of OA or help with pain control measures, particularly for the nonsteroidal anti-inflammatory intolerant patient. Nutraceutical intervention comes in many forms from botanicals to nutritional enhancement; botanicals will be covered elsewhere in this issue. This overview of nutraceuticals will cover nonbotanical interventions including fish oil, glucosamine/chondroitin, avocado/soybean unsaponifiables, undenatured collagen, green lipped mussel, and egg shell membrane supplementation.

Joint Injection Techniques and Indications **959**

Chris W. Frye and Allison Miller

Indications for injecting synovial joints may include diagnostic, therapeutic, or combination. Diagnostic injectates aim to reduce or eliminate the contribution of pain to lameness and may be assessed both subjectively or objectively by the clinician. Diagnostic joint injections are not specific for a disease and their limitations must be remembered when interpreting a response—including false-negative results. Patient selection and sterile technique throughout the procedure minimize adverse effects. Risks of intra-articular (IA) injections may include transient soreness, cartilage damage, and, rarely, septic arthritis. Ultrasound guidance with a trained clinician may provide further benefits including the reduction of periprocedural discomfort, reduction in iatrogenic cartilage damage during needle insertion, and improvement in synovial fluid feedback. The removal of some synovial fluid before administering an IA injection should be considered to confirm needle placement, provide diagnostic sampling, and help accommodate injectate volume.

Intra-articular Injectates: What to Use and Why **967**

Peter J. Lotsikas

Intra-articular injections are a nonsurgical treatment modality that can be used to manage osteoarthritis, naturally occurring or surgically induced acute synovitis, and intra-articular ligamentous or tendon injury. This option may be assistive for patients in which other conservative modalities are ineffective, or in conjunction with other forms of treatment. It may also be used as the primary treatment. Injectates labeled for use in companion animal joints include corticosteroids and viscosupplements. Additional injectates, that are not specifically approved for use in companion animals are but are reported in the literature, include orthobiologics and a radioisotope of Tin-117m.

Platelet-Rich Plasma as an Orthobiologic: Clinically Relevant Considerations **977**

Brittany Jean Carr

Platelet-rich plasma (PRP) is an autologous blood-derived product processed to concentrate platelets and the associated growth factors. PRP has been shown to be relatively well-tolerated and safe to use for a number of conditions in humans, equines, and canines. There are multiple commercial systems that have been validated for canine use. These systems use a variety of methodologies to produce a PRP product. However, PRP products have been shown to differ greatly between systems. Further study is needed to fully elucidate optimal component concentrations for various indications.

Physical Rehabilitation for Small Animals **997**

Lauri-Jo Gamble

Physical rehabilitation incorporates several elements, including but not limited to therapeutic exercises, manual therapy, and physical modalities. Understanding of the effects, indications, contraindications, and precautions is essential for proper use, while understanding of the diagnosis, assessment of the stage of tissue healing and repair, and accurate clinical assessment of the functional limitations are essential when establishing a physical rehabilitation plan.

patient care solutions in many services within a hospital. After patient discharge, the team can then aid in the client and patient recovery at home with key home exercise programs and communications to bolster the patient's home recovery, ongoing rehabilitation, and eventual return to function.

VETERINARY CLINICS OF NORTH AMERICA: SMALL ANIMAL PRACTICE

FORTHCOMING ISSUES

September 2022
Telemedicine
Aaron Smiley, *Editor*

November 2022
Vector-Borne Diseases
Linda Kidd, *Editor*

January 2023
Clinical Pathology
Maxey L. Wellman and M. Judith Radin, *Editors*

RECENT ISSUES

May 2022
Hot Topics in Small Animal Medicine
Lisa Powell, *Editor*

March 2022
Soft Tissue Surgery
Nicole J. Buote, *Editor*

January 2022
Veterinary Dentistry and Oral Surgery
Alexander M. Reiter, *Editor*

SERIES OF RELATED INTEREST

Veterinary Clinics: Exotic Animal Practice
https://www.vetexotic.theclinics.com/

Preface
From Prevention to Injection: Exploring the Breadth of Orthopedic Medicine

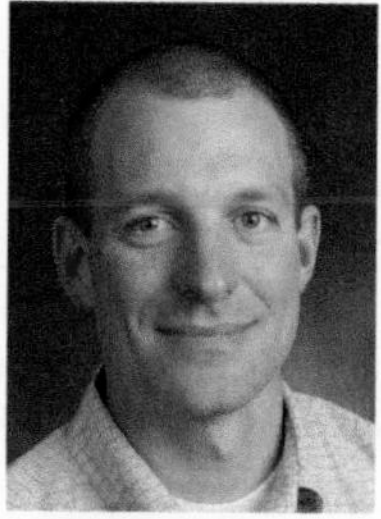

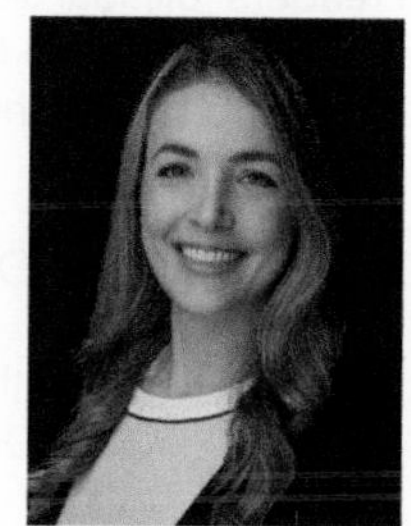

Felix Duerr, Dr. med. vet., MS, DACVS-SA, DECVS, DACVSMR

Lindsay Elam, DVM, MPH, DACVSMR

Editors

It is with great enthusiasm that we introduce this issue of *Veterinary Clinics of North America: Small Animal Practice* on "Orthopedic Medicine." Considerable advances in the realm of small animal orthopedics have transpired since the last *Veterinary Clinics of North America: Small Animal Practice* Orthopedics issue in 2005, including the establishment of the American College of Veterinary Sports Medicine and Rehabilitation (ACVSMR). The advent of this specialty has opened a variety of doors in enhancing patient care as well as in optimizing hospital efficiency. We have assimilated a breadth of topics written by some of the leaders in the ACVSMR field to present new and updated information in the evaluation, diagnosis, and medical treatment of small animal orthopedic mobility impairments. The articles in this issue systematically guide the reader through a patient evaluation: a comprehensive mobility assessment that transcends the standard orthopedic and neurologic examinations and diagnostic techniques inclusive of imaging and objective gait analysis. In addition, a breadth of common medical treatment strategies are reviewed, including evidence-based complementary and alternative medical techniques, nutritional considerations, joint injection therapies, physical rehabilitation, at-home therapeutic exercise, and extracorporeal shockwave therapy. Furthermore, there is a focus on prevention and maintenance of mobility to guide the reader through considerations and strategies ranging from conditioning a canine athlete to promotion of a healthy companion animal lifestyle.

While the focus of this issue is clinical, the final article discusses the myriad of benefits of orthopedic medicine and rehabilitation and strategies to implement this service in your practice. The article touches on the notion that an ACVSMR specialist as a

Vet Clin Small Anim 52 (2022) xi–xii
https://doi.org/10.1016/j.cvsm.2022.03.012
0195-5616/22/© 2022 Published by Elsevier Inc.

complement to an orthopedic surgeon has far-reaching benefits to a hospital that surpass the delivery of state-of-the-art patient care. We practice this paired ACVSMR and American College of Veterinary Surgery model at the James L. Voss Veterinary Teaching Hospital at Colorado State University. We are of the passionate opinion that the patients, clients, students, house officers, clinicians, and hospital alike are better for it.

We are sincerely grateful to the authors for their contributions on a variety of topics. The content of the articles represents their personal clinical impressions, interpretation of the literature, and opinions. As editors, we offered input and suggestions toward the goal of updating and enhancing the readers' clinical skills and knowledge base in this evolving field and are thankful for the opportunity to share more about our beloved specialty in the hopes of positively impacting the discipline of small animal orthopedics.

Felix Duerr, Dr. med. vet., MS, DACVS-SA, DECVS, DACVSMR
Associate Professor
Small Animal Orthopedic Medicine and Mobility
Department of Clinical Sciences
Colorado State University
Fort Collins, CO 80523, USA

Lindsay Elam, DVM, MPH, DACVSMR
Assistant Professor
Small Animal Orthopedic Medicine and Mobility
Department of Clinical Sciences
Colorado State University
Fort Collins, CO 80523, USA

E-mail addresses:
Felix.Duerr@colostate.edu (F. Duerr)
Lindsay.Elam@colostate.edu (L. Elam)

Canine Comprehensive Mobility Assessment

Christina Montalbano, VMD, DACVSMR, CCRP, CVA

KEYWORDS

- Mobility assessment • Stance • Posture • Gait • Movement
- Functional assessment

KEY POINTS

- A comprehensive mobility assessment is a valuable tool to aid in localization, the characterization of dysfunction, guide further advanced diagnostics, and provide information for the formulation of an appropriate treatment plan.
- A thorough assessment requires minimal equipment or special tools, relying on the clinician's visual observations, targeted palpation, and the assessment of a dog's function in the clinic or questioning of function in the dog's home environment.
- A detailed assessment of posture and gait, manual soft tissue evaluation, and the application of functional assessments complements a complete orthopedic and neurologic examination as part of a comprehensive mobility assessment.

 **Video content accompanies this article at http://www.vetsmall.theclinics.com.**

INTRODUCTION

A change in a dog's mobility is a common reason for seeking veterinary care. Changes to mobility may occur suddenly or have a history of chronicity and progression before presentation. Mobility issues may be attributable to injury or disease of specific joints, bones, or soft tissue structures affecting 1 or more limbs, or may be caused by neurologic disease to the spinal cord or peripheral nerves. Systemic diseases can also play a role in mobility and a systemic workup should be performed when indicated.

A thorough examination of the musculoskeletal and neurologic systems provides a wealth of information when assessing a dog with mobility impairment and can be paired with imaging and other diagnostics to identify the underlying cause. An orthopedic examination involves gait analysis and assessment of a dog's joints and long bones in a weight-bearing and a non–weight-bearing position. The clinician palpates for abnormalities, such as joint thickening and effusion, altered range of motion, and pain on joint manipulation or long bone palpation. A neurologic examination adds

NorthStar VETS, 315 Robbinsville-Allentown Road, Robbinsville, NJ 08691, USA
E-mail address: cmontalbano.vmd@gmail.com

Vet Clin Small Anim 52 (2022) 841–856
https://doi.org/10.1016/j.cvsm.2022.02.002

an assessment of spinal hyperalgesia, reflexes, conscious proprioception, and awareness of pain sensation. A systematic approach to examination is recommended to ensure thoroughness, and step-by-step procedures have been described for these examinations.[1,2] In the author's opinion, these conventional examinations may give an incomplete picture when considering the functional abilities and sources of pain in a patient. A comprehensive mobility assessment provides additional information to further aid in the localization and diagnosis of a joint, soft tissue, or neurologic injury or disease and in the formulation of a treatment plan.

Mobility refers to the ability and ease of a patient to move around the environment and participate in activities of daily living. In human medicine, there are several established tools available to guide mobility assessment. These tools have been used to predict success in independent living and identify fall risk in the elderly.[3,4] Although frailty indices have been used to quantify the risk of mortality in dogs,[5,6] no widely recognized assessment of mobility exists; much of what is performed clinically involves a subjective assessment by the clinician. Additionally, mobility is not only important in the geriatric population, but should be assessed in post-injury and post-operative patients or as a part of a fitness test for sporting and working dogs. An assessment of mobility aims to evaluate the patient with a systematic approach, both at a focal level (eg, a specific joint) and the body as a whole, in static and transitional postures, during various functional assessments, and by performing a detailed musculoskeletal palpation with a focus on specific soft tissue structures. With the information that follows, the author aims to provide the reader with a practical and systematic approach to the comprehensive mobility assessment to support the traditional orthopedic and neurological examinations.

POSTURE AND STANCE

Posture refers to how a dog holds or positions its body, with stance specifically referring to the posture of a dog standing upright on all limbs. A normal dog when standing with all limbs perpendicular to the floor should be weight bearing with approximately 30% of the body weight distributed to each forelimb and 20% to each hindlimb.[7] An abnormal stance may be apparent as significant weight shifting or holding up of a limb, creating visual asymmetry. Subtle displacements to weight bearing may be appreciated by lifting 1 limb at a time and identifying a limb that is consistently easier to displace than another, indicating resistance to bear weight; or a dog that is hesitant to allow picking up of one limb because further weight bearing through the contralateral limb induces pain. Observation of a dog from behind may demonstrate a larger visible surface of the paw pad in an affected limb that is not bearing as much weight as the remaining limbs. Similarly, if a dog is standing on a depressible surface (foam, inflated fitness disc, etc), alterations in weight bearing may be observed as greater and lesser depressions of the surface by the unaffected and affected limbs, respectively. A quantifiable stance analysis can be performed with 2 or 4 commercial bathroom scales, with a single limb placed on each scale and the results reported or with a commercial stance analyzer. Because the center of gravity and thus weight distribution may be altered depending on head position and voluntary shifting, a stance analysis can be considered a subjective measure, even with these quantitative measures.[7] The position of the limbs in relation to the rest of the body may aid in relief of pain while standing; therefore, the dog should also be observed for limb abduction and adduction as well as cranial or caudal displacement.

Posture can also be assessed in other static positions, such as a sit or down. Postural preferences may be behavioral, although abnormalities or changes to proper posture may indicate an injury or a lack of strength to hold a certain position. An assessment of posture at a sit should observe whether the hindlimbs are tucked squarely under the dog's torso or turned out to the side. Sitting places the stifle and hip in flexion angles nearing that reported for complete passive stifle flexion assessed via goniometry[8–10]; it is, therefore, common for dogs with stifle pain to resist full stifle flexion and adopt an abnormal sitting posture. Hindlimb position at a down should be assessed similarly. Changes in posture during urination and defecation are often readily noted by owners, either that the dog is no longer able to maintain a squat or is no longer lifting a leg to urinate. Leg lifting in male dogs is common, with up to 70% of males adopting this posture for urination regardless of castration status,[11] so it can be helpful information as a part of the assessment for mobility in male dogs.

Targeted Examination

Posture can be assessed at the level of individual joints of a weight-bearing limb, observing for changes such as joint hyperextension and limb rotation. The normal standing angles of joints have been reported for comparison,[12] or the contralateral limb can be assessed for asymmetry. Certain appearances can be characteristic for specific injuries or diseases, whereas others are nonspecific but remain noteworthy to complete the clinical picture. Postural abnormalities should be assessed further during non–weight-bearing palpation to determine whether they are joint related or localizing to soft tissues. Specific stresses applied as an isolated stretch against the action of the soft tissues or direct manual pressure may be applied with assessment of the pain response to aid in localization of soft tissue injury. Direct manual pressure to individual muscle bellies can be performed by a flat-handed or pincer technique. A flat-handed technique involves the application of pressure through the fingers to the muscle, compressing the muscle against an underlying firm surface, often bone. A pincer technique involves a grasping motion to compress the muscle between the examiners' thumb and fingers when there are no underlying structures to apply pressure against.[13]

Muscular tone can also be assessed both during stance and during a non–weight-bearing examination. A fullness or lack thereof of muscular substance in a particular region may be observed visually, especially evident if there is asymmetry compared with the contralateral aspect. A lack of muscularity may be due to muscle atrophy, or may appear as such owing to altered neurological input and muscle activity. Focal muscle atrophy can be characterized quantitatively by limb circumference measurements using a Gulick II measuring tape. Furthermore, tone can be assessed on the basis of an entire limb, with abnormalities most commonly of neurologic origin. Increased tone results from upper motor neuron lesions, causing a loss of neural inhibition preventing muscle relaxation, whereas decreased tone results from lower motor neuron lesions causing a loss of neural input.

The joint capsule

The joint capsule and other periarticular soft tissues are altered frequently as a component of degenerative joint disease, undergo changes when a limb is immobilized or during decreased weight bearing, and are occasionally sites of primary injury. These structures can be assessed during joint range of motion by appreciating the "end feel" of a movement. Various classification systems have been designed to describe joint end feel.[14,15] A simplification of joint end feels describes movement as capsular, soft, hard, and empty. A capsular end feel is created by the normal constraints from the joint capsule to stretch beyond maximal range of motion, with a firm but slightly elastic character. A soft end feel occurs when soft tissue (muscles, tendons, or ligaments) impedes further joint range of motion; this finding is normal in some joints (eg, the stifle, where the hamstrings can limit stifle flexion), but can also indicate pathology, such as a mass impeding joint movement. A hard end feel is often pathologic and can occur when osseous articular changes impede normal joint motion or fibrosis occurs to the joint capsule, creating a firm stop during passive joint movement. An empty end feel occurs when pain precludes assessment through the end of the range of motion.

The paws

Changes to the digits and paws may be accentuated in a weight-bearing position and the appearance alone may suggest localization. Injuries to the superficial and deep digital flexor tendons create characteristic changes to the shape of the digit in a weight bearing position, based on the unique insertion site and function of these tendons (**Fig. 1**). Injury to the superficial digital flexor tendon results in a flattened appearance of the toe in which the proximal interphalangeal joint loses control of flexion and the digit is held parallel to the ground. Injury to the deep digital flexor tendon results in dorsal elevation of the distal phalanx. Injury to both structures results in a combination of these appearances. Digital flexor injuries are expected to manifest as pain on extension of the interphalangeal or metacarpophalangeal or metatarsophalangeal joints, whereas pain on flexion may indicate injury to the digital extensors. Swelling or thickening of individual tendons may be appreciated on the palmar or plantar surfaces of the paw. Degenerative joint disease or enthesopathies affecting joints of the paw may be appreciated by visible thickening around the proximal and distal interphalangeal joints or metacarpophalangeal or metatarsophalangeal joints, with pain on direct palpation and/or with focused range of motion. Digital luxations, particularly of the second and fifth digits, may be visibly evident as a medial or lateral deviation of the toe from the sagittal plane. Applying varus and valgus stress to digital joints assesses the integrity of the collateral ligaments for further assessment in suspected luxation or laxity.

The forelimb

Carpal abnormalities may be evident as joint varus or valgus, hyperextension, or less commonly hyperflexion during weight bearing (**Fig. 2**). Swelling of the medial or lateral aspect of the carpus may indicate an injury to the collateral ligaments and may be

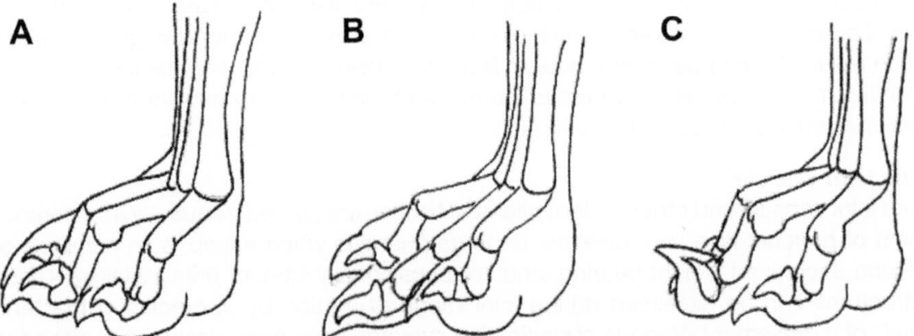

Fig. 1. (*A*) Drawing of a normal paw for comparison with (*B*) a flattened appearance of a proximal interphalangeal joint characteristic of a superficial digital flexor tendon injury versus (*C*) dorsal elevation of the distal phalanx characteristic of injury to the deep digital flexor tendon injury.

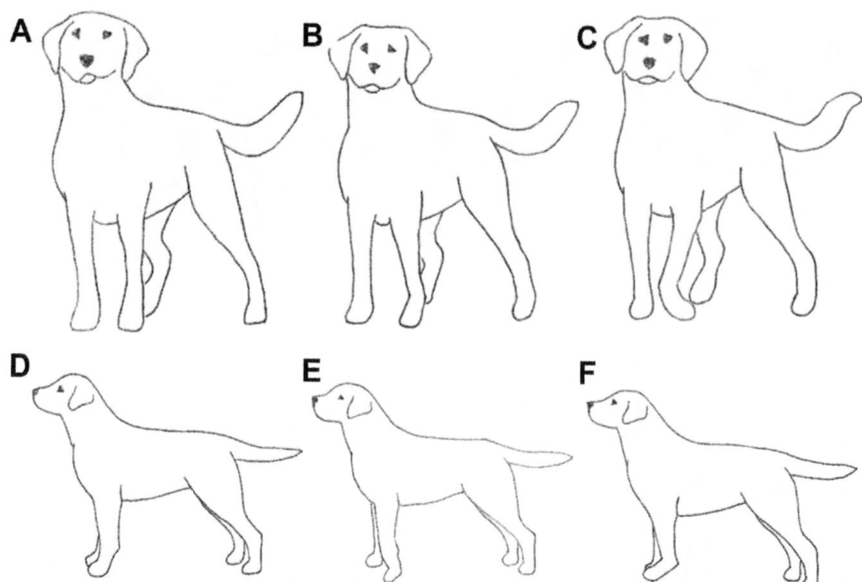

Fig. 2. (*A*) Drawing of a normal dog viewed from the front for comparison with (*B*) carpal varus and (*C*) carpal valgus. (*D*) Drawing of a normal dog viewed from the side for comparison with (*E*) carpal hyperflexion and (*F*) carpal hyperextension.

associated with pain and joint instability on direct palpation or upon application of valgus and varus stresses, respectively. Stenosing tenosynovitis to the abductor pollicis longus tendon as it courses medially over the carpus to insert on the first digit may be identified as focal swelling and pain on manipulation of the first digit.[16] Carpal extensor injuries (eg, to the extensor carpi radialis) may appear as swelling and pain affecting the soft tissues on the craniolateral aspect of the antebrachium and discomfort on carpal flexion, although this finding has only been reported in 2 cases to date.[17] Carpal and digital flexor injuries (eg, to the flexor carpi ulnaris) result in swelling and pain to the caudomedial structures of the antebrachium and pain on carpal extension. Discrete thickening may be appreciated if the injury is focal.

Pain localizing to the elbow often results in external rotation of the joint and abduction of the limb away from the sagittal plane (**Fig. 3**), with changes in the standing joint angle. If abnormalities are present bilaterally, this positioning may cause a wide-based stance of the thoracic limbs. Most abnormalities localizing to the elbow region are joint-related issues (eg, arthritis) and should be evident on conventional orthopedic examinations.

Shoulder pain is commonly caused by soft tissue injuries, often owing to chronic repetitive stress. Postural changes are often limited to decreased weight bearing on the affected limb and do not aid in further localization. An exception to this is infraspinatus contracture, which causes a characteristic external rotation of the shoulder with lateral deviation of the limb. Severe medial shoulder instability may result in abduction of the limb during stance owing to an inability to maintain the limb in the sagittal plane, with laxity and pain identified on shoulder abduction or medial shoulder palpation, furthering clinical suspicion. Supraspinatus insertion and biceps brachii origin injuries both may cause pain on shoulder flexion and palpation of the cranial aspect of the shoulder joint; these entities may be differentiated by the biceps stretch test, which

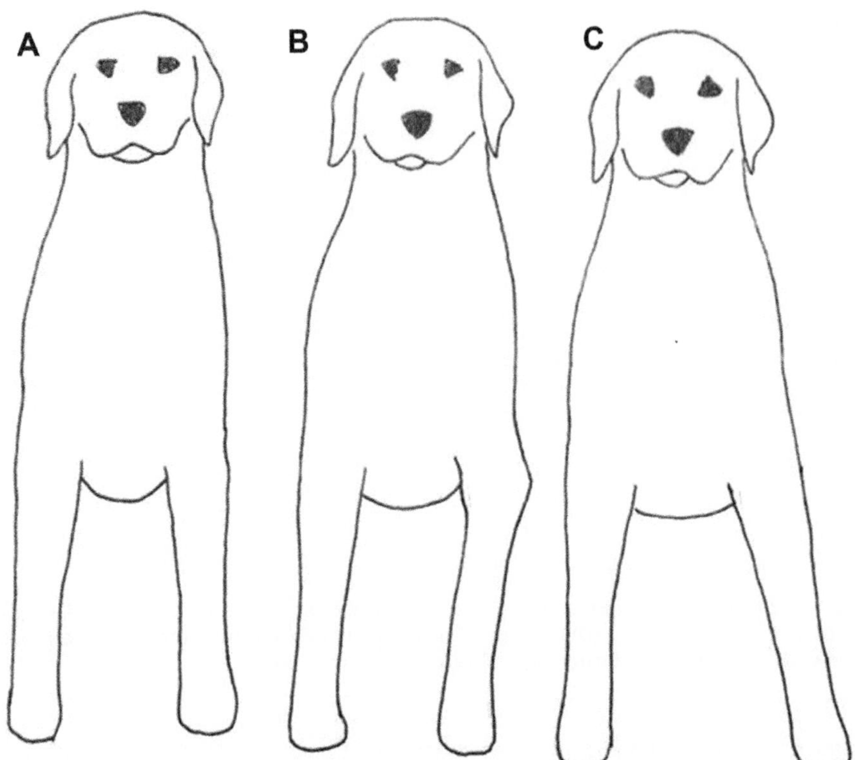

Fig. 3. (*A*) Drawing of a normal dog viewed from the front for comparison with (*B*) elbow abduction versus (*C*) abduction of the entire limb.

adds concurrent elbow extension during shoulder flexion, which should increase the pain response in a biceps injury compared with a supraspinatus injury. Musculoskeletal ultrasound examination or MRI is recommended for definitive localization and diagnosis.

Traumatic rupture of the triceps is one of the most common sites of skeletal muscle injury in racing greyhounds.[17] Triceps tears primarily occur in the long head of the triceps brachii muscle. They can be observed visually as well as on palpation as a lack of muscular substance near the normal origin site on the caudal aspect of the scapula with swelling distally in the brachium. Shoulder extension with elbow flexion may elicit a pain response.

The hindlimb

Like the carpus, injury to the tarsus can appear as hyperextension, hyperflexion, varus, or valgus postural abnormalities (**Figs. 4–6**). Tarsal hyperextension may occur owing to primary tarsal pain (eg, osteochondritis dissecans) or secondary to pain proximally in the limb (eg, the hip). Tarsal hyperflexion may occur owing to injury of the calcaneal tendon, which presents variably, depending on the affected structures and severity of injury. A complete rupture of the common calcaneal tendon (including the conjoined tendon of the biceps femoris, semitendinosus, and gracilis; gastrocnemius, as well as the superficial digital flexor) results in a complete plantigrade stance, whereas

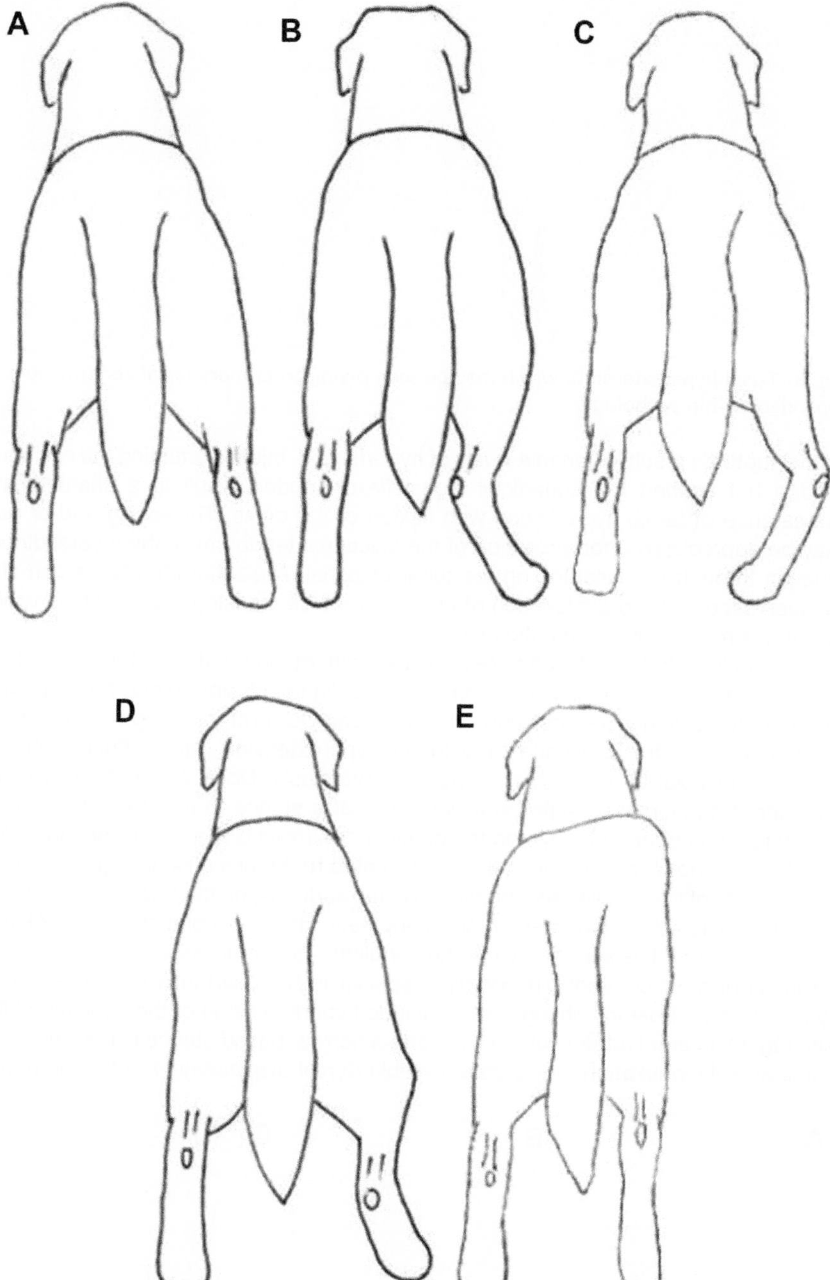

Fig. 4. (*A*) Drawing of a normal dog viewed from behind for comparison to (*B*) tarsal valgus versus (*C*) tarsal varus, (*D*) stifle abduction, and (*E*) craniodorsal displacement of the hip.

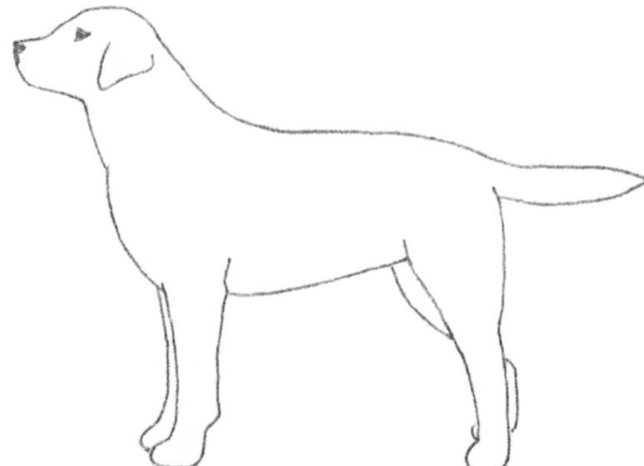

Fig. 5. Tarsal hyperextension, which may be seen owing to primary tarsal abnormalities or secondary to hip pathology.

partial ruptures result in variable levels of hyperflexion. Injuries affecting the calcaneal tendon but sparing the superficial digital flexor tendon result in a characteristic appearance of tarsal hyperflexion with flexion of the digits. Thickening and/or pain may be appreciated upon palpation of the calcaneal tendon from the myotendinous junction through the insertion on the tuber calcanei. A plantigrade stance can also be seen secondary to dysfunction of the sciatic nerve, causing a lack of innervation to the gastrocnemius as an antigravity muscle.

Abnormalities to the stifle often result in external rotation of the joint and lateral deviation of the limb (see **Fig. 4**D). A cranial cruciate ligament rupture may be suspected owing to decreased stifle extension at a stance and visible cranial displacement of the tibial tuberosity; the presence of pain on hyperextension, stifle effusion, cranial drawer, and tibial thrust further support the diagnosis. Dogs with patellar luxation may adopt an increased stifle extension angle at a stance to maintain activation of the quadriceps apparatus to keep the patella from luxating in a weight-bearing position. In some dogs, pain on palpation may localize to the pes anserinus (the common insertion site of the gracilis, semitendinosus, and sartorius) on the craniomedial aspect of the tibia; it is not known whether this phenomenon may be a primary cause of lameness in dogs or if it is secondary to other hindlimb abnormalities.

Hip pain is most commonly due to hip dysplasia and osteoarthritis, or can be caused by hip luxation. Postural changes may include hyperextension of the tarsi and stifles (see **Fig. 5**), internal rotation of the limb, and a narrow-based stance in the hindlimbs. Craniodorsal hip luxation may create a visible dorsal displacement of the femur and

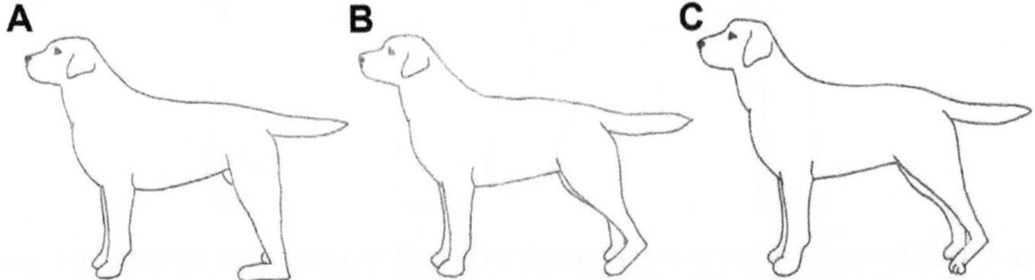

Fig. 6. (*A*) Drawing of a plantigrade stance owing to complete common calcaneal tendon rupture versus (*B*) partial tarsal hyperflexion owing to partial rupture and (*C*) partial tarsal hyperflexion with digital flexion due to partial rupture that spares the superficial digital flexor tendon.

asymmetric appearance of the gluteal musculature (see **Fig. 4**E). Ilioposas pain also localizes to the hip region; this pain may be secondary to other pathologies or a source of primary injury (as with avulsion of the lesser trochanter and iliopsoas tendon of insertion). Iliopsoas pain may be differentiated from hip pain by applying stress to the soft tissues through hip extension with concurrent internal rotation, typically with a sudden and sharp pain response in dogs with iliopsoas pain, but not in those with hip joint pain.[18] The muscle and tendon can also be palpated manually in a neutral hip joint position. Lumbosacral and stifle pathology must be differentiated from hip pain when presented with an abnormal hip extension and abduction. Indirect motion of the lumbosacral spine and stifle results when the hip is extended and further localization using direct palpation or special tests (eg, tibial thrust for the stifle) are indicated. Sacroiliac pathology may similarly present as pain on hip abduction and may be localized by direct palpation.

Gracilis pathology creates several characteristics that can differentiate it readily from other hindlimb issues. Gracilis rupture, most common in racing greyhounds,[19] may be identified as a soft swelling of the muscle at the site of the acute tear. A gracilis injury may precede fibrotic myopathy. Fibrotic myopathy can also affect the semitendinosus, and prior trauma is not always documented. It creates a characteristic change to the dog's gait (elastic external rotation of the tarsus with concurrent internal rotation of the stifle during the swing phase) and can be identified as a palpably firm and thickened muscle belly.

The axial skeleton

Spinal kyphosis, lordosis, or scoliosis may indicate pain and/or weakness of the spine or supporting soft tissues; postural changes to the spine may also indicate orthopedic pain and chronic weight shifting off a painful limb (**Fig. 7**). It is important to differentiate these abnormal postures from conformational variations among dogs, such as the sloped back commonly seen in German Shepherd dogs.[20] Palpation of a spine with abnormal posture may elicit pain or abnormal mobility of spinal segments (hypomobility or hypermobility) to aid in the differentiation of spinal versus orthopedic abnormalities. The latter enters the realm of chiropractic assessment, which can be a useful tool in identifying anatomic abnormalities at the level of individual joints. The position of the head and neck can aid in the identification of cervical discomfort; dogs resistant to moving the neck may have a low head and neck carriage and move their eyes or entire bodies to track an object rather than turning their necks. Tail carriage may be low in dogs with lumbosacral spinal pain, owing to tail trauma, or owing to repetitive overuse injury (ie, swimmer's or limber tail).

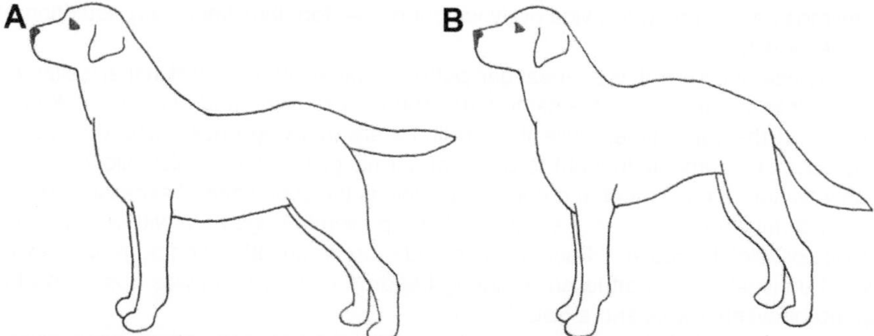

Fig. 7. (*A*) Drawing of a dog with spinal lordosis versus (*B*) spinal kyphosis.

The musculature supporting the cervical, thoracic, and lumbar spine may be more commonly identified as a site of compensatory or referred pain rather than a source of primary injury. These muscles should be palpated for tension, spasm, and sensitivity. Abnormalities appreciated here may be nonspecific for the underlying cause, but may be a significant source of ongoing discomfort if only the primary source of pain is addressed.

GAIT ANALYSIS

A gait analysis is a foundational component of the orthopedic and neurologic examination and should be included in every mobility assessment. A gait analysis allows the clinician to assess a dog through controlled and predictable movement patterns to identify when abnormalities occur during the gait pattern and localize a problem to a specific limb. It is performed frequently in a subjective manner using a series of descriptive terms or a sliding or categorical numerical scale for characterization.[21] Objective gait analysis systems including force platforms, temporospatial walkways, and 2-dimensional or 3-dimensional motion analysis, are superior in the identification and localization of lameness compared with subjective measures, especially in cases of mild lameness.[21,22] These kinetic and kinematic technologies can provide a wealth of additional information about a patient's gait when available, but require specialized equipment, dedicated space, and time, which make them less available outside of academic institutions, specialty practice, or research settings.

During a subjective gait analysis, a skilled assistant should control the dog on a leash. A quiet, flat area with good footing should be used to decrease distractions and slipping, which may complicate the assessment. The dog should be observed moving toward and away, as well as from both sides. The most common gaits for mobility assessment include the walk and trot, with the pace preferred over the trot by some dogs (Video 1).

The walk is the slowest of the gaits with a 4-beat pattern, meaning that each paw strikes the ground individually. As the dog moves forward, the hindpaw lands preceding the ipsilateral forepaw, then the same pattern is repeated on the contralateral limbs. Moderate to severe lameness may be visible at the walk and is easy to localize owing to the slow, 4-beat nature of the gait. Because the forces on each limb at any given time are minimal, subtle lameness may not be evident during the walk.

The trot is a 2-beat gait pattern in which diagonal paws strike the ground at the same time. A hindpaw and contralateral forepaw will land together, while the opposite set of limbs is in swing phase, then switch to the other diagonal. During the trot, forces on the forelimbs can reach up to twice body weight of the dog, thus improving detection of subtle lameness.

The pace, like the trot, is a 2-beat gait pattern. It differs from the trot in that ipsilateral paws strike the ground at the same time. The right forepaw and hindpaw strike the ground at the same time, while the left limbs are in swing phase, and vice versa. The pace is commonly thought to be an abnormal gait pattern, which allows for the conservation of movement and energy, as well as the avoidance of excessive forces on a painful limb. However, a study identified pacing in dogs both with and without musculoskeletal disease.[23] Pacing was noted more frequently when dogs were evaluated on leash versus off leash or during treadmill exercise and was observed at a speed between a walk and a trot.[23]

Faster gaits include the canter and gallop, a 3- and 4-beat gait pattern, respectively. Although these gaits of the dog are natural and abnormalities to the gait pattern may be noted in dogs with mobility issues, these gaits tend to be more challenging as a tool for the detection of lameness owing to the speed of movement. Changes to these gaits may, therefore, indicate a mobility concern but not clearly point to where the problem lies.

Lameness may be detected at the walk and trot by several characteristic features. During a gait cycle, each limb moves through a stance and swing phase. Stance occurs when the paw is in contact with the ground; the swing phase occurs when the limb is not in contact with the ground. As a limb moves through the stance phase of gait, weight bearing results in increased forces on the limb and lameness is detected most readily owing to the resulting pain. The patient attempts to divert weight from the affected limb, which results in an upward displacement of the proximal segment of the limb, and either head or hip motion in an upward direction for a forelimb or a hindlimb lameness, respectively. The common saying "down on sound" refers to the opposite observation that the head (or hip) will move downward as the contralateral limb enters stance phase and the affected limb moves into a non–weight-bearing swing phase.

Changes to the stride length or the path of limb movement may also be observed. The cranial or caudal portion of the stride may be visibly decreased in dogs attempting to minimize the weight-bearing forces and stance duration on an affected limb. Limb circumduction may also be noted during the swing phase of gait, with the limb displaced laterally during swinging movement and returning to the sagittal plane for stance as a means of avoiding active joint range of motion.

Video recording may aid in subjective gait analysis, allowing a review of the dog's gait multiple times without causing fatigue in the patient; this video can serve as a reference over time as well. Although a study showed no significant difference in lameness detection using real speed versus a slow motion video assessment,[24] the extent of lameness severity was not mentioned in this study and it is the author's opinion that a slow motion video can be a useful tool in the detection of subtle lameness.

Neurological gait abnormalities are most commonly evaluated at the walk. Ataxia and weakness may be noted in one or more limbs as an uncoordinated gait (unpredictable where the paw will land with each step), limbs crossing over midline, and scuffing or knuckling of the paws.

FUNCTIONAL ASSESSMENTS

Functional assessments observing the dog during complex movements beyond static observations or gaiting across even ground aid in the comprehensive examination. Success or failure in the completion of these tasks provide an indication of the dog's ability to coordinate movements, overall or targeted muscular strength, and joint and soft tissue comfort. The movements described herein incorporate common motions required of companion animals as activities of daily living. High-level sporting and working dogs may be required to perform more complex tasks beyond the scope of this discussion; a functional assessment test specific to working dogs has been proposed.[25]

The 6-minute walk test assesses the distance a patient walks within 6 minutes. In humans, the distance walked has been shown to be decreased by arthritis, other musculoskeletal diseases, advancing age, decreasing muscle mass, and impaired cognition.[26] Owing to the simplicity of this test, it is one of the most frequently used functional assessment tools in dogs, evaluating a variety of diseases including muscular dystrophy, centronuclear myopathy, and cardiopulmonary diseases.[27–31] Validation testing for other mobility impairments has not been performed.

The timed up and go test in humans assesses a patient rise from a chair, walk 3 m, turn, then return to sitting in the chair. This test has been found to predict a patient's independent mobility and fall risk, with established reference values for various age groups.[32–34] Assessing a dog's ability to change recumbency and rise from recumbency or from sitting into a stand is frequently used as a subjective tool of a dog's strength, comfort, and coordination of movements. A canine timed up and go test has been proposed, but not validated.[35] A timed up and go test could be useful to provide quantitative data to serve as an outcome measure after therapeutic interventions or to monitor for progressive dysfunction over the course of a disease.

In humans, 1-legged standing time assesses static lower limb stability and proprioception and can serve as a screening tool for low functionality and frailty and, more specifically, as a predictor of falls resulting in injury in the elderly.[36,37] Moving from weight bearing on 2 legs to 1 leg is required for everyday human activities such as walking and stair climbing and requires an initial change in center of mass and decrease in force variability, most critical for balance within the first 5 seconds.[38] A comparable assessment in quadrupeds includes a 3- or 2-legged stand; neither assessments have been studied for potential usefulness as a functional assessment tool in dogs. However, one may gather helpful information on individual patients comparing ease of performing a 3-legged stand on the forelimbs versus hindlimbs or between contralateral limbs, a 2-legged stand comparing ipsilateral or diagonal limb pairs, and changes to these tests over time.

Traversing a set of stairs or an incline or standing statically on an inclination are activities of daily living common for many dogs. In humans, the number of steps climbed in a specified time or the duration required to climb a certain number of stairs have been used as an indication of lower extremity power, a scale of functional impairment, as well as an outcome measure after therapeutic interventions of various lower limb pathologies.[39,40] Postural stability has been found to be greater in humans standing or walking down an incline compared with uphill, with age and the gradation of the incline affecting stability.[41] An adaptation period is required for return of postural control upon return to a horizontal surface.[42] Comparable studies have not been performed in quadrupeds, with studies instead focusing on kinetics and kinematics. Joint range of motion is altered compared with walking on flat ground in quadrupeds. In horses, the triceps brachii and brachiocephalicus were found to have prolonged muscular activity during uphill walking and variable activation of hindlimb musculature has been found in both dogs and horses.[43–46] Force redistribution shifts more weight to the hindlimbs during 10% incline movement in horses.[47] A timed in-clinic and at-home trial of stair climbing has demonstrated potential as a component of a canine frailty assessment tool.[48] Subjectively, scuffing or tripping of a particular limb may indicate a joint abnormality or muscular weakness, and circumduction may indicate a reluctance to move a joint through the necessary range of motion.

Stepping over an object is a common task of daily living; obstacles may be present constantly in the environment (eg, a threshold) or appear suddenly (eg, object falling in path). Cavaletti obstacles are commonly used as a therapeutic exercise during a rehabilitation program and can aid in assessing active joint flexion and limb coordination. The range of motion, particularly in flexion of the elbow, carpus, stifle, and tarsus, was found to be increased in normal dogs walking over cavalettis,[45] as well as elbow flexion in dogs with elbow osteoarthritis.[49] Muscle activation of the gluteus medius varies during Cavaletti exercises compared with walking over land.[42] This movement can be a useful tool to observe for dysfunction localizing to a specific joint or the limb as a whole. Abnormal joint movement can be assessed subjectively as incomplete active flexion or extension of the affected joint, hitting of the obstacles, and limb circumduction. In humans, advancing age and decreasing available response time (for a suddenly appearing object) increased risk of obstacle contact; these factors have not been assessed in dogs.[50]

Circling has been used as a movement for the assessment of horses to observe for lameness, flexibility of the spine, and limb coordination; although there are not comparable studies in dogs, the concepts are thought to be similar. Lateral bending of the equine thoracolumbar spine occurs in the same direction as the circle.[51] The center of mass of the body as a whole, as well as the head and neck segments, changes during circling in horses with leaning toward the inside of small circles.[52] In the forelimb, the peak vertical force is decreased on the inside limb of normal horses, whereas the stance phase is increased.[53] Trotting in a circle produced greater hindlimb asymmetry in sound horses ,which may be confused for inside hindlimb lameness.[54] The ease of movement, appearance of lameness, and limb coordination when compared in the clockwise and counterclockwise directions may serve as a helpful aid in the mobility assessment of the dog.

Backward walking requires coordinated neuromuscular control and proprioceptive feedback and is used in humans to assess fall risk and balance in various disease states.[55–57] It has not been assessed as a functional mobility tool in dogs, but has been shown to increase weight bearing to the hindlimbs and particularly activates the gluteal and hamstring musculature.[58] A kinematic study of backward walking revealed no alterations in trunk or joint motions compared with forward walking, aside from a decreased carpal flexion through the swing phase of a backward step.[59]

A video assessment of the dog navigating its home environment is a valuable addition to in-clinic functional assessments. Although much can be learned from simulating obstacles common in a household or assessing various movements, dogs may be anxious and perform differently in the clinic or dysfunctional mobility may be situational and unable to be replicated.

SUMMARY

A comprehensive mobility assessment provides thorough investigation through a visual, hands-on, and functional examination to complement the conventional orthopedic and neurological examination. It should be performed in a systematic manner, although additions or omissions from what has been discussed may be appropriate for an individual patient. This practice can aid in the localization of the problem, guide a further diagnostic workup, and identify problem areas requiring focused attention during formulation of a treatment plan.

CLINICS CARE POINTS

- A mobility assessment is commonly used in humans, particularly assessing fall risk in the elderly; a comparable assessment in dogs is not widely performed beyond a basic orthopedic and neurological examination.
- Functional tests are a major component of mobility assessment in humans and may be modified for canine assessment.
- Observation of the overall stance and posture paired with hands-on joint and soft tissue examination provide complementary information to further understand mobility impairments.

DISCLOSURE

The author has nothing to disclose.

SUPPLEMENTARY DATA

Supplementary data related to this article can be found online at doi:10.1016/j.cvsm.2022.02.002

REFERENCES

1. Von Pfeil DJF, Duerr FM. The orthopedic examination. In: Duerr FM, editor. Canine lameness. Hoboken, NJ: Wiley-Blackwell; 2020. p. 31–40.
2. Bartner L. The neurologic examination. In: Duerr FM, editor. Canine lameness. Hoboken, NJ: Wiley-Blackwell; 2020. p. 41–66.
3. Paulisso DC, Schmeler MR, Schein RM, et al. Functional mobility assessment is reliable and correlated with satisfaction, independence and skills. Assist Technol 2019;33(5):264–70.
4. Zijlstra W, Aminian K. Mobility assessment in older people: new possibilities and challenges. Eur J Ageing 2007;4:3–12.
5. Banzato T, Franzo G, Di Maggio R, et al. A frailty index based on clinical data to quantify mortality risk in dogs. Sci Rep 2019;9(1):1–9.
6. Hua J, Hoummady S, Muller C, et al. Assessment of frailty in aged dogs. Am J Vet Res 2016;77:1357–65.
7. Roy WE. Examination of the canine locomotor system. Vet Clin N Am 1971;1:53–70.
8. Feeney LC, Lin CF, Marcellin-Little DJ, et al. Validation of two-dimensional kinematic analysis of walk and sit-to-stand motions in dogs. Am J Vet Res 2007;68:277–82.
9. Jaegger G, Marcellin-Little DJ, Levine D. Reliability of goniometry in Labrador Retrievers. Am J Vet Res 2002;63:979–86.
10. Reusing M, Brocardo M, Weber S, et al. Goniometric evaluation and passive range of joint motion in chondrodystrophic and non-chondrodystrophic dogs of different sizes. Vet Comp Orthop Traumatol 2002;3:e66–71.
11. Bennet MD. Male dog urination posture preference: a survey of owner observations. J Vet Behav 2020;39:37–40.
12. Milgram J, Slonim E, Kass PH, et al. A radiographic study of joint angles in standing dogs. Vet Comp Orthop Traumatol 2004;17:82–90.
13. Wall R. Introduction to myofascial trigger points in dogs. Top Companion Anim Med 2014;29(2):43–8.
14. Marcellin-Little DJ, Levine D. Principles and application of range of motion and stretching in companion animals. Vet Clin Small Anim 2015;45:57–72.
15. Petersen CM, Hayes KW. Construct validity of Cyriax's selective tension examination: association of end-feels with pain at the knee and shoulder. J Orthop Sports Phys Ther 2000;30(9):512–27.
16. Grundmann S, Montavon PM. Stenosing tenosynovitis of the abductor pollicis longus muscle in dogs. Vet Comp Orthop Traumatol 2001;14(2):95–100.
17. Anderson A, Stead AC, Coughlan AR. Unusual muscle and tendon disorders of the forelimb in the dog. J Small Anim Pract 1993;34(7):313–8.
18. Breur GJ, Blevins WE. Traumatic injury of the iliopsoas muscle in three dogs. J Am Vet Med Assoc 1997;210(11):1631–4.
19. Iddon J, Lockyer RH, Frean SP. The effect of season and track conditions on injury rate in racing greyhounds. J Small Anim Pract 2014;55:399–404.
20. Humphries A, Shaheen AF, Gomez Alvarez CB. Different conformations of the German shepherd dog breed affect its posture and movement. Sci Rep 2020;10:16924.

21. Waxman AS, Robinson DA, Evans RB, et al. Relationship between objective and subjective assessment of limb function in normal dogs with an experimentally induced lameness. Vet Surg 2008;37:241–6.
22. Quinn MM, Keuler NS, Lu Y, et al. Evaluation of agreement between numerical rating scales, visual analogue scoring scales, and force plate gait analysis in dogs. Vet Surg 2007;36:360–7.
23. Wendland TM, Martin KW, Duncan CG, et al. Evaluation of pacing as an indicator of musculoskeletal pathology in dogs. J Vet Med Animhealth 2016;8(12):207–13.
24. Lane DM, Hill SA, Huntingford JL, et al. Effectiveness of slow motion video compared to real time video in improving the accuracy and consistency of subjective gait analysis in dogs. Open Vet J 2015;5(2):158–65.
25. Farr BD, Ramos MT, Otto CM. The Penn Vet Working Dog Center Fit to Work Program: a formalized method for assessing and developing foundational canine physical fitness. Front Vet Sci 2020. https://doi.org/10.3389/fvets.2020.00470.
26. Enright PL. The six-minute walk test. Respir Care 2003;48(8):783–5.
27. Acosta AR, Van Wie E, Stoughton WB, et al. Use of the six-minute walk test to characterize golden retriever muscular dystrophy. Neuromuscul Disord 2016; 26:865–72.
28. Boddy KN, Roche BM, Schwartz DS, et al. Evaluation of the six-minute walk test in dogs. Am J Vet Res 2004;65(3):311–3.
29. Cerda-Gonzalez S, Talarico L, Todhunter R. Noninvasive assessment of neuromuscular disease in dogs: use of the 6-minute walk test to assess submaximal exercise tolerance in dogs with centronuclear myopathy. J Vet Intern Med 2016;30:808–12.
30. Rajyalakshmi S, Venkatesakumar E, Vijayakumar G, et al. Evaluation of six minute walk test to detect occult cardiomyopathy in apparently healthy Labrador retrievers. Indian Vet J 2020;97(03):27–30.
31. Swimmer RA, Rozanski eA. Evaluation of the 6-minute walk test in pet dogs. J Vet Intern Med 2011;25:405–6.
32. Bohannon RW. Reference values for the timed up and go test: a descriptive meta-analysis. J Geriatr Phys Ther 2006;29(2):64–8.
33. Podsiadlo D, Richardson S. The timed "up & go": a test of basic functional mobility for frail elderly persons. J Am Geriatr Soc 1991;39(2):142–8.
34. Shumway-Cook A, Brauer S, Woollacott M. Predicting the probability for falls in community-dwelling older adults using the timed up & go test. Phys Ther 2000; 80(9):896–903.
35. Hesbach AM. A proposed canine movement performance test: the canine timed up and go test (CTUG). Orthopaed Phys Ther Pract 2003;15(2):26.
36. Vellas BJ, Rubenstein LZ, Ousset PJ, et al. One-leg standing balance and functional status in a population o 512 community-living elderly persons. Aging Clin Exp Res 1997;9:95–8.
37. Vellas BJ, Wayne SJ, Romero L, et al. One-leg balance is an important predictor of injurious falls in older persons. J Am Geriatr Soc 1997;45:735–8.
38. Jonsson E, Seiger A, Hirschfeld H. One-leg stance in healthy young and elderly adults: a measure of postural steadiness? Clin Biomech 2004;19:688–94.
39. Bean JF, Kiely DK, LaRose S, et al. Is stair climb power a clinically relevant measure of leg power impairments in at-risk older adults? Arch Phys Med Rehabil 2007;88:604–9.
40. Bennell K, Dobson F, Hinman R. Measures of physical performance assessments. Arthritis Care Res 2011;63(S11):s350–70.

41. Barbosa RC, Vieira MF. Postural control of elderly adults on inclined surfaces. Ann Biomed Eng 2017;45(3):726–38.
42. Choi SD. Postural balance and adaptations in transitioning sloped surfaces. Int J Constr Edu Res 2008;4:189–99.
43. Breitfuss K, Franz M, Peham C, et al. Surface electromyography of the vastus lateralis, biceps femoris, and gluteus medius muscle in sound dogs during walking and specific physiotherapeutic exercises. Vet Surg 2014;44(5):588–95.
44. Hodson-Tole E. Effects of treadmill inclination and speed on forelimb muscle activity and kinematics in the horse. Equine Comp Exerc Physiol 2006;3(2):61–72.
45. Holler PJ, Brazda V, Dal-Bianco B, et al. Kinematic motion analysis of the joints of the forelimbs and hind limbs of dogs during walking exercise regimens. Am J Vet Res 2010;71:734–40.
46. Miro F, Galisteo AF, Garrido-Castro JL, et al. Surface electromyography of the longissimus and gluteus medius muscles in Greyhounds walking and trotting on ground flat, up, and downhill. Animals 2020;10(6):968.
47. Dutto DJ, Hoyt DF, Cogger EA, et al. Ground reaction forces in horses trotting up an incline and on the level over a range of speeds. J Exp Biol 2004;207(20): 3507–14.
48. Morgan EM, Heseltine JC, Levine GJ, et al. Evaluation of a low-technology system to obtain morphological and mobility trial measurements in dogs and investigation of potential predictors of canine mobility. Am J Vet Res 2019;80:670–9.
49. Bockstahler B, Fixl I, Dal-Bianco B, et al. Kinematic motion analysis of the front legs of dogs suffering from osteoarthritis of the elbow joint during special physical therapy exercise regimes. Winer Tierärztliche Monatsschrift. 2011;98(3/4):87–94.
50. Chen HC, Ashton-Miller JA, Alexander NB, et al. Effects of age and available response time on ability to step over an obstacle. J Gerontol 1994;49(5): M227–33.
51. Bystrom A, Hardeman AM, Serra Braganca FM, et al. Differences in equine spinal kinematics between straight line and circle in trot. Sci Rep 2021;11:1–13.
52. Clayton HM, Sha DH. Head and body centre of mass movement in horses trotting on a circular path. Equine Vet J Suppl 2006;36:462–7.
53. Chateau H, Camus M, Holden-Douilly L, et al. Kinetics of the forelimb in horses circling on different ground surfaces at the trot. Vet J 2013;e20–6.
54. Greve L, Pfau T, Dyson S. Thoracolumbar movement in sound horses trotting in straight lines in hand and on the lunge and the relationship with hind limb symmetry or asymmetry. Vet J 2017. https://doi.org/10.1016/j.tvjl.2017.01.003. In press.
55. Carter VA, Farley BG, Wing K, et al. Diagnostic accuracy of the 3-meter backward walk test in persons with Parkinson disease. Top Geriatr Rehabil 2020;36(3): 140–5.
56. Kocaman AA, Arslan SA, Ugurlu K, et al. Validity and reliability of the 3-meter backward walk test in individuals with strokes. J Stroke Cerebrovasc Dis 2021; 30(1):1–6.
57. Unver B, Sevik K, Yarar HA, et al. Reliability of 3-m backward walk test in patients with primary total knee arthroplasty. J Knee Surg 2019;33(6):589–92.
58. McLean H, Millis D, Levine D. Surface electromyography of the vastus lateralis, biceps femoris, and gluteus medius in dogs during stance, walking, trotting, and selected therapeutic exercises. Front Vet Sci 2019. https://doi.org/10.3389/fvets.2019.00211.
59. Vilensky JA, Cook JA. Do quadrupeds require a change in trunk posture to walk backward? J Biomech 2000;33(8):911–6.

Objective Gait Analysis: Review and Clinical Applications

Nina R. Kieves, DVM

KEYWORDS

• Canine • Gait analysis • Kinetics • Kinematics • Objective clinical assessment

KEY POINTS

- Kinetic gait analysis gathers data on the forces created during the stance phase of the gait cycle. It can be obtained using force platforms or pressure-sensitive walkways. These ground reaction forces are used to evaluate canine gait in both research and clinical settings.
- Objective gait analysis can be used clinically to assess subtle lameness in the patient and to objectively evaluate improvement with therapy over time.
- Kinematic gait analysis is the study of the motion of gait without regard to the forces acting to create the motion. Unlike kinetic assessment of gait, kinematics enables assessment of motion of the entire body, a single limb, or even a specific joint. It is primarily used for research purposes.

INTRODUCTION

Gait analysis has been used in veterinary medicine for decades. Objective gait analysis is most commonly used for research purposes to objectively assess outcome of a treatment over time. However, it can also be used for clinical evaluation of patients, particularly for dogs with a subtle lameness that may be hard to detect visually. Although gait analysis can provide a tremendous amount of information for the clinician or clinician scientist, it is operator dependent in regards to accuracy of data collected and evaluation of data. Therefore, it is imperative that it be obtained in a methodical manner and analyzed with equal meticulous discipline.

There are 2 main categories of gait analysis, kinetics and kinematics. Kinetics relates to the assessment and study of forces generated while the dog is moving, whereas kinematics is the study of the mechanics of gait without reference to the forces or masses causing the motion. It is used to record joint angles, and position and orientation of body segments relative to one another. One full gait cycle is defined

Small Animal Orthopedic Surgery, The Ohio State University, 601 Vernon L Tharp Street, Columbus, OH 43210, USA
E-mail address: kieves.1@osu.edu

Vet Clin Small Anim 52 (2022) 857–867
https://doi.org/10.1016/j.cvsm.2022.03.009
0195-5616/22/

as a complete stance phase and swing phase. When the foot is in contact with the ground, this is deemed the stance phase, and as the foot is in the air, it is the swing phase.

Kinetic gait analysis gathers data on the forces created during the stance phase of the gait cycle. This data is called a ground reaction force and is the force an animal's paw exerts on the ground when the paw makes contact during stance. The ground exerts an equal and opposite force as dictated by Newton's third law. Depending on the system used to gather data, this can be done in several ways. Practically, this equates to the use of a force plate system or a pressure-sensitive walkway and gives information regarding the magnitude, and for some systems, also the direction, and the location (also called the center of pressure).

Kinetic Gait Evaluation

Force platform

Force plates have been the historical gold standard for obtaining objective kinetic gait data. They are composed of load cells that contain either piezoelectric elements, strain gauges, or beam load cells.[1] With strain gauges, as the force plate is loaded, the metal foil in the gauge produces an electric output. With loading, the material changes in electric resistance proportional to the deformation caused by the paw strike. Over time, the gauges will undergo some deflection and therefore require recalibration along with adjustment of the bridge excitation voltage to maintain accuracy. If they are overloaded, strain gauges will undergo permanent damage and thus some caution must be used in operating them. Piezoelectric systems, however, are more forgiving and do not require recalibration over time. They are built from quartz crystals, and when deformed, the crystals respond by generating an electric charge. As the paw hits the force plate, the crystal is deformed, which produces a proportional voltage that is collected by electrodes and transmitted via software into useable data.[2] Piezoelectric systems are very sensitive and accurate, less susceptible to damage due to their extreme rigidity, and can measure over a large frequency. Higher frequency enables the system to collect more data over time. Beam load cells act similar to transducers and convert force or weight into an electrical signal using strain gauges. The load cell flexes as the paw makes contact and causes a change in the electrical resistance leading to a change in the voltage across the circuit.

Force plates can be used as a single force plate or can be laid in-line to create a system with multiple force plates (**Fig. 1**). Using more than one force plate enables the researcher to collect data of multiple footfalls during a single pass of the dog.

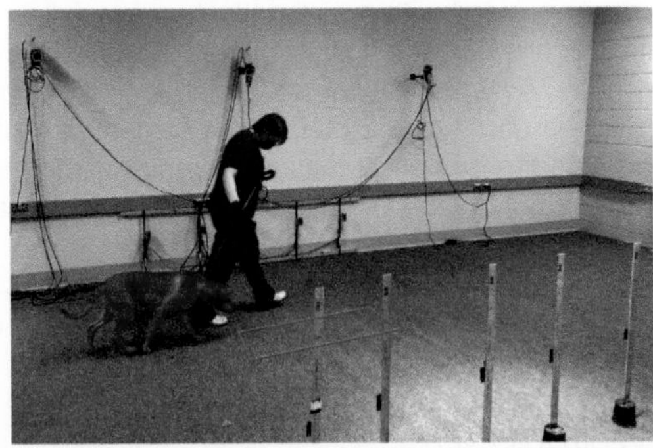

Fig. 1. The set-up of an indwelling force plate system (force platform outlined in *red*) with cameras mounted on the wall for recording. (*Courtesy of* Michael G. Conzemius.)

By placing the load cells in different orientations within the force platform, the direction and magnitude of forces can be obtained in a 3-dimensional manner. The load cell is distorted when the dog steps down on the force plate causing changes in voltage that are proportional to the force applied by the paw. The measured force vector can be broken down into 9 measurements; 3 orthogonal components describing direction of the force, 3 spatial components describing the location of the force vector, and 3 orthogonal moments (**Fig. 2**). These are defined as follows:

- Orthogonal components: F_x, F_y, F_z = direction
- Spatial components: x, y, z = location
- Orthogonal moments: M_x, M_y, M_z[3]

Associated computer software will report the 3 orthogonal ground reaction forces with F_x describing mediolateral force, F_y describing craniocaudal or braking/propulsion forces, and F_z describing vertical forces. The data are collected over time at a designated frequency and as such is displayed as a force versus time curve by the computer software. The resultant graphic represents the ground reaction forces generated during the stance phase of stride. Typically, force is reported as newtons or kilograms of force, and time is reported in seconds. Many additional forces can be reported including coefficient of friction, center of pressure, center of force, the moment around each axis including vertical torque; however, these are not commonly reported in veterinary gait analysis.

Data are frequently reported as a force versus time curve, from which numerous specific data points can be assessed. The force versus time curve varies in shape dependent on the velocity of the dog during data collection; at a walk, the graph seems like an M shape, whereas at a trot, it seems bell shaped. The largest force measured is the F_z or the vertical force. The second largest force measured is F_y, the craniocaudal force, or the braking/propulsion portion of the stance phase. This

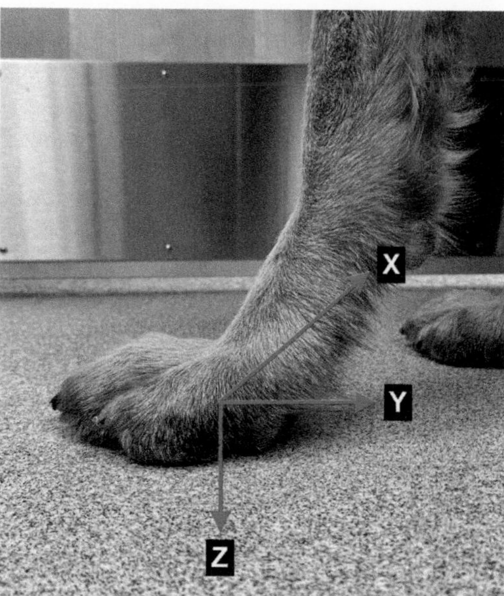

Fig. 2. The three forces measured by a force platform are shown here: X = mediolateral force, Y = craniocaudal force, and Z = vertical force.

can be further defined as deceleration seen at the start of the stance phase or braking as forward momentum decreases, and then propulsion or acceleration as the dog pushes off at the end of the stance phase as they prepare to begin the swing phase of the gait cycle. During braking, the force is a positive value, whereas during propulsion, it is a negative force value. Impulse is the area under the curve and represents force over time.

Data are reported in Newtons but then commonly normalized by converting it as a percent of body weight. This enables data between different weight dogs to be more easily compared. However, for dogs with different morphology, height may also affect ground reaction force values and so normalizing to dog height at the withers has also been recommended, particularly when evaluating vertical impulse data.[4] Another method of standardizing data between a heterogenous population of dogs is to assess data as percentage of body weight distribution (%BWD). This eliminates some factors, such as dog size and leg length, that can make comparison between a heterogenous population challenging. Kano and colleagues reported that using %BWD can be highly accurate.[5]

Pressure-sensitive walkway systems

Temporospatial data such as velocity, acceleration, stance, and stride time cannot be determined by use of only a force plate; it must be coupled with additional equipment. Pressure-sensitive walkways however, are able to obtain both ground reaction force data as well as temporospatial data all at once (**Fig. 3**). Pressure mats are available in various lengths and are much more portable than force plate systems. They have been validated for analyzing gait data in both normal and abnormal dogs.[6–11]

A major benefit of pressure-sensitive walkway systems is their ability to enable data of all limbs and multiple gait cycles to be obtained on one pass. This enables symmetry of limbs to be evaluated. Normal symmetry has not been well evaluated and has been reported to be as low as less than 3.2% between left and right limbs and as high as 6%.[12,13] Additionally, normal dogs have been reported to have some degree of asymmetry.[12]

There are several pressure-sensitive walkway systems commercially available for purchase dependent on your geographic location. Sensors are embedded within

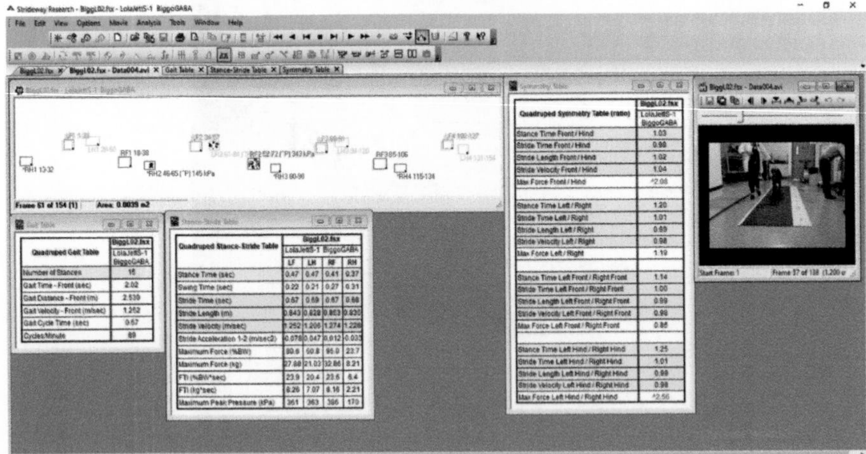

Fig. 3. Pressure-sensitive walkway set up with corresponding data output acquired by the system.

the walkway, which are triggered when the paw contacts the mat. This data are communicated to a computer where software converts them to calculate various gait parameters.

These systems can be covered with protective mats. However, it must be noted that data collected with or without a cover, or with different types of covers, do not correlate.[14,15] Therefore, care must be taken when performing multi-institutional studies to use the same cover. Additionally, direct comparison of data from different studies that do not report, or report the use of different covers, cannot be done accurately. Although one study did show that reference intervals for some gait evaluation variables can be transferrable between locations.[16] It must be noted that this study used the same model of pressure-sensitive walkway, the same cover, and ensured that calibration and equilibration were preformed in the same manner.[16]

In addition to force platforms and pressure-sensitive walkways, ground reaction forces can be measured using static platforms and instrumented treadmills. Static platforms are not used as commonly as other systems and can obtain static measurements in addition to dynamic moving data. However, they have been shown to be accurate for assessment of lameness.[17,18] Even bathroom scales have been reported as a method to crudely assess symmetry of hind limb static weight-bearing.[19] Instrumented treadmills have the benefit of being able to obtain a tremendous amount of data in a short period of time at a defined velocity. However, this set velocity also constrains the natural gait of dogs, which is a negative in many cases. It should be noted that data collected on an instrumented treadmill does vary compared with that collected on a pressure-sensitive walkway.[20] Comparing force plates embedded in a treadmill with those on land, vertical forces were comparable but other forces could not be consistently acquired.[21]

In selecting to use a force plate system versus a pressure-sensitive walkway system, there are several considerations to make. Due to their varying lengths and portability, if space is a constraint, or the clinician and/or researcher plans to obtain data at multiple locations, a pressure-sensitive walkway system may be more ideal (although not all systems are portable).

For small breed dogs and cats, the standard force plate size does not always enable only 1 paw strike to be obtained at a time. If multiple simultaneous paw strikes occur on a force plate, the data cannot be effectively differentiated. For this reason, pressure-sensitive walkways can be more versatile for evaluating dogs (and even cats) of varying sizes. One of the most beneficial elements of a pressure-sensitive walkway is the ability to obtain data on multiple gait cycles in one pass. You can also assess a single limb at a time if needed. By evaluating multiple gates cycles at a time, it allows for stance time, stride time, and stride length to be directly reported.

Force plate systems obtain data in raw newtons (N) in 3 directions as previously described (vertical, craniocaudal, and mediolateral), whereas pressure-sensitive walkways report pressure data in the vertical direction and as a total pressure index (craniocaudal and mediolateral forces cannot be measured). The vertical force can be calculated in pressure-sensitive walkways if they are able to be calibrated. However, although this data is consistent and repeatable, it is not comparable to vertical force obtained directly by a force plate and thus they cannot be directly compared.[8] If direct vertical force is needed by a researcher, then a force plate must be used rather than a pressure-sensitive walkway system.

Data collection

It is imperative that anyone who is going to perform objective gait analysis, regardless of what system is used, is trained well in appropriate data collection. This is to best decrease variability in data collected. Numerous sources of variability have been reported in the literature with most variations being attributed to the dog itself rather than external factors such as the handler.

Before data collection, the dog should be allowed to habituate to the room because this has been shown to affect data collection.[22] Although it was once thought that handlers contributed significantly to variability in data collected, it has been shown that this is not true.[23] In fact, Jevens and colleagues showed that variance attributable to handlers was only 0% to 7% for ground reaction forces measured, leading them to conclude that multiple handlers can participate in studies without significantly affecting the results. Similar to force platforms, there are minor variations in data acquisition using a pressure sensitive walkway in regards to handler variability, but it is still low at 8% and unlikely to alter overall data interpretation in a study, especially if only evaluating the hindlimb.[24] One study did note that if the forelimb is of interest, particularly in smaller breed dogs, some walks should be performed with the handler on the left of the dog and some on the right of the dog as smaller breed dogs tended to shift their weight toward the side opposite the leash, which may affect data collection.[24] It is unknown if this is true for large breed dogs.

A valid trial is very distinctly defined and involves the following:

- The dog walking or trotting at a consistent velocity
- No significant acceleration (+/– 0.5 m/s^2)[25]
- No pulling on the leash
- No movement of the dog's head from side to side/veering from midline
- The dog maintaining a straight line walk or trot throughout the trial
- For force plate collection only, a distinct front and hind foot strike on the platform should be seen

The dog's velocity needs to be defined during the study design and then be consistent throughout the study as velocity has a significant effect on peak forces recorded.[26,27] Studies can either choose to obtain trials with the dog at a walk, a trot or both. Velocity for these speeds has been defined previously in the literature. A walk has been reported as being between 0.8 and 1.3 m/s (14,28) with trotting velocity being much wider ranging from 1.7 to 3.0 m/s.[26,28,29] In some cases, allowing the dog to walk at their preferred speed may be most prudent as dogs of varying sizes can have significantly different chosen velocity for a given gait, that is, a great Dane versus a dachshund preferred walking speed. If this is the case, the dogs chosen speed can be recorded and then moving forward that individual dog can be walked/trotted at its individually chosen speed for all follow-up time points.[25]

Chosen gait velocity may be dependent on what the evaluator is assessing. For instance, one study found that trotting dogs was more sensitive and accurate compared with walking dogs when evaluating for a low-grade hind limb lameness.[28] Conversely, if assessing a population with severe lameness, such as postoperatively, a walk may be more appropriate as dogs with severe lameness may not be able to trot.[29] Regardless of velocity chosen, it is well documented that as velocity increases, so do peak vertical forces, whereas stance time decreases.[25,30] Therefore, data obtained at a walk cannot be directly compared with that of a trot. In addition to overall dog velocity, limb velocity can affect data obtained and needs to be controlled for as well.

If using a pressure-sensitive walkway, velocity is calculated by the software automatically if 2 full gait cycles are captured and can be assessed rapidly to determine if the trial falls within the specified speed. If using a force platform system, velocity can be measured with a stop watch as a crude method of assessing dog speed, or more accurately, a laser or a photocell can be set up before and another after the platform that are triggered by the subjects' torso as they pass by it that is also reported by system software. To calculate velocity, a minimum of 2 photocells or lasers must be used because velocity is a measure of distance over time.

In addition to controlling velocity, acceleration must also be evaluated. An acceleration of less than 0.5 m/s^2 is recommended because acceleration can affect primarily data in the craniocaudal plane.[31] Similar to velocity, acceleration is measured automatically by pressure-sensitive walkways, or can be measured with a laser system for force platform analysis. Unlike velocity, 3 sequential lasers are required to measure acceleration, and 3 full gait cycles must be captured by the pressure-sensitive walkway system.

The number of valid trials used for statistical analysis is most commonly 5 trials. The maximum number of trials to be attempted should also be defined (ie, maximum 10 trials attempted even if 5 valid trials are not acquired), so that a dog is not asked to perform an overtly large number of trials to get 5 valid trials, possibly exacerbating their lameness and making their condition worse.[32] Recently, an article detailing best practices for measuring and reporting ground reaction forces in dogs was published with several consensus statements on data collection and evaluation.[25]

Kinematic Gait Evaluation

Kinematic gait analysis is the study of the motion of gait without regard to the forces acting to create the motion. Unlike kinetic assessment of gait, kinematics enables assessment of motion of the entire body, a single limb, or even a specific joint. This includes determining the velocity and acceleration/deceleration of a limb/joint and the angles a joint creates during motion (eg, maximum flexion and extension). Motion can be assessed in 2 dimensions or 3 dimensions depending on the type of equipment being used. A 2-dimensional assessment only allows evaluation of one plane motion, that is, the sagittal, transverse, or frontal plane, whereas a 3-dimensional assessment evaluates the motion in all 3 planes at once.

Kinematic gait analysis is not performed as frequently as kinetic evaluation because it requires very specific and often costly equipment, particularly if 3-dimensional systems are used, although 2-dimensional analysis is easier and less costly to obtain. Reflective markers or light-emitting diodes markers are placed over specific landmarks on the limb(s) to be evaluated (**Fig. 4**), and high-speed cameras are used to capture the dog in motion. The cameras capture the markers, and computer software is able to determine their relative position in 2-dimensional or 3-dimensional space depending on the set-up of the laboratory. If a force plate system or pressure-sensitive walkway is set up where the animal is walking, concurrent kinetic data can be captured.

Several parameters can be determined from the data captured including range of motion, angular velocity, and displacement. Several factors have been determined to affect kinematic data captured included skin motion, and accuracy of marker placement, which can be affected by the person applying the marker.[33,34] Normal motion of the pelvic limb has been previously published,[35] and the use of kinematic data to evaluate limb and joint motion is becoming increasingly popular with research groups. To date, kinematic analysis has limited clinical utility as compared with kinetic evaluation, which is used by clinicians to assist in diagnosis of subtle lameness as well as to objectively follow improvement with treatment over time.

The most accurate method of assessing joint kinematics has been to use single-plane or biplanar fluoroscopic analysis.[36–38] Recently, normal data for the canine hind limb in multiple breeds assessed via biplanar fluoroscopic evaluation has been

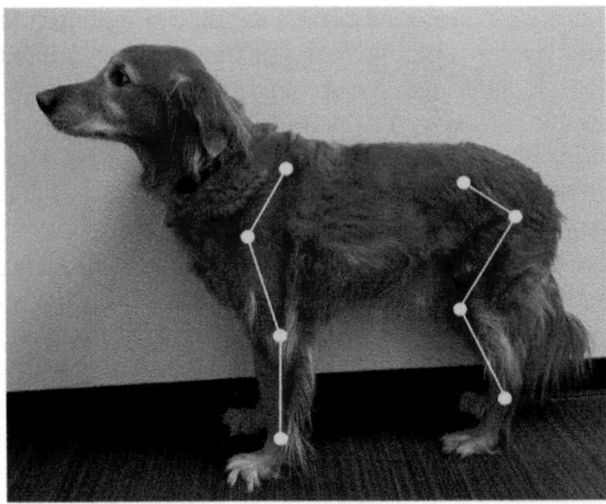

Fig. 4. Common locations of skin markers used for kinematic gait analysis. In the thoracic limb this includes the dorsal scapular spine, acromion/greater tubercle, lateral humeral epicondyle, and ulnar styloid process. In the pelvic limb common marker locations include the iliac crest, femoral greater trochanter, femorotibialjoint, and lateral malleolus of the distal tibia.

published.[39] Unfortunately, this type of assessment is only available at a few locations globally due to the investment of equipment needed to perform such analysis.

SUMMARY

Substantial objective data can be obtained on canine gait using kinetic and kinematic processes. This data has been shown to be repeatable in both normal and abnormal dogs. The use of such equipment requires training to ensure that accurate data is obtained and that the evaluation of the data is done appropriately. Force plate and pressure-sensitive walkway systems both offer the clinician the ability to obtain useful kinetic data. Which system is preferred depends on what specific data the researcher or clinician hopes to acquire, both are accurate and consistent but each offers pros and cons compared with the other that must be considered to best fit the individual's needs. Kinetic gait analysis can be used as an objective measure of treatment intervention over time but can also be used to evaluate progress of clinical patients. Kinematic data is unnecessary for most clinical situations but offers additional valuable insight into joint motion for researchers. This equipment is significantly more expensive to obtain and requires more advanced training to use effectively.

CLINICS CARE POINTS

- Plan protocols ahead of time (ie, trot vs walk, set velocity vs preferred velocity)
- Ensure person(s) involved in data collection are trained to acquire and interpret data appropriately
- Kinematics can provide different and more detailed information regarding joint angles but may not be as practical to acquire data as kinetics

DISCLOSURE

The author has no conflicts of interest to disclose in regards to this article.

REFERENCES

1. Lamkin-Kennard KA, Popovic MB. Sensors: natural and synthetic sensors. In: Popovic Marko B, editor. Biomechatronics. Cambridge (Massachusetts): Elsevier BV; 2019. p. 81–107.
2. McLaughlin RM. Kinetic and kinematic gait analysis in dogs. Vet Clin North Am 2001;31(1):193–201.
3. Torres BT. Gait Analysis. In: Johnston Spencer A, Tobias Karen M, editors. Veterinary surgery: small animal. St. Louis (Missouri): Elsevier, Inc; 2018. p. 1385–96.
4. Voss K, Galeandro L, Wiestner T, et al. Relationships of body weight, body size, subject velocity, and vertical ground reaction forces in trotting dogs. Vet Surg 2010;39(7):863–9.
5. Kano WT, Rahal SC, Agostinho FS, et al. Kinetic and temporospatial gait parameters in a heterogeneous group of dogs. BMC Vet Res 2016;12:2. https://doi.org/10.1186/s12917-015-0631-2. Available at.
6. Light VA, Steiss JE, Montgomery RD, et al. Temporalspatial gait analysis by the use of a portable walkway system in healthy Labrador retrievers at a walk. Am J Vet Res 2010;71(9):997–1002.
7. Besancon MF, Conzemius MG, Derrick TR, et al. Comparison of vertical forces in normal greyhounds between force platform and pressure walkway measurement systems. Vet Comp Orthop Traumatol 2003;16(3):153–7.
8. Lascelles BD, Roe SC, Smith E, et al. Evaluation of a pressure walkway system for measurement of vertical limb forces in clinically normal dogs. Am J Vet Res 2006;67(2):277–82.
9. Webster KE, Wittwer JE, Feller JA. Validity of the GAITRite walkway system for the measurement of averaged and individual step parameters of gait. Gait Posture 2005;22:317–21.
10. Gordon-Evans WJ, Evans RB, Conzemius MG. Accuracy of spatiotemporal variables in gait analysis of neurologic dogs. J Neurotrauma 2009;26:1055–60.
11. LeQuang T, Maitre P, Roger T, et al. Is a pressure walkway system able to highlight a lameness in dog? J Anim Vet Adv 2009;8:1936–44.
12. Budsberg SC, Jevens DJ, Brown J, et al. Evaluation of limb symmetry indices, using ground reaction forces in healthy dogs. Am J Vet Res 1993;54(10):1569–74. PMID: 8250378.
13. Fanchon L, Grandjean D. Accuracy of asymmetry indices of ground reaction forces for diagnosis of hind limb lameness in dogs. Am J Vet Res 2007;68(10):1089–94.
14. Kieves NR, Hart JL, Evans RB, et al. Comparison of three walkway cover types for use during objective canine gait analysis with a pressure-sensitive walkway. Am J Vet Res 2019;80(3):265–9.
15. Kozlovich TE, Jones SC, Kieves NR. Use of a protective cover affects ground reaction force measurements obtained from dogs walking on a validated pressure-sensitive walkway. Am J Vet Res 2021;1–4. Epub ahead of print. PMID: 34941563.
16. Olsen AM, Lambrechts NE, Weng HY, et al. Transference of reference intervals for variables of instrumented gait analysis in walking dogs. Am J Vet Res 2020;81(10):790–5.

17. Wilson ML, Roush JK, Renberg WC. Single-day and multiday repeatability of stance analysis results for dogs with hind limb lameness. Am J Vet Res 2019;80(4):403–9.
18. Clough WT, Canapp SO. Assessing clinical relevance of weight distribution as measured on a stance analyzer through comparison with lameness determined on a pressure sensitive walkway and clinical diagnosis. Vet Comp Orthop Traumatol 2018;31(S 02):A1–25.
19. Hyytiäinen HK, Mölsä SH, Junnila JT, et al. Use of bathroom scales in measuring asymmetry of hindlimb static weight bearing in dogs with osteoarthritis. Vet Comp Orthop Traumatol 2012;25(5):390–6. Epub 2012 Jul 25. PMID: 22828919.
20. Assaf ND, Rahal SC, Mesquita LR, et al. Evaluation of parameters obtained from two systems of gait analysis. Aust Vet J 2019;97(10):414–7. Epub 2019 Jul 8. PMID: 31286488.
21. Bockstahler BA, Skalicky M, Peham C, et al. Reliability of ground reaction forces measured on a treadmill system in healthy dogs. Vet J 2007;173(2):373–8. Epub 2005 Dec 1. PMID: 16324859.
22. Rumph PF, Steiss JE, Montgomery RD. Effects of selection and habituation on vertical ground reaction force in greyhounds. Am J Vet Res 1997;58(11):1206–8. PMID: 9361879.
23. Jevens DJ, Hauptman JG, DeCamp CE, et al. Contributions to variance in force-plate analysis of gait in dogs. Am J Vet Res 1993;54(4):612–5. PMID: 8484583.
24. Keebaugh AE, Redman-Bentley D, Griffon DJ. Influence of leash side and handlers on pressure mat analysis of gait characteristics in small-breed dogs. J Am Vet Med Assoc 2015;246(11):1215–21.
25. Conzemius MG, Torres BT, Muir P, et al. Best practices for measuring and reporting ground reaction forces in dogs. Vet Surg 2022. https://doi.org/10.1111/vsu.13772. Epub ahead of print. PMID: 35083759.
26. McLaughlin RM, Roush JK. Effects of subject stand time and velocity on ground reaction forces in clinically normal Greyhounds at the trot. Am J Vet Res 1994;55:1666–71.
27. Renberg WC, Johnston SA, Ye K, et al. Comparison of stance time and velocity as control variables in force plate analysis of dogs. Am J Vet Res 1999;60(7):814–9.
28. Voss K, Imhof J, Kaestner S, et al. Force plate gait analysis at the walk and trot in dogs with low-grade hindlimb lameness. Vet Comp Orthop Traumatol 2007;20(4):299–304.
29. Evans R, Gordon W, Conzemius M. Effect of velocity on ground reaction forces in dogs with lameness attributable to tearing of the cranial cruciate ligament. Am J Vet Res 2003;64(12):1479–81.
30. Roush JK, McLaughlin RM Jr. Effects of subject stance time and velocity on ground reaction forces in clinically normal greyhounds at the walk. Am J Vet Res 1994;55(12):1672–6. PMID: 7887509.
31. Budsberg SC, Rytz U, Johnston SA. Effects of acceleration on ground reaction forces collected in healthy dogs at a trot. Vet Comp Orthopaed 1998;12:20–4.
32. Mickelson MA, Vo T, Piazza AM, et al. Influence of trial repetition on lameness during force platform gait analysis in a heterogeneous population of clinically lame dogs each trotting at its preferred velocity. Am J Vet Res 2017;78(11):1284–92.
33. Kim SY, Kim JY, Hayashi K, et al. Skin movement during the kinematic analysis of the canine pelvic limb. Vet Comp Orthop Traumatol 2011;24(5):326–32. Epub 2011 Aug 5.

34. Torres BT, Gilbert PJ, Reynolds LR, et al. The effect of examiner variability on multiple canine stifle kinematic gait collections in a 3-dimensional model. Vet Surg 2015;44(5):581–7.
35. Fu YC, Torres BT, Budsberg SC. Evaluation of a three-dimensional kinematic model for canine gait analysis. Am J Vet Res 2010;71(10):1118–22. Erratum in: Am J Vet Res. 2011 Mar;72(3):416-1122. PMID: 20919895.
36. Jones SC, Kim SE, Banks SA, et al. Accuracy of noninvasive, single-plane fluoroscopic analysis for measurement of three-dimensional femorotibial joint poses in dogs. Am J Vet Res 2014;75(5):477–85.
37. Jones SC, Kim SE, Banks SA, et al. Accuracy of noninvasive, single-plane fluoroscopic analysis for measurement of three-dimensional femorotibial joint poses in dogs treated by tibial plateau leveling osteotomy. Am J Vet Res 2014;75(5): 486–93.
38. Fischer MS, Schilling N, Schmidt M, et al. Basic limb kinematics of small therian mammals. J Exp Biol 2002;205(Pt 9):1315–38. PMID: 11948208.
39. Fischer MS, Lehmann SV, Andrada E. Three-dimensional kinematics of canine hind limbs: in vivo, biplanar, high-frequency fluoroscopic analysis of four breeds during walking and trotting. Sci Rep 2018;8(1):16982.

Orthopedic Imaging

A Practical Clinical Guide

Jennifer Brown, DVM

KEYWORDS

• Orthopedic imaging • Radiography • Musculoskeletal ultrasound
• Computed tomography • Magnetic resonance imaging

KEY POINTS

- Imaging is an important component of a complete orthopedic medicine evaluation to accurately diagnose musculoskeletal injury.
- The most practical imaging modality in practice is radiography, but it is important to assure a complete study with at least orthogonal views with accurate positioning to optimize its value in making a diagnosis.
- Additional views (eg, oblique, stress, or skyline views) can further aid in accomplishing a diagnosis using radiography.
- Musculoskeletal ultrasound can be helpful for the diagnosis of soft tissue injury and response to treatment.
- Arthroscopy can provide direct visualization of the articular structures.
- Computed tomography and magnetic resonance imaging may be necessary to ultimately make a diagnosis for some conditions.

INTRODUCTION

To appropriately treat musculoskeletal injuries, establishing an accurate diagnosis is key. This can only be accomplished using diagnostic imaging. Practically speaking, the choice of imaging modality will often be dictated by availability and cost, which can be a challenging factor when the most ideal diagnostic option is not easily accessible or affordable. However, when the basic imaging modalities are not yielding answers, it is important to know what other options to present to owners that are most likely to make the diagnosis. Pet insurance and mobile imaging services for ultrasound and computed tomography (CT) have increased affordability and access for some clients and practices, making some options more practical.

The goal of this article is to guide the practitioner through the selection of imaging modalities that should be considered to establish a diagnosis for appendicular musculoskeletal injuries using a location-based approach. While bone and joint tumors and

---

The author has nothing to disclose.
Florida Veterinary Rehabilitation and Sports Medicine, 11016 North Dale Mabry Highway #202, Tampa, FL 33618, USA

Vet Clin Small Anim 52 (2022) 869–906
https://doi.org/10.1016/j.cvsm.2022.03.010

fractures will also be encountered, they will not be a focus of this section. Emphasis will be on radiography as it is the most practical and accessible imaging modality. Other options discussed include diagnostic ultrasound, CT, needle/nano arthroscopy, and magnetic resonance imaging (MRI).

SHOULDER

The shoulder is a common site of forelimb lameness in the dog, with soft tissue injuries one of the more frequent sources. The diagnosis of soft tissue injuries in the shoulder can be challenging. To achieve a complete understanding of all structures that are involved, multiple diagnostics are often required.[1] This is especially true in the forelimb whereby it can be difficult to differentiate between shoulder and elbow joints as the site of lameness and it can be very worthwhile when performing diagnostics to evaluate both joints concurrently.

RADIOGRAPHY

While radiography is typically unrewarding for soft tissue injuries, they remain a baseline diagnostic to document the presence of arthritis, soft tissue mineralization, enthesopathies, rule out other differential diagnoses. Radiography can help guide the next steps in the diagnostic plan. Arthritic changes are characterized by periarticular osteophytes of the caudal humerus and glenoid of the scapula. One of the more common soft tissue mineralization in the shoulder is at the cranial aspect of the shoulder joint and humerus. On the lateral view of the shoulder joint, it can be difficult to ascertain whether this mineralization is within the supraspinatus or the biceps tendon/groove. Therefore, another view to consider is a skyline view of the shoulder to isolate the greater tubercle and intertubercular groove. The skyline view is easily achieved in the dog and can be performed in both the sedated and a cooperative nonsedated patient. The dog is placed in sternal recumbency with the shoulder and elbow flexed and the distal limb angled away from the body (**Fig. 1**).[2] When mineralization is seen in the cranial aspect of the shoulder the skyline view can be considered as part of a complete radiographic study. In the skyline view, one can more readily determine if that mineralization is associated with the greater tubercle (more cranial and lateral) and therefore, the supraspinatus tendon versus the intertubercular groove and biceps tendon (**Fig. 2**). Although less common, enthesopathy at the insertion of the infraspinatus tendon can also be identified on the craniocaudal shoulder extended view.

In young dogs that present with lameness that is isolated to the shoulder, especially with discomfort on end range maximal flexion, osteochondrosis dissecans (OCD) of the caudal humeral head will need to be ruled out. Radiography has good sensitivity for the identification of OCD lesions.[3] Lesions typically are obvious radiographically (**Fig. 3**) but they can be in locations whereby they might be missed with a standard lateral view. When there is a suspicion of OCD and lateral radiographs are inconclusive, both supinated and pronated laterals may help define the lesion. It is also important that lateral films are well positioned with the shoulder extended so that the joint is not superimposed over the thorax or sternum if possible. The opposite front limb should be pulled back and slightly abducted to eliminate superimposition. In some cases, extension of the neck also helps prevent superimposition over the cervical vertebrae.

ULTRASONOGRAPHY

As soft tissue injuries are a frequent source of lameness associated with the shoulder, ultrasound is particularly useful for evaluation. It also can play an important role in

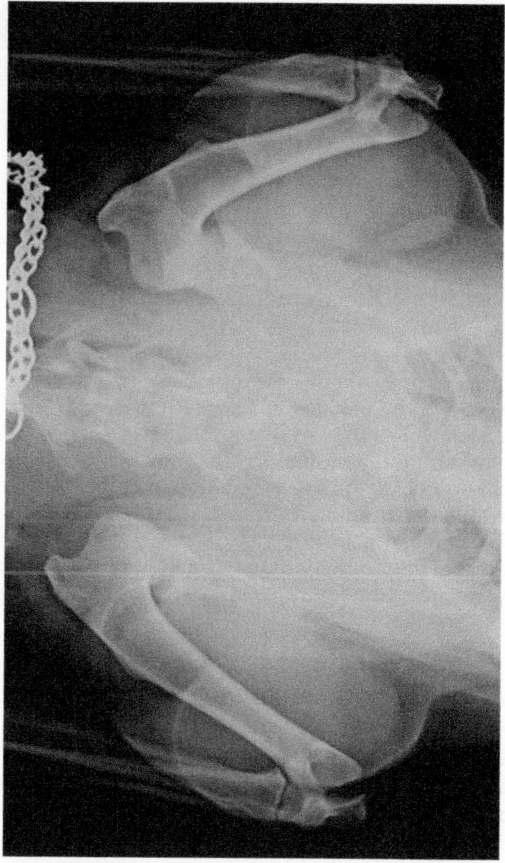

Fig. 1. Skyline view of the shoulder. Dog is placed in sternal recumbency and the shoulders and elbows flexed with the distal limb slightly pulled away from the body. This view allows a complete view of the intertubercular groove and greater tubercle of the humerus.

following the healing of tissues after treatment and rehabilitation. Ultrasound is relatively accessible, but the biggest obstruction to obtaining a good musculoskeletal ultrasound examination is a steep learning curve, limited training opportunities, and, on a referral basis, radiologists proficient in performing or reading musculoskeletal ultrasound. Essential equipment includes a linear musculoskeletal probe with a recommended minimum frequency of 12 to 13 MHz, which is available with most console and laptop machines. In many cases, it can be performed without sedation. As this is becoming a more sought-after modality for orthopedic imaging, more specialists in radiology, sports medicine, and rehabilitation are gaining and delivering training in this area, which should make it more accessible.

In the shoulder, the structures that can be most reliably evaluated include the supraspinatus, biceps tendon, and infraspinatus tendon and their associated musculature. The joint and biceps sheath can be evaluated for signs of inflammation with effusion, synovial proliferation, and thickening of the joint capsule. The medial joint structures including the medial glenohumeral ligament and subscapularis tendon cannot be reliably imaged for pathology, making ultrasound ineffective for definitively diagnosing cases of medial shoulder instability/syndrome (MSI/MSS).[1,4] Description of both

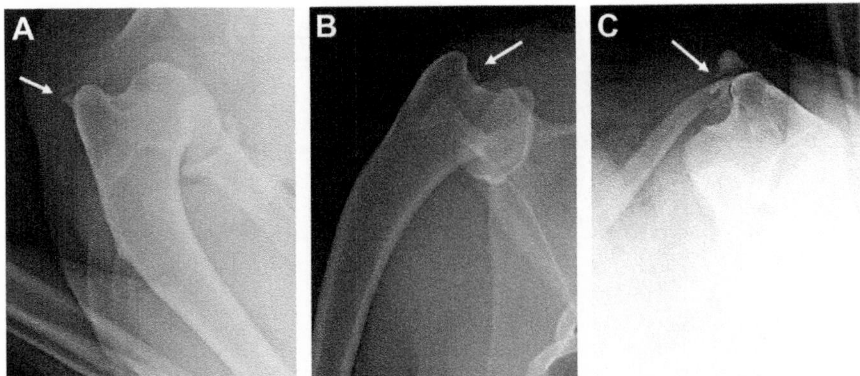

Fig. 2. Skyline of the view of the shoulder in 3 dogs. This view is helpful in determining the location of mineralization when observed on the lateral view and what structures are more likely involved. Mineralization is indicated by white arrows. In panel *A*, mineralization is discretely of the greater tubercle with the mineralization of the insertion of the supraspinatus. Mineralization within the intertubercular groove as with panel *B* implicates the biceps tendon as a potential source of pain. In panel *C* there is significant mineralization of the supraspinatus insertion down into the intertubercular groove that implicates both the severe supraspinatus mineralizing tendinopathy as well as possible impingement of the biceps tendon as a source of lameness.

normal and abnormal findings in the shoulder have been published along with comparisons of findings between symptomatic and asymptomatic dogs.[5–11]

The supraspinatus tendon is identified at the level of the acromion extending from its large muscle cranial to the scapular spine down the insertion on the greater tubercle of the humerus. On longitudinal view, it has an ovate shape and becomes diffusely hypoechoic compared with the surrounding tissue with a hyperechoic peritenon (**Fig. 4**). Some acoustic shadowing by the greater tubercle may be noted on the caudal aspect of the tendon. On tangential views, it is ovoid at the insertion. It is uniformly hypoechoic without the typical recognizable linear fiber pattern of other tendon/ligament

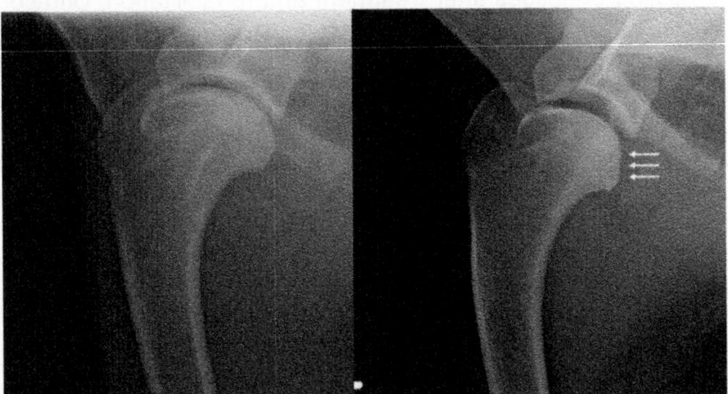

Fig. 3. Radiographs of a 11-month-old Border Collie presenting for a 3-month history of LF lameness. In the first image taken, the OCD lesion of the caudal humeral head is not easily identified. With the pronation of the shoulder in the second radiograph, the flattening and irregularity of the caudal humeral head are more easily recognized (*white arrows*).

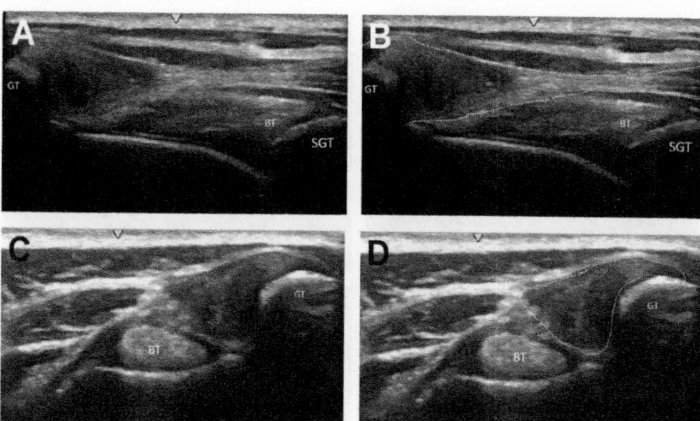

Fig. 4. Longitudinal (panels A and B) and transverse (panels C and D) ultrasounds of the supraspinatus tendon. The supraspinatus tendon is ovate in shape and becomes diffusely hypoechoic compared with the surrounding and other tendon tissue as it widens at the insertion on the greater tubercle in longitudinal scans. In transverse it wraps around the greater tubercle in a comma-shape and continues to be hypoechoic especially compared with the adjacent biceps tendon. A hyperechoic peritenon delineates the margins of the tendon. The biceps tendon can be visualized deep to the supraspinatus but will be out of the plane in most dogs. BT, tendon; GT, greater tubercle of the humerus; SGT, supraglenoid tubercle of the scapula. In panels B and D the supraspinatus tendon is outlined (*dashed line*).

structures (**Fig. 5**). Size (cross-sectional area in the transverse plane, width in the longitudinal plane) will vary with the size of the dog and has been documented by weight and breed.[5,11] Abnormalities of the supraspinatus tendon include mineralization, disruption of the homogenous fiber pattern with hyper- or hypoechoic regions, bony remodeling of the greater tubercle, and enlargement that sometimes compresses or displaces the biceps tendon in the intertubercular groove (**Fig. 6**). Clinically the difficulty with the identification of supraspinatus abnormalities using any modality, including ultrasound, is the interpretation of the clinical significance in the lame dog. Supraspinatus changes have been noted in dogs without evidence of lameness and in the unaffected limb in several studies.[7,11,12] Any finding of supraspinatus abnormalities should be interpreted in conjunction with other diagnostic findings in the shoulder joint. Often supraspinatus injury does not happen in isolation from other soft tissue injuries including the biceps tendon, MSI/MSS, or elbow disease, therefore, with any finding of supraspinatus tendinopathy, these other areas should be explored as well.[1,13,14]

Within the shoulder joint and biceps tendon sheath, evaluation for effusion, and disruption to the biceps tendon should be performed. The biceps tendon can be evaluated from the origin of the supraglenoid tubercle down to the proximal musculotendinous junction. The biceps tendon in general is hyperechoic and unlike the supraspinatus tendon, has the typical fiber pattern and echogenicity of tendon tissue (see **Fig. 6**). Changes will include hypoechoic lesions indicative of acute tears or a more mottled and/or hyperechoic appearance with chronic injury. The presence of a significant increase in fluid surrounding the tendon is indicative of synovitis and/or biceps tenosynovitis. Often when significantly increased, especially circumferentially, other joint pathology such as MSI/MSS is more likely to be present (**Fig. 7**).[7]

The infraspinatus tendon on the lateral aspect of the shoulder is identified from the large infraspinatus muscle that arises on the scapula caudal to the spine. Similar to the

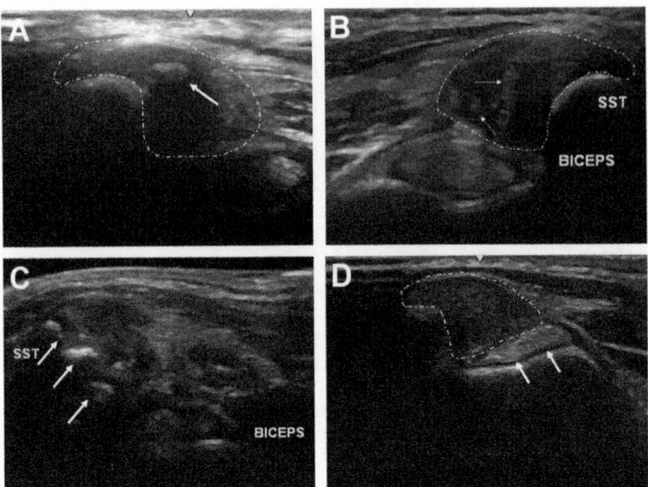

Fig. 5. Examples of ultrasonographic abnormalities noted on ultrasound of the supraspinatus tendon. Panel *A*–mineralization within the supraspinatus tendon (*white arrow*). Mineralization causes acoustic shadowing which obscures the visualization of structures deep into the mineralization. Panel *B*- disruption of the homogenous fiber pattern with hyper- or hypoechoic regions as indicated by the arrows. Panel *C*-bony remodeling (*white arrows*) of the greater tubercle. This dog also has severe disruption of the fiber pattern of the SST with both hyper and hyperechoic regions, discrete mineralization, and loss of normal margins on the craniolateral aspect. Panel *D*-enlargement of the supraspinatus tendon causing compression of the biceps tendon in the intertubercular groove. SST, supraspinatus tendon.

supraspinatus, it can be evaluated from the musculotendinous junction to the insertion on the caudal distal aspect of the greater tubercle can be evaluated in transverse and longitudinal planes. No different than other tendon injuries, pathology may include mineralization, abnormal fiber pattern, tendon enlargement, and boney remodeling at the insertion. Ossification or inflammation infraspinatus bursa may also be noted. Infraspinatus tendinopathy may be identified in conjunction with other shoulder soft tissue injuries (eg, supraspinatus or biceps tendon) or as an isolated injury. When occurring as an isolated injury it is typically noted with infraspinatus contracture and its characteristic physical examination findings.[15]

Osteochondrosis lesions can also be identified with ultrasound, but should be used with caution as sensitivity, specificity, and accuracy are low compared with other options and false positives can occur.[3]

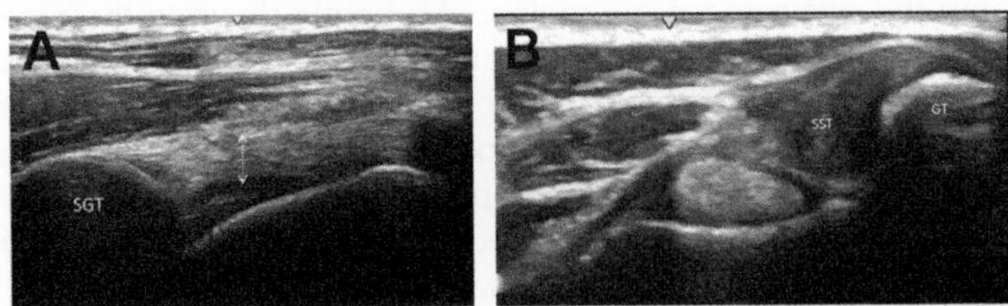

Fig. 6. Longitudinal (*A*) and transverse (*B*) ultrasound images of the biceps tendon. On longitudinal scan, the biceps (between arrow heads) has a typical linear fiber pattern and is hyperechoic. On transverse, the biceps is oval in shape and diffusely hyperechoic. GT, greater tubercle of the humerus; SGT, supraglenoid tubercle; SST, supraspinatus tendon.

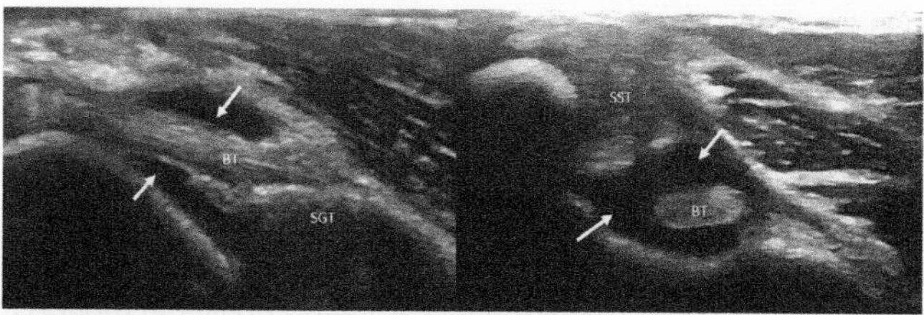

Fig. 7. Ultrasound of a 3-year-old Labrador Retriever showing significant effusion (white arrows) in the shoulder joint and proximal biceps sheath. BT, Biceps tendon; SGT, supraglenoid tubercle; SST, supraspinatus tendon.

COMPUTED TOMOGRAPHY

Computed tomography is a cross-sectional x-ray modality that can be used to create multiplanar three-dimensional images of the area of interest. As it is an x-ray modality it is primarily used for suspected bony lesions in orthopedic evaluations.[16] In the shoulder CT has been used to evaluate shoulder pathology and is readily able to identify osteochondral lesions that may have been missed on conventional radiography (**Fig. 8**).[14,16] While OCD lesions can be identified via ultrasound, CT will be a superior modality due to the limitations of ultrasound relative to lesion location within the joint.[3] It can also be used to further characterize soft tissue mineralization in the supraspinatus, infraspinatus, biceps, and subscapularis tendons.[14] The disadvantage compared with ultrasound is that it gives little detailed information of other aspects of tendon injury and structure.

NEEDLE/NANO ARTHROSCOPY

Arthroscopy can be a highly effective modality for the diagnosis of intraarticular diseases of the shoulder joint. This is especially true for medial shoulder instability/medial shoulder syndrome whereby the subscapularis tendon and medial glenohumeral ligament cannot be fully assessed by radiography, ultrasound, or CT. It can also be used to evaluate the biceps tendon and the surface of the humeral head and glenoid for cartilage defects and OCD lesions. Needle arthroscopy is generally described as arthroscopy using a small arthroscope (1.9 mm or less) and is frequently performed under sedation. Arthroscopy as a diagnostic tool allows direct visualization of the structures within the joint and the ability to assess for soft tissue and cartilage damage.

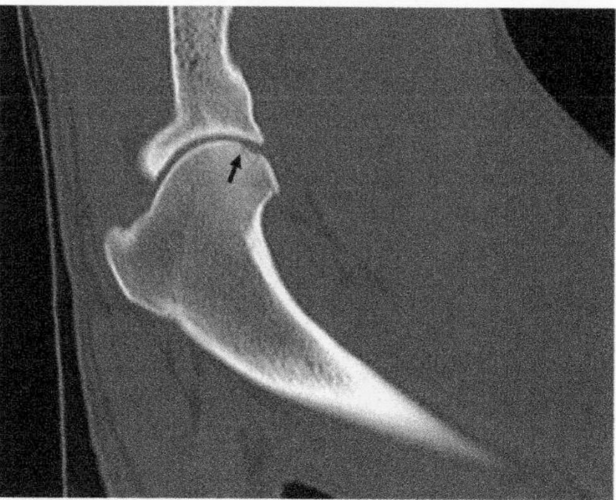

Fig. 8. CT of the shoulder of a 13-month-old Labrador showing a defect in the caudal humeral head (*black arrow*). This defect was not obvious on radiographs of the shoulder.

Disadvantages are the evaluation is confined to the intraarticular structures only and additional imaging modalities such as ultrasound or MRI would be necessary for extra-articular structures. Advantages of needle arthroscopy over classic arthroscopy include the ability to perform the procedure under sedation, shorter procedure time, and cost.[17] Disadvantages include inferior image quality compared to traditional arthroscopy and the inability to treat possible lesions when identified. The intent of needle arthroscopy is as a diagnostic, rather interventional modality so it should be approached with that in mind. Despite a lesser image quality in most cases images are sufficient to make a diagnosis (**Figs. 9** and **10**). Accessibility to needle arthroscopy is growing in the veterinary field; however, specific training is limited. Board-certified surgeons that receive training and perform classic arthroscopy are easily able to perform needle arthroscopy but may not choose to have needle arthroscopy in addition to their surgical equipment. Outside the surgical specialty, specialists in sports medicine and rehabilitation are increasingly adding this modality into their diagnostic repertoire with training and education. Insertion of an arthroscope into the joint can cause cartilage damage and iatrogenic damage to the joint needs to be carefully considered before the utilization of this technique.[18,19] Knowledge of patient/limb positioning, portal placement, and identification of anatomic structures and pathology are key components to successful utilization of needle arthroscopy.

MAGNETIC RESONANCE IMAGING

MRI is the gold-standard imaging modality of soft tissue injury in human patients and over the past 2 decades has become increasingly used in dogs. With a good study, it can provide good anatomic and pathologic definitions in multiple planes. It is the single imaging modality that will allow the evaluation of both the intra and extraarticular structures of the shoulder. In one study it was found to be in strong agreement and concordance for most of the intraarticular soft tissues.[20] Despite its increased use, access to MRI can be limited in some regions, requires general anesthesia, and costs can be high. So practically it may not be an ideal modality for some clients.

KEY POINTS-SHOULDER

- Radiography is reliable for the identification of shoulder OCD, but one may need to include pronated and supinated views to identify the lesion

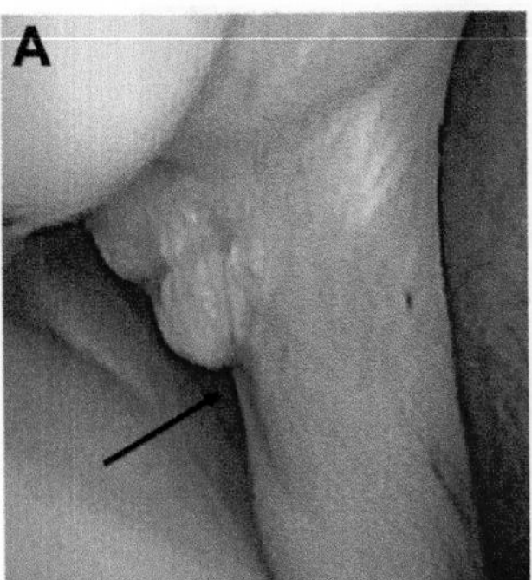

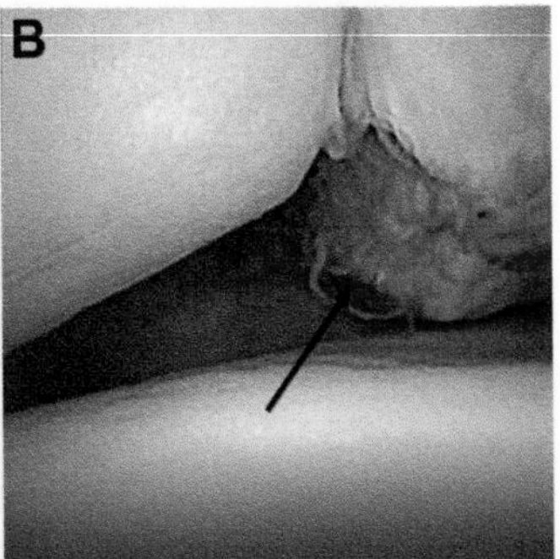

Fig. 9. Needle/nano arthroscopy of the shoulder joint in the dog using the Arthrex Nanoscope. Panel *A* shows a normal biceps tendon (*black arrow*) from the origin down to the intertubercular groove. In panel *B* there is a partial biceps tear affecting about 50% of the tendon (*black arrow* indicating the region of tear). (Images courtesy of Dr. Peter Lotsikas.)

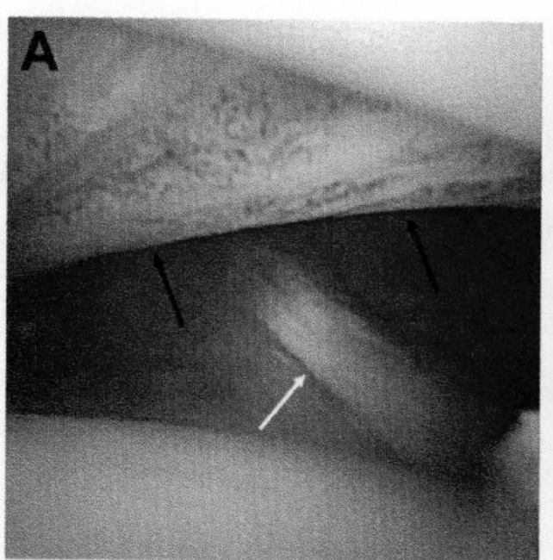

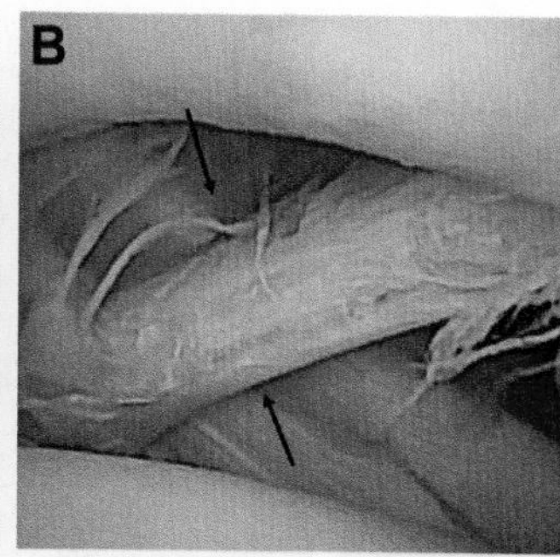

Fig. 10. Needle/Nano arthroscopy of the shoulder joint in a dog using the Arthrex Nanoscope. In panel *A* the normal medial glenohumeral ligament (MGL) is indicated by the black arrow and the subscapularis tendon by the white arrow. In Panel B a torn MGL is seen (*black arrows*). (Image in panel B courtesy of Dr. Peter Lotsikas.)

- Radiography is limited for diagnosing soft tissue injury but can provide some information when calcified tendinopathies are present. Additional radiographic views are often necessary to accurately identify existing pathology
- Ultrasound is a good diagnostic method for the evaluation of soft tissue structures in and around the joint, apart from the medial shoulder structures
- The utility of CT is ideal to detect osseous changes including soft tissue mineralization, enthesopathy, and OCD.
- Classic arthroscopy and needle/nano arthroscopy can be valuable in the evaluation of intraarticular structures, especially for the detection of pathology of the medial aspect of the shoulder
- MRI can be used to evaluate both intra and extraarticular bony and soft tissue structures

ELBOW

The primary conditions of concern in the elbow joint is elbow dysplasia, most commonly medial compartment disease and associated arthritis. Elbow dysplasia is a constellation of developmental conditions within the joint including coronoid disease, ununited anconeal process (UAP), OCD, and joint incongruity. Medial compartment disease, with severe cartilage loss in the medial compartment, is thought to be associated with either elbow dysplasia or trauma. Soft tissue injury is an infrequent source of lameness in the elbow.

RADIOGRAPHY

The secondary degenerative changes associated with medial compartment disease are frequently identifiable with radiography, particularly in older dogs. However, it is important for a full assessment that a properly positioned series is performed in all suspected cases. The elbow is a complex joint and superimposition of the humerus, radius and ulna require multiple views to assess the joint. A complete study will include mediolateral extended, mediolateral flexed 45°, craniocaudal (Cr-Cd), and cranial-caudal to craniolateral 15° oblique (**Fig. 11**). Performing a complete series will optimize the likelihood of the diagnosis of elbow disease as a single lateral view will not always identify pathology. UAP is the only condition that can be reliably diagnosed with radiography. It is typically readily identified on the mediolateral views, especially the flexed view (**Fig. 12**). In the case of coronoid disease, multiple views are needed, especially

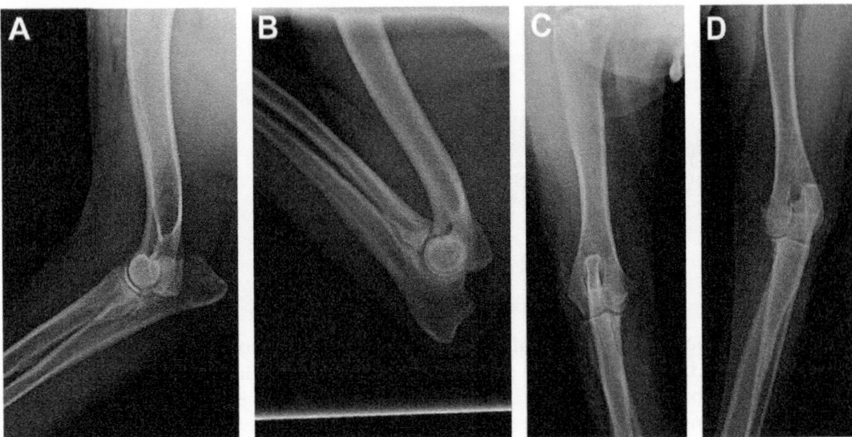

Fig. 11. Standard radiographic views for elbow dysplasia and medial compartment disease. (*A*)-mediolateral extended, (*B*)-mediolateral flexed 45°, (*C*)-craniocaudal, and (*D*)- cranial-caudal to craniolateral 15° oblique.

the Cr-Cd and Cr-Cd oblique views (**Fig. 13**). Alternatively, a CT may be considered (see later in discussion). Osteophytes associated with elbow dysplasia can be identified on all projections and will be located on the dorsoproximal radius, medial and lateral condyles, medial coronoid, and the anconeal process. In the case of elbow joint incongruity, whereby there is malalignment of the articulation between the ulna,

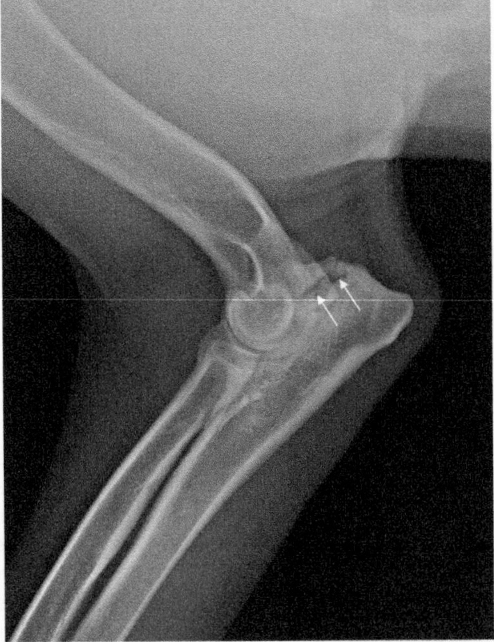

Fig. 12. Radiographic appearance of an ununited anconeal process on the neutral medial to lateral projection. White arrows are indicating the fissure of the united anconeal process. It would have less superimposition with the humerus with the elbow flexed to 45°.

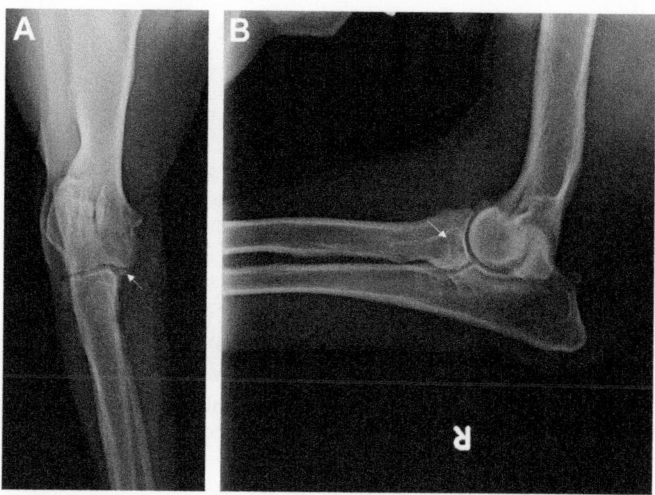

Fig. 13. Cranial-caudal to craniolateral 15° oblique (panel A) and mediolateral (panel B) radiographs of a 22-month-old intact male German Shepherd. In panel *A*, abnormal conformation and fragmentation of the medial coronoid (*white arrow*) are observed. On the mediolateral projection once again you can see the irregular coronoid along with osteophyte formation on the dorsoproximal radius.

radius, and humeral condyle, radiographs can be used to determine the presence and degree of radioulnar and humeroulnar incongruity. However, the sensitivity and specificity can be quite variable and significantly influenced by the position of the elbow during image acquisition.[21]

Flexor enthesopathy may be noted and is characterized by the calcification of the medial epicondyle of the humerus, they are found as discrete lesions and can occur concurrently with other signs of elbow disease.[22,23] The mineralization is associated with the origin of the flexor muscles on the medial epicondyle (flexor carpi ulnaris, superficial, and deep digital flexors) and may occur as a discrete calcified body or enthesophyte of the medial humeral epicondyle.[23] (**Fig. 14**)

Radiography can frequently identify elbow joint pathology but acquiring a complete series is an important factor in the success of using this modality. Experience in reading a complete elbow series can play a role in making a diagnosis, so sending for a radiologist review may be helpful before moving on to more advanced imaging options in dogs with elbow pain.[24]

ULTRASONOGRAPHY

Several studies have been performed describing the ultrasonographic anatomy of the canine elbow to provide a guide for complete examination.[25–27] However, the utility of ultrasound for elbow dysplasia/medial compartment syndrome is questionable. Ultrasound examination of the pathologies associated with elbow dysplasia have been described and include coronoid disease, osteophytes, and ununited anconeal process.[28,29] However, compared with the arthroscopy, ultrasound had a 45% false negative for free fragments, 91% for nondisplaced fragments, and was only 77% accurate for identifying abnormalities of the coronoid.[30] It is not surprising that it does not compare favorably, and likely would not against other imaging options, as ultrasound is limited in the comprehensive evaluation of the elbow joint due to its small size and the inability of ultrasound to image beyond the bone surface.

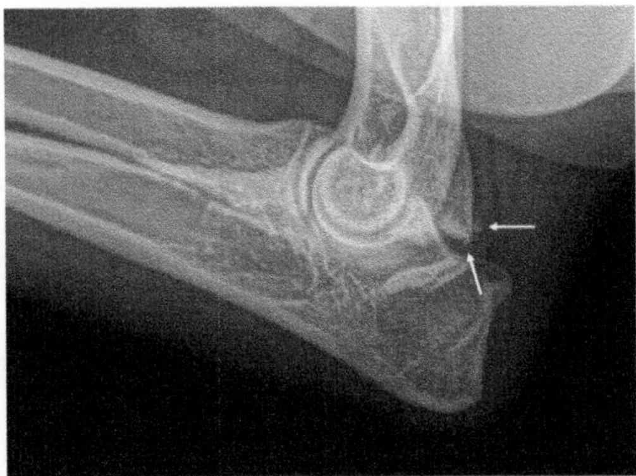

Fig. 14. Primary flexor enthesopathy with a discrete calcified body and enthesophyte - "bone spur" - (white arrows) of the medial humeral epicondyle.

Soft tissue injuries around the elbow are uncommon, but ultrasound can play a role in the evaluation of the involved structures including the collateral ligaments, triceps insertion, and flexor enthesopathy.[22,29]

COMPUTED TOMOGRAPHY

Computed tomography has been shown in multiple studies to be highly specific and sensitive for identifying medial coronoid lesions as well joint incongruity and degenerative joint pathology associated with elbow dysplasia.[31,32] Fragments of the coronoid process are readily identified, with a 100% sensitivity and 93% specificity against the gold standard of arthroscopy (**Fig. 15**).[31] There are some limitations in the identification of nonosseous medial coronoid fragments and cartilage erosions and slice thickness of 1 mm or less helps improve lesion identification and improve image quality.[32,33]

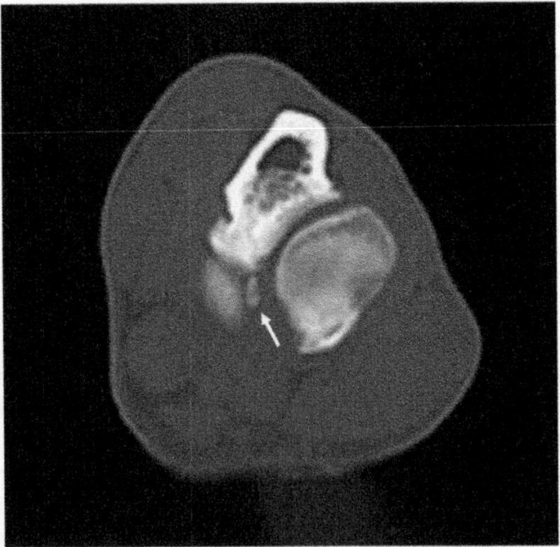

Fig. 15. CT of the elbow showing a fragment (*white arrow*) of the medial coronoid in a 1-year-old mixed breed dog.

NEEDLE/NANO ARTHROSCOPY

Needle arthroscopy has been compared with classic arthroscopy and CT for the evaluation of medial compartment disease in 27 dogs.[34] For identifying cartilage lesions needle arthroscopy was equivalent to traditional arthroscopy, but in fragment identification traditional arthroscopy had a higher sensitivity and specificity but was not found to be statistically superior to needle arthroscopy.[34] Both traditional and needle arthroscopy were inferior to the detection of fissures when compared with CT, but this also was not statistically signficant.[34] Based on this work it appears that needle arthroscopy has diagnostic value in the identification of cartilage damage and fragment/fissure identification with some limitations. As stated above, caution should be used when considering this technique to avoid iatrogenic joint damage.

MRI - Magnetic resonance imaging The size of the elbow joint does create some issues for use of MRI to make a diagnosis of coronoid fragmentation and was inferior to arthroscopy in identifying the degree of cartilage damage in one study.[35] Use of MRI-arthrography does improve the visualization of cartilage defects, but is not necessary for defining coronoid disease.[36,37] Its advantage over CT is unknown.

KEY POINTS–ELBOW

- Evaluation of the elbow joint for elbow dysplasia/medial compartment disease with radiography should include multiple views including the mediolateral extended, mediolateral flexed 45°, craniocaudal (Cr-Cd), and cranial-caudal to craniolateral 15° oblique, if radiography is used as the only diagnostic imaging modality
- Ultrasonography is unreliable for identifying medial coronoid disease and its use is confined to soft tissue injury (specifically flexor enthesopathy)
- Computed tomography has a very high sensitivity and specificity for medial coronoid disease and incongruity but will not reliably identify cartilage lesions.
- A combination of radiography (or ideally CT) and arthroscopy are likely to be the most rewarding for the identification of elbow dysplasia and medial compartment disease
- Needle/nano arthroscopy has some promise to diagnose medial coronoid disease, joint incongruency, and cartilage damage but iatrogenic cartilage damage may occur

Carpus

Injury to the carpus occurs less frequently than shoulder and elbow. Sprains are the most common and can affect the flexor carpi ulnaris, extensor tendons, and the carpal ligaments, but all these occur infrequently. In the case of significant damage to the palmar carpal structures, carpal hyperextension can occur. Injury can be acute or chronic and arthritis is a common sequela of chronic disease and instability. Fractures in the carpus are common in Greyhound racing dogs.

RADIOGRAPHY

Standard radiographic views of the carpus include the dorsal-palmar (DP) and medial-lateral views. As the carpus is a complex joint with 3 joints and 14 bones, standard views may not always readily identify bony pathology. Therefore, oblique and flexed medial-lateral views should then be added for a complete evaluation. Stressed views may also be helpful to diagnose collateral ligament and subtle hyperextension injury. To assess collateral ligament integrity, stressing the joint medially or laterally to identify

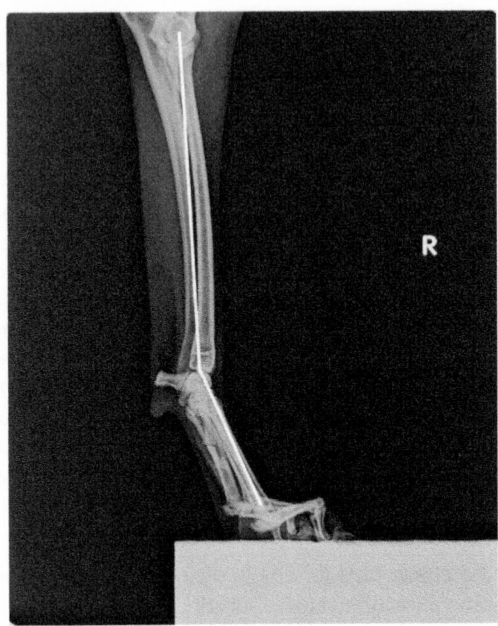

Fig. 16. Lateral radiograph of the carpus in a standing dog. The LF is elevated to encourage maximal weight bearing. The joint angle is then measured and compared with the contralateral limb and against published normal values to assess for carpal hyperextension.

an abnormal widening of the joint space on the DP view is used.[38,39] For carpal hyperextension, lateral standing or simulated weight-bearing radiographs can be used to measure the joint angle of the carpus. Comparison to both the normal limb and against previously determined normal values (**Fig. 16**) can be performed.[40,41] Avulsion fragments, enthesopathy, and bony remodeling at the origin/insertions and sclerosis of the distal radial groove can be noted with soft tissue injury (**Fig. 17**).

ULTRASOUND

Due to the anatomic structures overlying the palmar aspect, evaluation of the palmar carpal ligaments is difficult. It is routinely used for the evaluation of the extensor tendons, flexor carpi ulnaris, and collateral ligaments and normal ultrasonographic anatomy of the dorsal aspect of the carpus was recently described.[42] Ultrasound was shown to successfully characterize changes associated with stenosing tenosynovitis of the abductor pollicis longus tendon and follow treatment, but otherwise clinical reports for diagnosing carpal pathology are scant.[43,44] The author has found it useful in acute and chronic injuries with carpal swelling to help differentiate between joint and tendon/tendon sheath injury (**Fig. 18**). As the tendons and ligaments of the carpus are superficial and small in size, visualization can be improved by the utilization of an ultrasound stand-of pad.

COMPUTED TOMOGRAPHY

The use of CT in the carpus is limited to the identification of fractures and other bony abnormalities and surgical planning. It has not been shown to be superior to MRI and is not enhanced by CT-arthrography for the identification of soft tissue structures.[45]

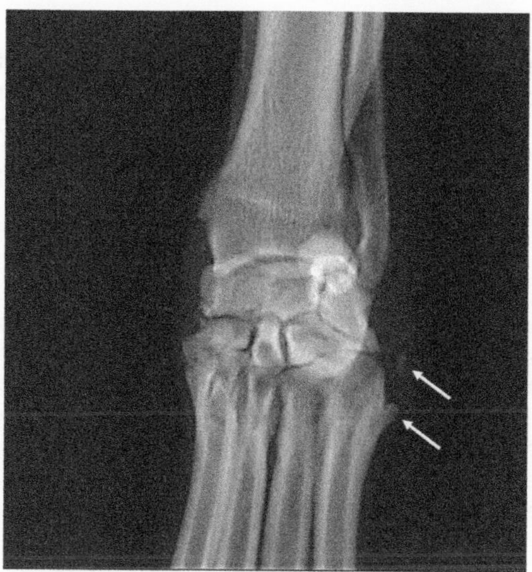

Fig. 17. DP radiograph of an 11-year-old Australian Shepherd with lateral collateral desmitis. Note the soft tissue swelling and mineralization of the lateral collateral ligament and enthesophyte of the 5th metatarsal head (*white arrows*).

MAGNETIC RESONANCE IMAGING

Despite the small size of the structures, MRI can be used to evaluate the palmar carpal ligaments in normal dogs and MRI arthrography seems to be superior to MRI alone.[45,46] High-field MRI will be necessary for the carpus and 3 T machines will provide ideal image quality. No studies have been published on the clinical application of MRI for common carpal injuries.

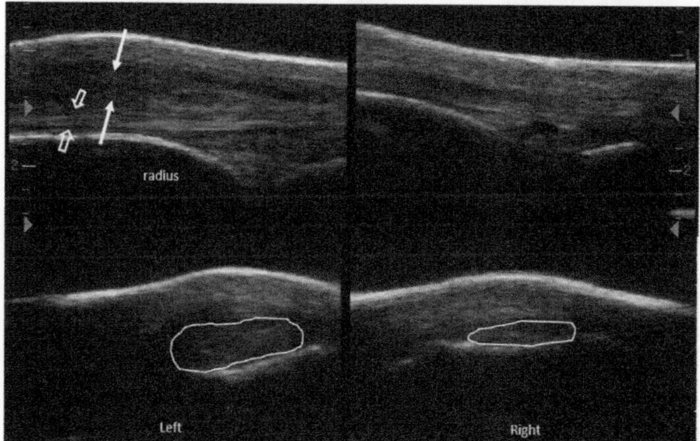

Fig. 18. Ultrasound of the dorsal aspect of the left carpus, with the right as a comparison, in an 8-year-old Labrador Retriever who developed lameness and carpal swelling after a fall during a Field Trial competition. Ultrasonographic examination shows soft tissue swelling (*solid arrows*) overlying and surrounding the common digital extensor tendon (*open arrows*) which is also enlarged.

KEY POINTS–CARPUS

- In addition to standard projections, stressed views may be helpful to evaluate the integrity of the collateral ligaments and palmar carpal ligaments
- Ultrasound is most useful to evaluate structures on the dorsal aspect of the carpus, collateral ligaments, and the flexor carpi ulnaris tendon
- MRI, specifically MR arthrography, is likely to be more rewarding than CT for carpal injury

Digits

Digit injuries are well-recognized as a source of lameness in the canine athlete. In racing Greyhounds, sprain of the digits was the most frequent injury reported in one study.[47] Based on survey analysis completed by handlers of dogs that compete in agility, injury to the digits was the most common area reported after shoulder and spine.[48,49] There is little information in the literature on imaging of the digits, but the identification of fractures, arthritis, sprains, strains, and sesamoid pathology will be the primary targets of the diagnostic modalities.

RADIOGRAPHY

When taking radiographs of the digits they must be positioned to eliminate superimposition and overcome the natural joint angles. When the paw is placed in a neutral position, the normal angle of the proximal interphalangeal joint is at 135° and the distal interphalangeal joint at 90° making it difficult to fully assess the bones and joints in their entirety.[50] To get a complete evaluation of these structures, it is important to pull the digits into full extension and can be accomplished by placing tape around the nail(s) and applying traction. Additionally, the digits can be fanned out individually on both the DP and lateral views to facilitate the assessment of the individual phalanges and associated soft tissues (**Fig. 19**). Using the tape, one can also assess medial or lateral instability by stabilizing the upper portion of the foot and then lateralizing the digit to see

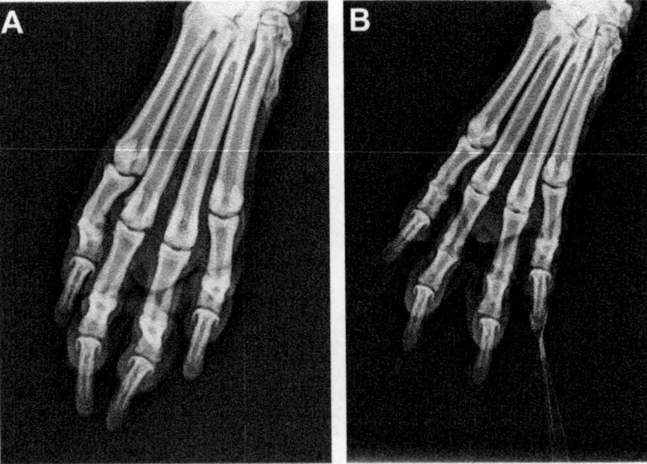

Fig. 19. Radiographic positioning for the digit. A DP view of the foot with the digits in neutral (*A*) and extended and separated with tape (*B*). Using tape to extend and separate the digits allows the reviewer to better assess the joints and for the presence of bone abnormalities.

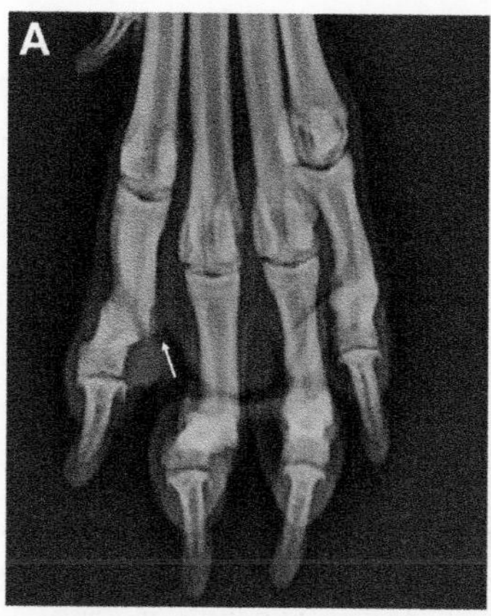

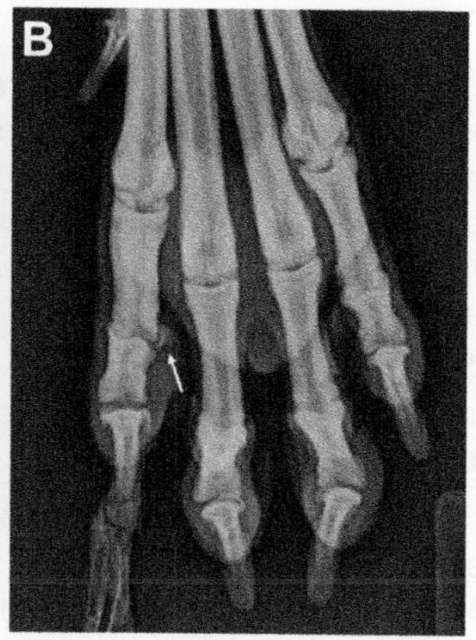

Fig. 20. DP radiograph with (*B*) and without (*A*) the 2nd digit pulled into extension with tape to facilitate visualization of a fragment (white arrow) of the axial aspect of proximal P2 and associated soft tissue swelling.

if the joint space opens due to the lack of collateral ligament integrity. Radiographs can identify soft tissue swelling, arthritic changes, fractures, and in the case of collateral ligament avulsions a bony fragment from the site of the avulsion from the phalanx (**Fig. 20**).

ULTRASOUND

Ultrasound has limited application in the digit. On the palmar/plantar surface of the foot the flexor tendons can be evaluated in the metacarpal/tarsal region, but distally the digital pads do not allow for the evaluation of the flexor tendons down into the digits. The author has used ultrasound to assess the collateral ligaments, fractures/avulsions and for joint effusion in a few cases (**Fig. 21**).

COMPUTED TOMOGRAPHY/MAGNETIC RESONANCE IMAGING

Normal anatomy of osseous and soft tissue structures has been published and showed that both bones and the major tendons and ligaments of the foot could be identified with some limitations for smaller structures and vasculature.[51] These advanced techniques have been used in isolated cases, typically to identify foreign bodies or characterize tumors. For bone and soft tissue injuries, they may be useful for a complete diagnosis, but no current studies are available on clinical applications for these injuries.

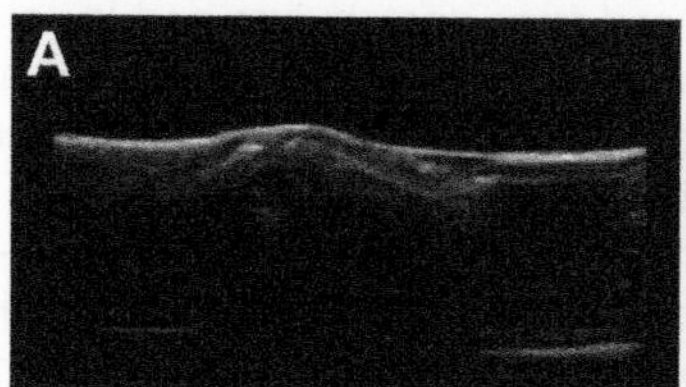

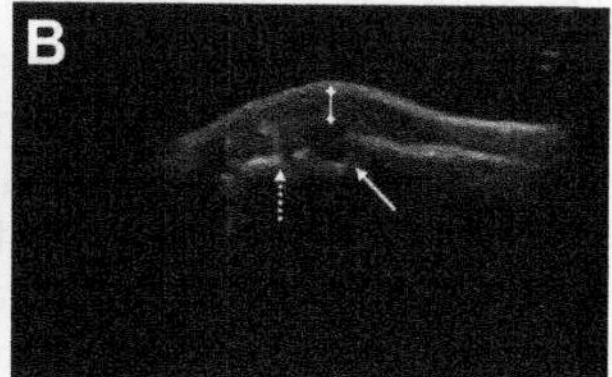

Fig. 21. Ultrasound of the PIP joint. In panel *A* is the normal appearance of the abaxial aspect of the joint. In panel *B* there is significant effusion (*solid arrow*) within the joint, bony remodeling at the insertion of the collateral ligament (*dashed arrow*) and thickening of the soft tissue and collateral ligament (between *diamonds*).

KEY POINTS–DIGITS

- To fully evaluate the digits radiographically it is critical that the affected phalanges be pulled into full extension on the DP view and fanned out in the DP and lateral views
- Ultrasound can be used, but structures that may be contributing to the lameness may not be accessible
- Little information is available on the clinical utility of CT and MRI for digit injuries, but could be considered in difficult cases

Hip/iliopsoas

Traumatic injury and dysplasia with associated arthritis are the typical hip-related orthopedic issues encountered in practice. The iliopsoas is also becoming a more widely suggested source of pain and lameness in the pelvic limbs. The iliopsoas starts as the psoas major originating of the ventral aspect of L2 and L3, joins the iliacus at the level of L7, and ultimately terminates on the lesser trochanter of the femur as a common tendon of insertion. This structure can suffer a primary strain of the muscle(s), fibrotic myopathy, or a tendon injury including acute strain, avulsion, or chronic tendinopathy.[52–54] Both hip dysplasia/arthritis and iliopsoas injury may cause pain on examination of the hip region. Differentiation between hip joint, primary iliopsoas injury, and secondary adaptive shortening of the iliopsoas due to other pathology can be a diagnostic challenge. Other soft tissue injuries to the large muscles of the thigh can also occur (muscle strains, tears, fibrotic myopathy) and may be identified on examination and be amenable to imaging.

RADIOGRAPHY

A ventral-dorsal (VD) projection of the pelvis with the hips extended is the standard radiographic view for the evaluation of the conformation of the hip joints and for signs of arthritis. It is especially important to make sure the limbs are extended straight from the hip joint symmetrically and patellae rotated dorsally to optimize evaluation (**Fig. 22**). Radiographic signs of hip dysplasia include shallow coverage of the femoral head by the acetabulum, subluxation, peri-articular osteophytes, flattening of the femoral head, and thickening of the femoral neck. Other more subtle radiographic signs include the caudal curvilinear osteophyte (Morgan Line) and circumferential femoral head osteophyte/rimming. In a young dog, hip joint laxity, which is positively correlated with the development of osteoarthritis, may not be obvious radiographically or accompanied by other signs of hip dysplasia.[55,56] In the US PennHip screening is the method used for the evaluation of passive hip joint laxity and gives a quantitative objective measurement called the Distraction Index (DI). The distraction index measures the displacement of the femoral head from acetabulum and is calculated by dividing the distance between the geometric center of the femoral head and the geometric center of the acetabulum by the radius of the femoral head.[57,58] PennHip certification is currently free and available to both veterinarians and veterinary technicians. There are 3 radiographs in the PennHip series: VD pelvis hip-extended, hip joint compression, and passive distraction using the PennHip distraction device. Radiographs are submitted for evaluation and a DI is calculated by PennHip and a formal report is generated (**Fig. 23**). The Distraction Index indicates the risk of development of arthritis with a DI close to 0.30 at low risk and an increasing risk as this number increases (see **Fig. 23**). In cases where there is a concern for possible hip dysplasia despite a normal VD radiograph, a PennHip study should be considered

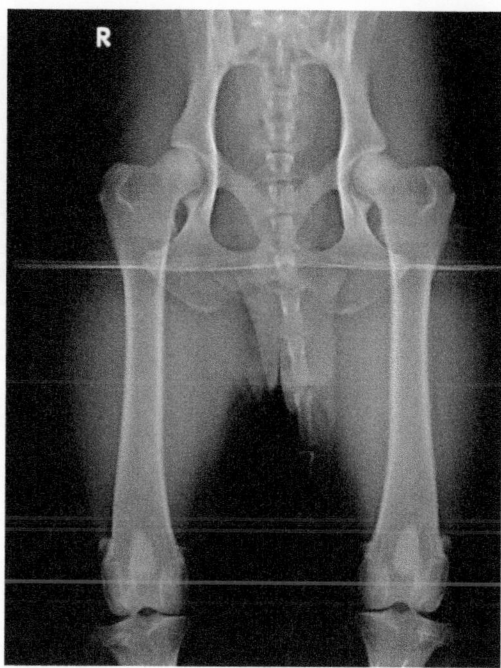

Fig. 22. A well-positioned ventrodorsal hip extended radiograph to assess the hip joint conformation. Note the femurs extend straight from the hip joint with equal coverage of the tuber ischii by femurs, patella are centered, and obturator foramen are equal indicating the pelvis is straight.

to evaluate laxity and risk of arthritis. This is especially true in dogs intended for sport or breeding.

The use of radiographs for iliopsoas injury will be limited to chronic tendinopathy and avulsion fractures. In these cases, changes to the lesser trochanter may be observed (**Fig. 24**).

ULTRASOUND

Ultrasound can be used to detect muscle strain of the psoas major and iliacus as well as changes to the iliopsoas.[52,59] Most dogs with pain on palpation or on iliopsoas stretch often won't tolerate the deep pressure of the probe and sedation is recommended for a good ultrasonographic examination. Normal ultrasonographic anatomy of the iliopsoas from the muscle origin to the insertion has been described.[59] With the dog in dorsal recumbency and the leg extended and slightly abducted, the tendon can be evaluated in longitudinal and transverse views (**Fig. 25**). Ultrasonographic changes will be typical of other tendon injuries, with a change in fiber pattern and/or echogenicity and bony changes associated with insertionopathy or avulsion (**Fig. 26**). A grading scale for characterizing injury of the iliopsoas has been proposed.[52] Within the muscle of the iliacus or psoas major there may be changes indicative of both acute and chronic damage. A grading scale for ultrasonographic changes associated with muscle injury was introduced by Tomlinson that describes the features of muscle injury that can be applied to the iliopsoas and is presented in **Table 1**.[60] In addition to the muscles of the iliopsoas this can also be applied to any muscle injury such as the one shown in **Fig. 27** of the gracilis.

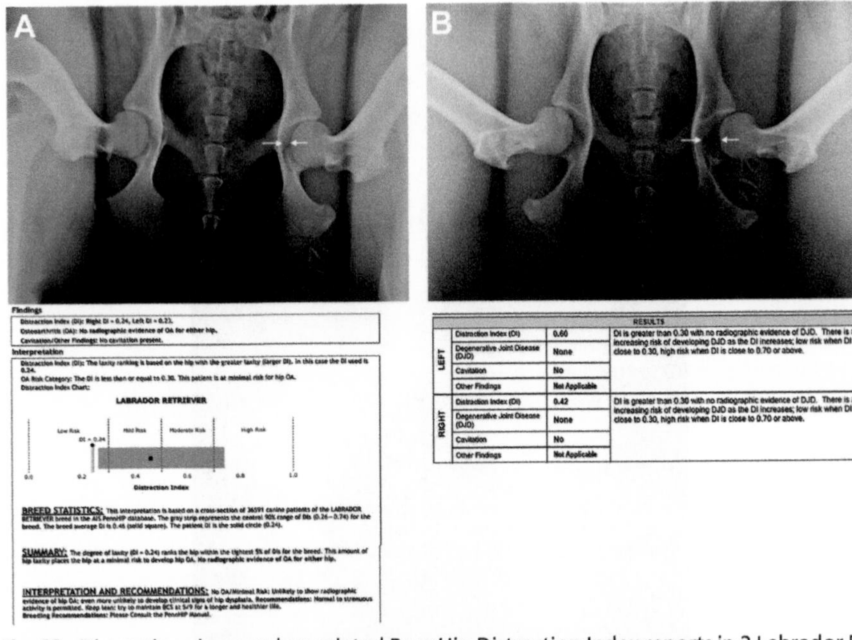

Findings

Distraction Index (DI): Right DI = 0.24, Left DI = [illegible].
Osteoarthritis (OA): No radiographic evidence of OA for either hip.
Cavitation/Other Findings: No cavitation present.

Interpretation

Distraction Index (DI): The laxity ranking is based on the hip with the greater laxity (larger DI). In this case the DI used is 0.24.
OA Risk Category: The DI is less than or equal to 0.30. This patient is at minimal risk for hip OA.
Distraction Index Chart:

BREED STATISTICS: This interpretation is based on a cross-section of 36591 canine patients of the LABRADOR RETRIEVER breed in the AIS PennHIP database. The gray strip represents the central 90% range of DIs (0.26–0.74) for the breed. The breed average DI is 0.46 (solid square). The patient DI is the solid circle (0.24).

SUMMARY: The degree of laxity (DI = 0.24) ranks the hip within the tightest 5% of DIs for the breed. This amount of hip laxity places the hip at a minimal risk to develop hip OA. No radiographic evidence of OA for either hip.

INTERPRETATION AND RECOMMENDATIONS: No OA/Minimal Risk: Unlikely to show radiographic evidence of hip OA; even more unlikely to develop clinical signs of hip dysplasia. Recommendations: Normal to strenuous activity is permitted. Keep lean: try to maintain BCS at 5/9 for a longer and healthier life.
Breeding Recommendations: Please Consult the PennHIP Manual.

RESULTS			
LEFT	Distraction Index (DI)	0.60	DI is greater than 0.30 with no radiographic evidence of DJD. There is an increasing risk of developing DJD as the DI increases; low risk when DI is close to 0.30, high risk when DI is close to 0.70 or above.
	Degenerative Joint Disease (DJD)	None	
	Cavitation	No	
	Other Findings	Not Applicable	
RIGHT	Distraction Index (DI)	0.42	DI is greater than 0.30 with no radiographic evidence of DJD. There is an increasing risk of developing DJD as the DI increases; low risk when DI is close to 0.30, high risk when DI is close to 0.70 or above.
	Degenerative Joint Disease (DJD)	None	
	Cavitation	No	
	Other Findings	Not Applicable	

Fig. 23. Distraction views and associated PennHip Distraction Index reports in 2 Labrador Retrievers. The dog in A has a low DI in both hips with low risk of development of arthritis in either hip. This dog was OFA Excellent. In panel B the dog's Distraction Index was 0.42 in the R hip and 0.60 in the L hip. This dog has a much higher risk of arthritis in both hips, especially the L due to its significant laxity. This dog was OFA Good. The distance between white arrows highlights the difference in passive joint laxity between the 2 dogs (but *arrows* are not associated with the PennHip evaluation).

Ultrasound has not been found to be a useful tool to determine hip joint laxity and as a predictor for hip dysplasia in dogs.[55,61] It can be helpful to guide intraarticular injections for treatment of arthritis in the dysplastic dog.[62]

COMPUTED TOMOGRAPHY/MAGNETIC RESONANCE IMAGING

In general CT and MRI will not be necessary to help identify pathology in routine orthopedic cases involving the hip joint. In isolated cases, MRI may be valuable

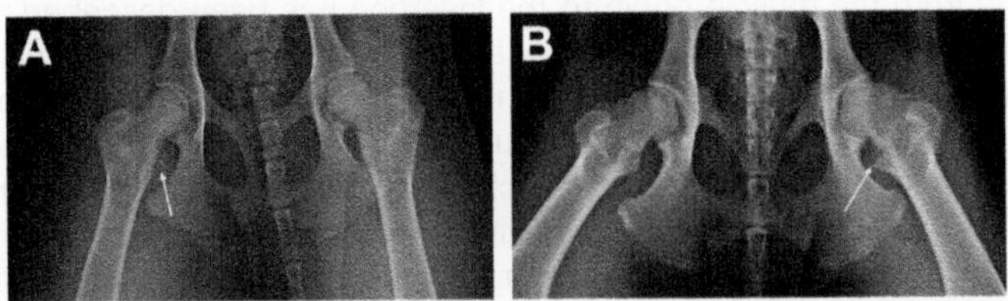

Fig. 24. Changes to the lesser trochanter with iliopsoas tendinopathy. (*A*): 8-month-old German Shorthaired Pointer with an avulsion of the lesser trochanter (*arrow* indicating the avulsed fragment). (*B*): 7-year-old Border Collie with hip dysplasia and chronic iliopsoas tendinopathy. There is bony remodeling of the less trochanter and mineralization of the iliopsoas tendon (*arrow*).

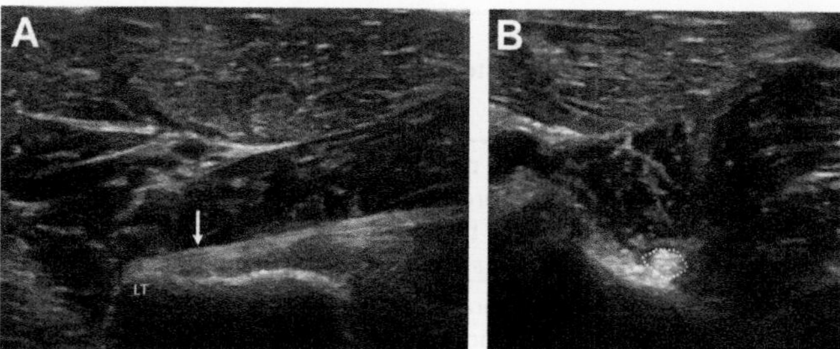

Fig. 25. Normal iliopsoas tendon in longitudinal (*A*) and transverse (*B*). LT, lesser trochanter of the femur which is the site of insertion of the tendon (*white arrow*). It can also be evaluated transverse by the rotation of the probe of the longitudinal plane and has a hyperechoic appearance with densely packed tendon fibers (*outlined*).

for soft tissue injury in the hip, iliopsoas, and surrounding musculature. This may be especially true when chronic injury to the psoas major muscle is affecting the femoral nerve, and other diagnostics have been unrewarding despite clear clinical signs.[63]

KEY POINTS–HIP/ILIOPSOAS

- Well positioned hip radiographs will give the clinician the ability to evaluate for hip dysplasia and arthritis
- PennHip evaluation should be considered when there is a concern for hip joint laxity, which is significantly correlated with the development of osteoarthritis
- Ultrasound can be used to identify acute and chronic injury to the muscle and tendon of the iliopsoas along with other muscle injuries

Stifle

Cranial cruciate ligament (CrCL) disease is the most common stifle pathology and cause of hind limb lameness encountered. Damage to the CrCL may include both complete and partial tears with partial tears often presenting a diagnostic challenge. In the case of partial tears, obvious instability may not be present on examination and in some cases overt pain on stifle examination may not be apparent and baseline radiographs only show minor changes (eg, joint effusion and early degenerative

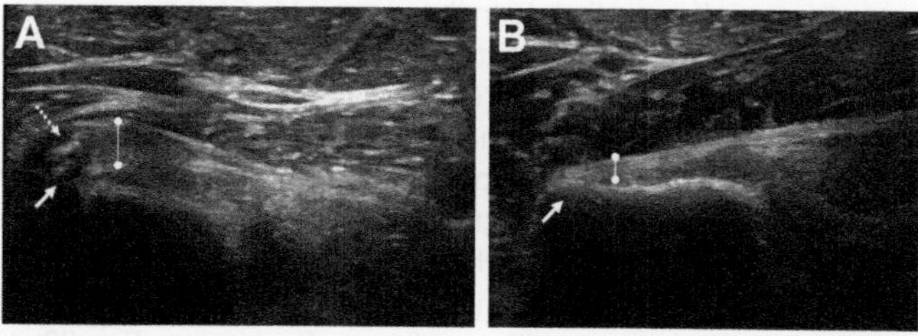

Fig. 26. Ultrasound of the 8-month-old German Shorthaired Pointer from **Fig. 24** (*A*) with an avulsion of the lesser trochanter and iliopsoas tendon. In the affected side (*A*) the iliopsoas tendon is markedly thickened (*white bar*) and the avulsed fragment (*dashed arrow*) is observed. The lesser trochanter (*solid arrow*) is irregular. In panel B is the opposite limb imaged for comparison.

Table 1
Grading muscle injury with diagnostic ultrasound

Grade of Injury	Description
1 – spasm, pain	• Weakening of muscle striations, increasing in speckling • Muscle structure still visible, clear and continuous boundaries • Striations may be close together due to muscle contraction • No significant swelling or increase in muscle thickness
2 - no macrotearing	• Muscle structure is compromised with the loss of striations • Increased echodensity between striations consistent with infiltrate • No significant swelling or increase in muscle thickness • Some areas of muscle contraction
3 - small tear	• Incomplete muscle boundaries with localized anechoic areas (<25% of total) • Increased echodensity between striations consistent with infiltrate
4 - full tear	• Localized anechoic regions, 30%–90% of muscle belly • Swelling and increase in muscle thickness • Loss of boundaries with other muscles/surrounding tissues • Edema in surrounding tissues

Ultrasonographic appearance and grading scale for muscle injury in the dog (Table courtesy of Dr Julia Tomlinson DVM, PhD, DACVSMR).[60]

changes). Concurrent meniscal injury may be present in 33% to 77% of dogs with CrCL tears.[64,65] Medial and lateral patellar luxation, OCD are other issues that affect the stifle. Soft tissue injuries such as collateral ligament desmopathy, long digital extensor tendon pathology, and quadriceps tendon injury are less common. Primary patellar desmopathy is also uncommon but is encountered as a complication of TPLO surgery.

RADIOGRAPHY

Lateral and cranial-caudal (Cr-Cd) views are the standard baseline radiographs for all diseases of the stifle. While a lateral-only may be a common approach for screening for CrCL disease, a Cr-Cd will help define some of the other changes noted within the joint as well as identify other pathology that may be missed on a lateral alone. To improve the diagnostic accuracy of lateral radiographs, the stifles should be taken individually from medial to lateral and collimated to the stifle and the femoral trochleae should be superimposed. As dogs with CrCL injury are at a 50% to 60% risk of rupture of the contralateral limb, radiographs of the opposite limb are indicated to assess for early changes in the nonaffected limb.[66] In the cases of CrCL injury, the clinician will be looking for evidence of effusion and degenerative changes that are classic signs of the disease. While an increase in joint fluid is not easily characterized in other joints, in the stifle, mild to significant effusion can be noted due to the displacement of the infrapatellar fat pad ("fat pad sign").[66] In the normal stifle joint the fat pad is a radiolucent structure in the cranial aspect of the joint. It sits in the triangular region between the patellar ligament, femur, and tibia but when effusion is present it is seen as a more radiodense area pushed cranially by the joint effusion (**Fig. 28**). Caudal displacement of the fascia lines may also be seen with significant effusion (see **Fig. 28**). Other radiographic changes consistent with chronic CrCL include bony remodeling consistent with osteoarthritis. On the lateral view, these changes will include bony remodeling and osteophytosis of the proximal femoral trochlea, distal patella, caudal tibial plateau, fabellae, and enthesophyte or avulsion at the insertion of the CrCL

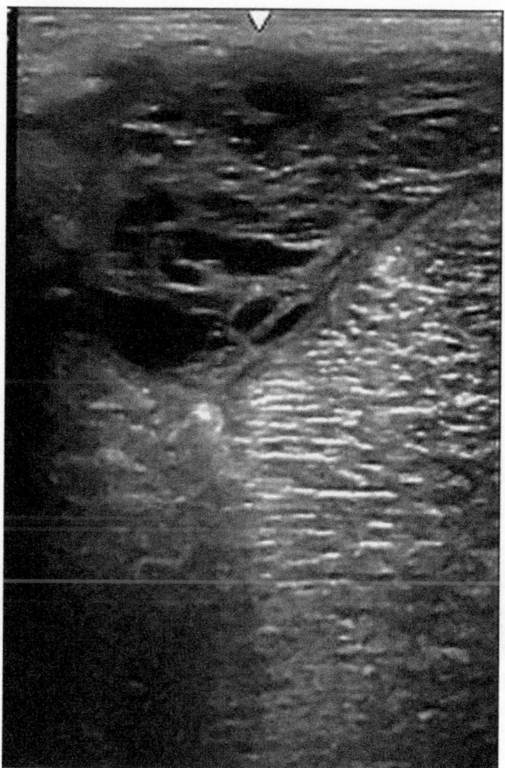

Fig. 27. Grade 4 acute muscle tear of the gracilis in an 8-year-old Giant Schnauzer. There is a significant disruption of normal muscle architecture with complete loss of normal striations, swelling, and loss of boundary with adjacent muscle on the caudal border. Anechoic regions are greater than 30% of the muscle belly.

(**Fig. 29**). Cranial tibial displacement may also be noted. In the Cr-Cd radiograph osteophytes, enthesophytes, and bony remodeling of the medial and lateral aspects of the tibial plateau, distal femur, origin of the long digital extensor and extensor fossa will be observed (see **Fig. 29**). In the case of early or low-grade partial tears, there may be very few radiographic changes and these cases are the ones that present a unique diagnostic challenge (**Fig. 30**).

Patellar luxation is readily identified on examination and radiographs may not provide any additional information other than to document the predisposing skeletal abnormalities. With chronic disease changes to the patella and mild arthritic changes associated with chronic inflammation may be present. When more substantial osteoarthritis and effusion are present, the dog should also be evaluated for CrCL disease. Concurrent CrCL rupture has been documented in up to 25% of dogs with medial patellar luxation and should be considered when evaluating a dog with a history of MPL who has persistent or acute worsening lameness.[67] Osteochondrosis lesions of the femoral condyles can be identified on radiographs. Both the medial to lateral and Cr-Cd projection should be obtained, but the medial to lateral may be more helpful diagnostically. To eliminate the superimposition of the femoral condyles and to help define lesions, oblique views may be helpful. Patellar ligament desmopathy is readily identified on radiographs due to the adjacent radiolucent infrapatellar fat pad helping

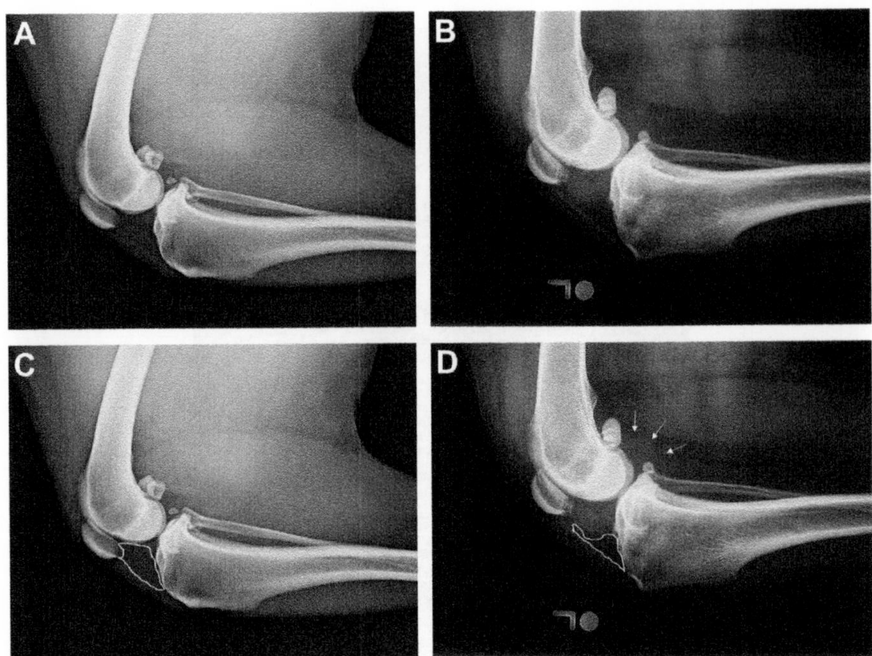

Fig. 28. Lateral radiograph of a normal stifle (*A*) and a joint with significant effusion associated with a chronic CCL injury (*B*). In panels C and D, the radiolucent infrapatellar fat pad is outlined to show the cranial displacement (fat pad sign) caused by the more radiodense effusion in D along with caudal displacement of fascial lines (*white arrows*).

to define the caudal border of the ligament. The thickening of the ligament is typically at the insertion on the tibia and mineralization or avulsed fragments may also be noted (**Fig. 31**).

ULTRASOUND

While ultrasound is a good imaging modality for identifying tendon and ligament pathology, the position of the cranial cruciate ligament in the joint does not allow for

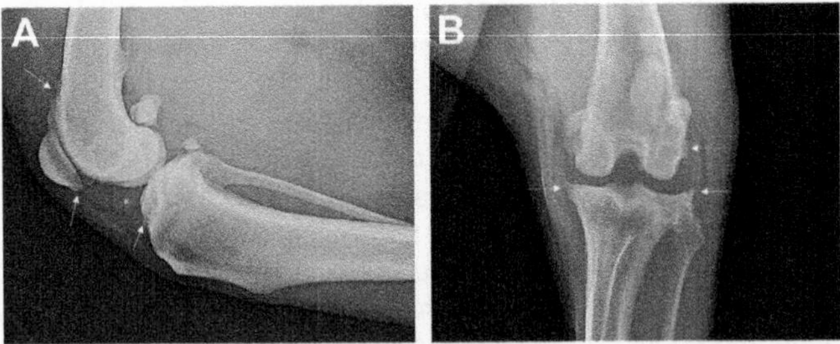

Fig. 29. Lateral (*A*) and cranial-caudal (*B*) radiograph of a 7-year-old Labrador Retriever with chronic CCL injury. Classic radiographic osteoarthritic changes are noted including osteophytosis of the proximal femoral trochlea, distal patella, caudal tibial plateau, and enthesopathy at CCL insertion on the tibia in the lateral view (*A–white arrows*). On the Cr-Cd view osteophytes, enthesophytes, and bony remodeling of the medial and lateral aspects of the tibial plateau, distal femur, origin of the long digital extensor and extensor fossa can be observed (*B–white arrows*).

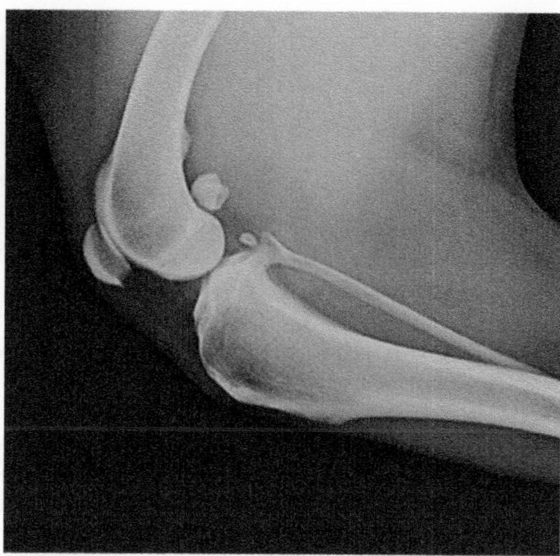

Fig. 30. Lateral radiograph of a 5-year-old intact male Labrador Retriever Field Trial dog with an intermittent hind limb lameness that worsens or recurs with exercise. At the time of the radiograph, which seems normal, he had a grade 1/5 lameness and no pain or instability noted on examination. Based on signalment and history arthroscopy was performed and tear encompassing approximately 20% of the cranial cruciate ligament was identified and a TPLO performed. This highlights the diagnostic challenge of early partial tears of the cranial crucial ligament can present.

accurate evaluation of the presence or degree of CrCL tears. In 2 studies CrCL damage was able to be identified in only 15.9% to 19.6% of cases.[68,69] Despite its dismal accuracy for the diagnosis of CrCL tears, patellar ligament, and meniscal pathology can be consistently identified. The meniscus appears as a wedge-shaped hyperechoic structure with a heterogenous speckled appearance (**Fig. 32**). Abnormalities

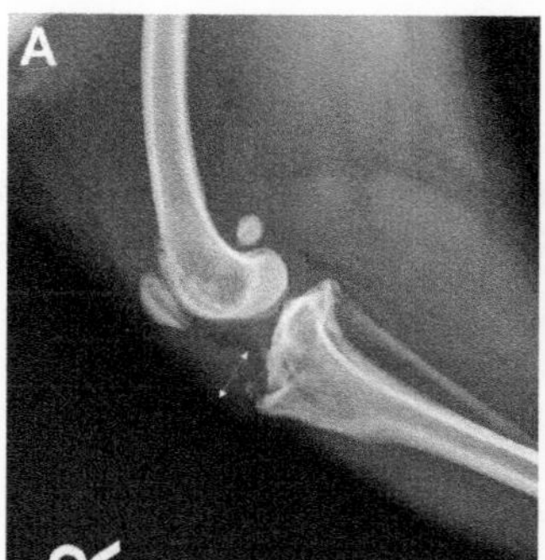

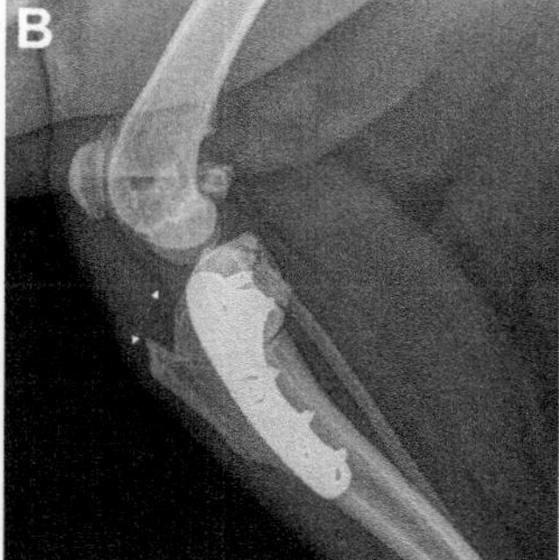

Fig. 31. Cases of primary (*A*) and secondary (*B*) patellar ligament desmopathy. In A is a 1.5-year-old French Bulldog with a grade 2/5 lameness and a history of medial patellar luxation. Radiographs show marked thickening of the patellar ligament (between *white arrows*) that is displacing the infrapatellar fat pad caudally along with mineral opacities just of the insertion on the tibial crest. In panel B is a 4 year mixed breed dog who is 8-weeks postop TPLO. At the time of radiographs, her lameness was more than expected and the patellar ligament was painful on palpation. Thickening (between *arrows*) and mineralization/avulsed fragments were noted.

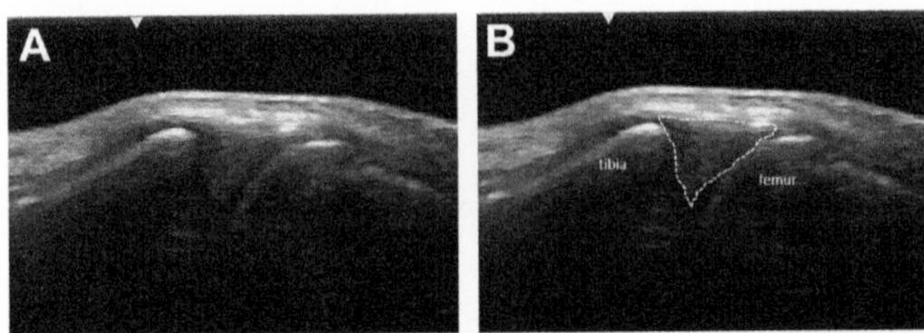

Fig. 32. Ultrasound of a normal meniscus. The normal meniscus has a wedge-shape (*B-dashed outline*) sitting between the tibia and femur on the medial or lateral aspect, deep to the collateral ligament. It is hyperechoic and has a heterogenous speckled appearance.

of meniscus include increased fluid signal around the meniscus, changes in fiber pattern and echogenicity, abnormal shape, and displacement (**Fig. 33**).[4,70] Ultrasound for meniscal injury has been shown to have very good sensitivity (from 82% to 95%) and specificity (80%–92%) for the experienced ultrasonographer.[64,68,70,71]

The normal patellar ligament is a flattened ovoid structure on transverse scan and in longitudinal it has a linear arrangement of fibers with a brighter white line of the periligamentous tissue demarcating it from the infrapatellar fat pad caudally and the skin and subcutaneous tissue cranially (**Fig. 34**). Desmopathy is characterized by enlargement and changes in fiber pattern and echogenicity and the presence of mineralization or fibrosis (**Fig. 35**).

NEEDLE/NANO ARTHROSCOPY

The use of needle/nano arthroscopy has not been described for use in the canine stifle, but has been used in equine patients to successfully identify cartilage and meniscal lesions.[72] The author has successfully used it in a few cases to assess the presence of partial CrCL tears when examination and routine radiographs were not conclusive. Peer-reviewed clinical reports are necessary to evaluate the value and limitations of this modality as a diagnostic, but it seems to have some promise.

COMPUTED TOMOGRAPHY

CT will have limited application for use in the stifle joint due to its limitations in providing good and accurate soft tissue detail. The application of CT arthrography (CTA) can improve the identification of CrCL injury with a good sensitivity and

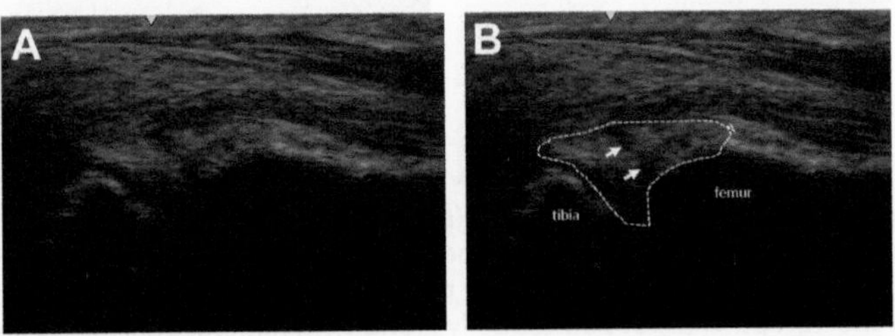

Fig. 33. Example of an abnormal medial meniscus on ultrasound (panel A). In panel B the meniscus is outlined and a bucket handle tear of the medial meniscus was confirmed with arthroscopy. There is a disruption in the fiber pattern (*white arrows*) due to a longitudinal tear in the meniscus. (Images courtesy of Dr. Julia Tomlinson).

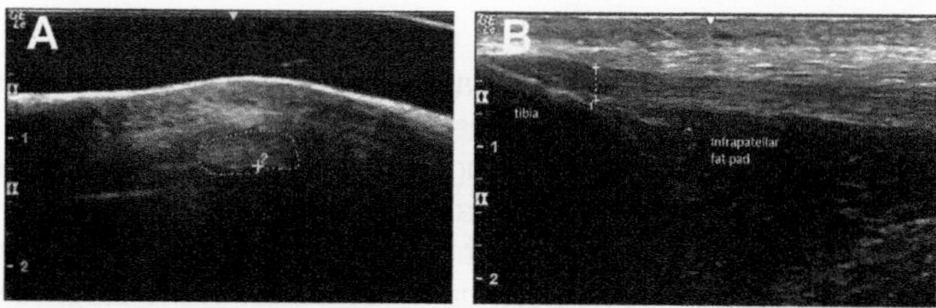

Fig. 34. Normal patellar ligament at the level of the insertion on the tibia in transverse (*A*) and longitudinal (*B*) planes.

specificity (96%–100%/75%–100%).[73] For meniscal tears sensitivity of CTA continues to be only fair in 2 studies with sensitivities only 13% to 73% and 57% to 64%.[73,74]

MAGNETIC RESONANCE IMAGING

MRI is the gold-standard diagnostic for CrCL disease in humans due to its exquisite soft tissue detail. In dogs normal anatomy has been described primarily using low-field (<0.5 T) units.[75,76] Pathology can be identified in both experimental and naturally occurring diseases including cranial and caudal cruciate ligament and meniscal tears, osteophyte development, and subchondral bone sclerosis.[77–82] The accuracy for lesion identification has varied among studies, but remains very good for the identification of CrCL lesions with a 93%-100% sensitivity and 100% specificity.[78,79] However, some caudal cruciate injuries may be misdiagnosed and some partial tears characterized as complete, which may not be clinically significant.[79] Identification of meniscal tears also seems to be reasonable across multiple studies using both low-field (<0.5 T) and high-field (>1.0 T) units. One would anticipate that low-field units to be inferior to high-field in lesion identification, however, in naturally occurring meniscal pathology using a 0.5 T machine the sensitivity and specificity were 64% and 90%.[80] 1.5 T MRI unit resulted in similar sensitivity and specificity in 2 studies, with both at 75%/100%.[70,83] Other studies show better results, all using high-field units, and have sensitivities from 90% to 100% and specificity from 94% to 100%.[77–79] While the differences between these studies may be technique, positioning, or experience related it seems that for meniscal injury that MRI may not be reliable in all cases, but high-field MRI may optimize diagnosis as they provide better image quality and higher resolution images.

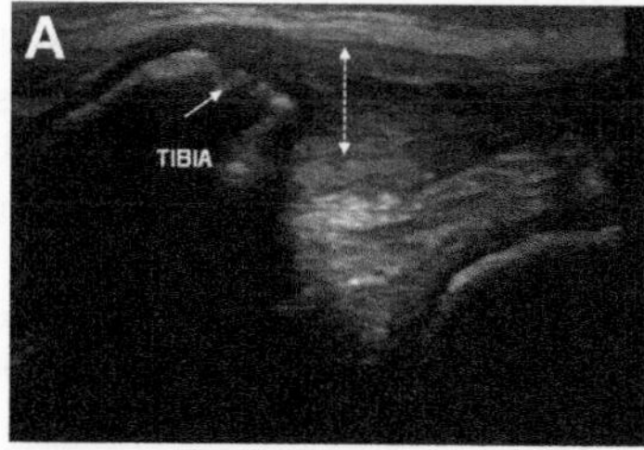

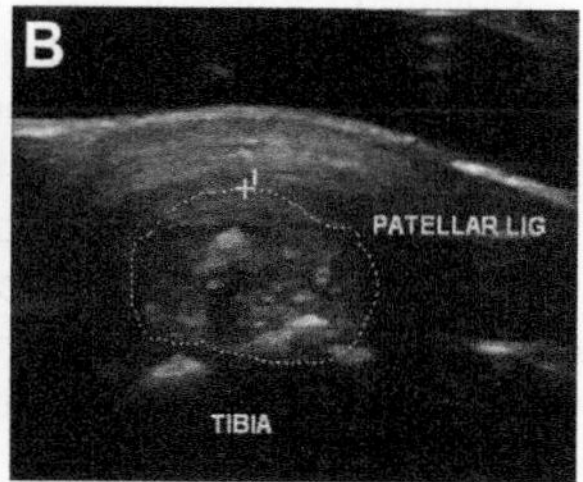

Fig. 35. Primary patellar ligament desmopathy of a 1.5 year French Bulldog (from radiographs in **Fig. 31**A) in longitudinal (*A*) and transverse (*B*) views. Ligament is between the arrowheads in A and dashed outline in B. Ligament is thickened and has an abnormal fiber pattern and loss of the normal homogenous echogenicity. In transverse sections, there is a mixture of hyper-and hypoechoic regions with some focal hyperintense regions signifying fibrosis and mineral densities. Bony irregularity of the tibia at the insertion of the patellar ligament is also noted (*white arrow*).

KEY POINTS–STIFLE

- Displacement of the infrapatellar fat pad is a reliable marker of effusion in the stifle joint and is an indicator of CrCL disease
- Ultrasound can be helpful in identifying meniscal injury but requires some experience. It is not useful for the identification of CrCL tears
- Ultrasound can readily be used to evaluate patellar ligament pathology
- Needle/nano arthroscopy has potential to be useful in the diagnosis of partial CrCL and potentially meniscal injury, but needs study
- CT arthrography can be used for CrCL injury, but is unreliable for meniscal injury
- Both low- and high-field MRI can diagnose pathology in the stifle, but the correct identification of meniscal injury is variable

Tarsus

Occurring as either an acute traumatic or chronic tendinopathy common calcaneal tendon (CCT) injury is the primary soft tissue injury encountered in the tarsal region.[84,85] On examination it will have thickening and potentially pain on palpation at the site of injury. A characteristic limb position may also be present and based on severity may include tarsal and digital hyperflexion to fully plantigrade stance. Other soft tissue injury includes superficial digital flexor tendon luxation, collateral ligament desmopathy, and deep digital flexor tendinopathy, but are rare. Osteoarthritis will typically be in response to other pathology in the joint such as collateral ligament injury, but primarily is seen as a consequence of OCD. The most common sites of OCD in the tarsus are the medial and lateral trochlear ridge of the talus.

RADIOGRAPHY

In addition to standard dorso-plantar and medial to lateral radiographs additional views are often necessary to help identify an OCD lesion as typical with a complex joint whereby superimposition and lesion location make identification difficult. The flexed dorsal-palmar skyline view and the oblique view (plantar medial-dorsolateral and plantar lateral-dorsomedial) have been to be the most successful in identifying lesions over standard views.[86,87] The skyline view is taken with the dog in dorsal recumbency with the stifles flexed and the tarsi resting on an elevated surface for acquisition. The tarsi can be flexed at varying angles up to 90° to highlight different areas of the trochlea, but approximately 75-degrees of flexion will achieve is recommended (**Fig. 36**).[87,88] Collateral ligament injury is typically associated with a traumatic event and associated with significant soft tissue swelling and effusion. Radiography in these cases can help identify avulsed fragments (**Fig. 37**). Oblique views are sometimes necessary to identify the avulsion and stressed medial to lateral views can be of value to assess ligament integrity and joint stability.[89] Radiographs will not typically provide additional information for common calcaneal tendinopathy unless there is a concern for other bony trauma. Soft tissue thickening, bony remodeling of the calcaneus, and dystrophic mineralization are typical radiographic findings associated with the disease (**Fig. 38**).

ULTRASONOGRAPHY

Several studies are available for reference describing the normal anatomy of the tarsus and common calcaneal tendon (CCT) along with associated pathology.[6,85,90,91] Easily accessible for ultrasound examination, the common calcaneal tendon from superficial to deep is made up of 3 tendons: superficial digital flexor tendon (SDFT),

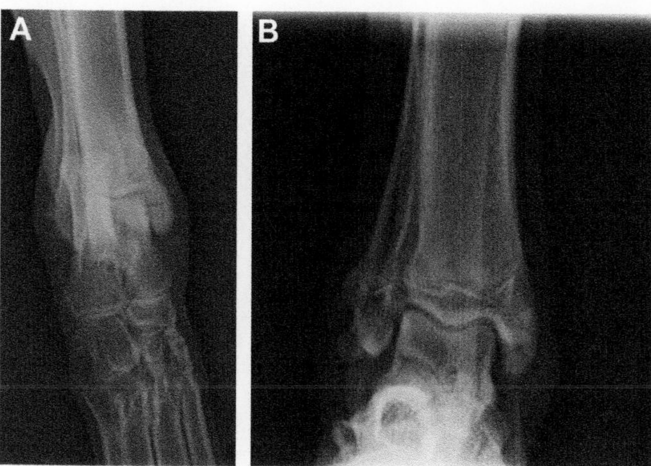

Fig. 36. Standard dorsoplantar (*A*) and a flexed dorsoplantar (skyline) using a horizontal beam radiograph (*B*). The skyline view eliminates the superimposition of the calcaneus and provides better visualization of the medial and lateral trochlea of the talus. Note the nondisplaced fragment of the medial malleolus which is better defined in the skyline view.

gastrocnemius tendon (GT), and the conjoined tendon (CT) (**Fig. 39**). The biceps femoris, gracilis, and semitendinosus combine to form the conjoined tendon. Despite several published works, there is some variation in structure identification via ultrasound across the studies.[6,29,85,91] This variation speaks to the potential difficulty of ultrasonographic assessment of the common calcaneal tendon. Some of these challenges may be due to the fact that the SDFT and GT run side by side until the distal one-third of their length whereby the SDFT wraps around to a more dorsal position and have a similar fiber pattern and echogenecity.[91] The conjoined tendon is slightly less echogenic than the SDFT and gastrocnemius but the visualization of the normal fibers can be lost at the insertion due to acoustic shadowing and should not be mistaken for pathology.[91] A bursa (calcaneal bursa) has been described lying between the SDFT and the gastrocnemius tendon based on dissection.[91,92] However, it has also been identified as sitting deep to the conjoined tendon in some of the literature.[29,85] In case reports anechoic fluid present deep to the gastrocnemius and/or conjoined tendons has been described as both the calcaneal bursa as well as an organizing hematoma at the site of the tear.[29,85,93] Based on these discrepancies it is difficult to know if fluid observed deep to the gastrocnemius and/or conjoined tendon is reflecting fluid accumulation in the calcaneal bursa or associated with soft tissue tearing (or both). Regardless, it is indicative of an active process associated with injury and/or inflammation. The goal of ultrasound assessment will be to identify the specific structures is involved and whether tears are partial or complete to guide conservative and surgical treatment options (**Fig. 40**). Ultrasound can also be used to follow tendon healing either postoperatively or after regenerative therapies.[93,94]

In addition to common calcaneal tendon lesions, ultrasound can be useful to characterize injuries to other soft tissues such as the deep digital flexor tendon, long and lateral digital extensor tendons, cranial tibial, and peroneus longus tendons.[90] Assessment of the collateral ligaments can also be performed but the medial collateral may be more challenging, especially in smaller patients.[90] Certainly when there is soft tissue swelling and effusion are present ultrasound is a good diagnostic to help make the diagnosis determine the best treatment (**Fig. 41**).

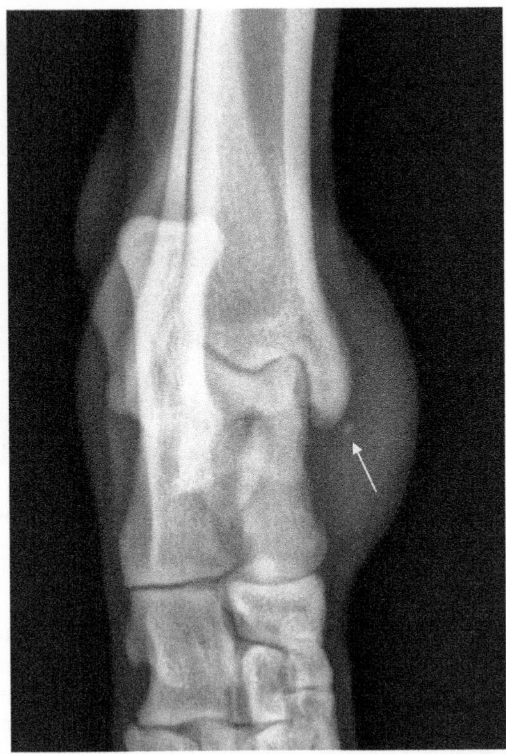

Fig. 37. Dorsoplantar projection of a 1-year-old Labrador Retriever with a traumatic injury to the tarsus that resulted in an avulsion of the short and long portions of the medial collateral ligament. Note the significant soft tissue swelling and avulsed fragment of the medial malleolus (*white arrow*).

COMPUTED TOMOGRAPHY/MAGNETIC RESONANCE IMAGING

The use of CT in the tarsus will be focused on those lesions difficult to identify with standard radiography, especially due to superimposition in this complex joint (**Fig. 42**). While a complete radiographic study with multiple orthogonal views

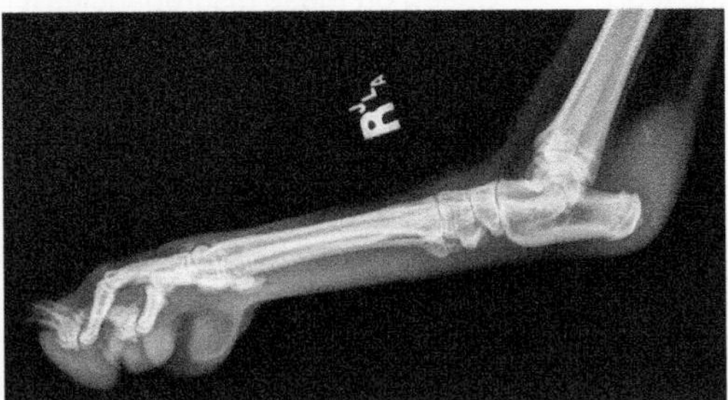

Fig. 38. Lateral radiograph of a 2-year-old Labrador Retriever with a partial common calcaneal tendon tear. There is soft tissue swelling proximal to the calcaneus, at the level insertion of the common calcaneal tendon on the calcaneus. There are multiple small mineralized ossicles within this soft tissue swelling. The cranial proximal margin of the calcaneus is irregular in shape with a focal, rough, concave defect.

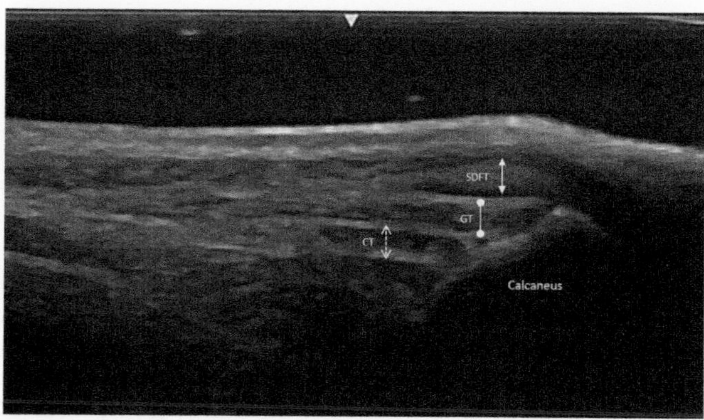

Fig. 39. Ultrasound of a normal common calcaneal tendon at the level of the insertion. The peritenon is a hyperechoic line defining tendon boundaries. From superficial to deep are the superficial digital flexor tendon (SDFT; between *solid arrow*), gastrocnemius tendon (GT; *round arrow heads*), and the conjoined (CT; *dashed arrow*) which is made up of the biceps femoris, gracilis, and semitendinosus.

may be successful in identifying OCD lesions, CT will identify the precise locations and presence of additional fragments.[95] The use of CT has been shown to be superior to standard radiographs in the identification of OCD lesions of the lateral trochlear ridge of the talus.[86] CT has a place as a diagnostic, prognostic, as well as a surgical planning tool not only for OCD, but for fractures of the tarsal bones.[95–98]

While normal MRI anatomy has been described, its use to assess the tarsus has been confined to a single case involving a partial tear of the common calcaneal tendon.[99,100] Certainly it could be used for any suspected soft tissue injury and to

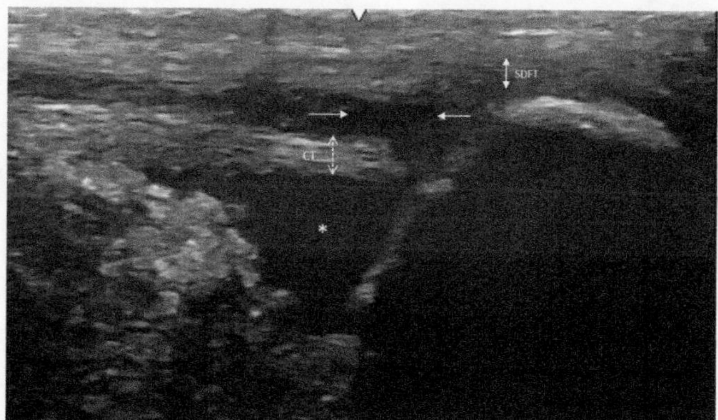

Fig. 40. Ultrasound images of a dog with a complete tear of the gastrocnemius tendon at the insertion. White arrows are indicating the ends of the torn tendon. There is anechoic fluid signal between the ends of the tendon. Superficial digital flexor tendon (SDFT) and conjoined tendon (CT) are intact. The CT has typical hypoechoic appears right at the insertion on the calcaneus due to acoustic shadowing, but should be evaluated in cross-section to assure integrity. Significant anechoic fluid is present (*asterisk*) deep in the CT.

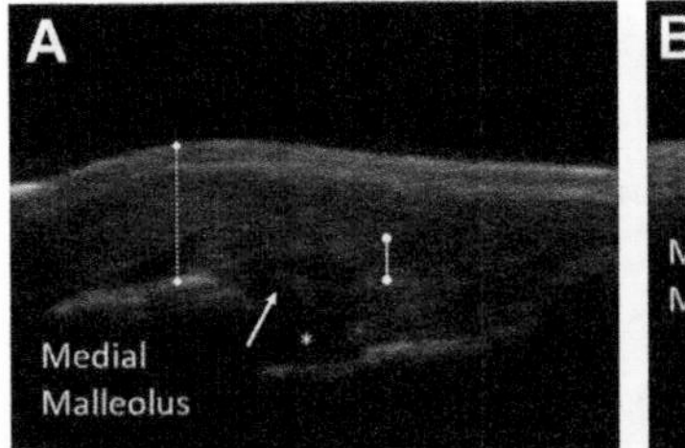

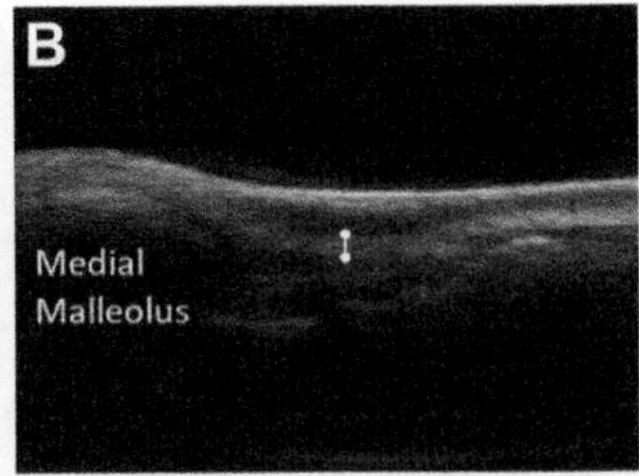

Fig. 41. Affected (*A*) and normal opposite limb (*B*) of a 2-year-old Labrador Retriever with a traumatic injury to the tarsus with significant soft tissue swelling (*dashed line*) along the medial aspect of the tibial tarsal joint. Based on ultrasound the osteochondral fragment noted on radiographs (see **Fig. 37**) was found to be an avulsion of the medial collateral ligament (*white line*). Effusion (*asterisk*) within the joint is also present, but as noted on the ultrasound a majority of the swelling is soft tissue in nature. Based on ultrasonographic findings surgery was recommended and the complete tear of the long and short portions of the collateral ligament was confirmed.

identify OCD lesions or fractures, but cost and access may limit its use over other imaging modalities.

KEY POINTS-TARSUS

- Multiple radiographic views are necessary to identify OCD lesions within the tarsus and should be performed when tarsal swelling/effusion is present
- Ultrasound can be used to identify full and partial tears of the common calcaneal tendon, but assessment can be difficult due to the anatomic arrangement of the tendons
- CT is superior to evaluate bony structures within the tarsus, especially in the case of OCD in some cases

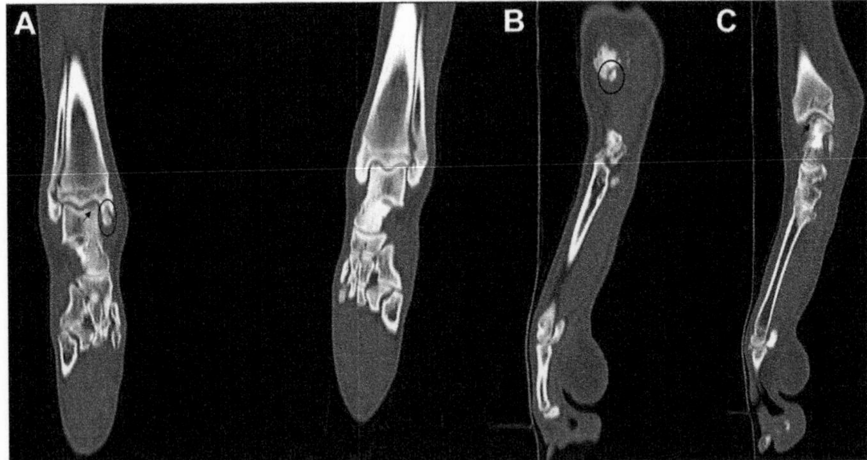

Fig. 42. Computed tomographic images from a 1-year-old Labrador Retriever with a non-displaced osteochondral fragment of the medial malleolus (within black circle) and a small osteochondrosis lesion on the medial trochlear ridge of the talus (indicated by black arrow). This is the same dog as in **Fig. 36**. Panel A is the Cr-Cd and panels B and C the lateral views.

REFERENCES

1. Cogar SM, Cook CR, Curry SL, et al. Prospective evaluation of techniques for differentiating shoulder pathology as a source of forelimb lameness in medium and large breed dogs. Vet Surg 2008;37(2):132–41.
2. Flo GL, Middleton D. Mineralization of the supraspinatus tendon in dogs. J Am Vet Med Assoc 1990;197(1):95–7.
3. Wall CR, Cook CR, Cook JL. Diagnostic sensitivity of radiography, ultrasonography, and magnetic resonance imaging for detecting shoulder osteochondrosis/osteochondritis dissecans in dogs. Vet Radiol Ultrasound 2015;56(1):3–11.
4. Cook CR. Ultrasound Imaging of the Musculoskeletal System. Vet Clin North Am Small Anim Pract 2016;46(3):355–71.
5. Spinella G, Loprete G, Musella V, et al. Cross-sectional area and mean echogenicity of shoulder and elbow tendons in adult German Shepherd dogs. Vet Comp Orthop Traumatol 2013;26(05):366–71.
6. Kramer M, Gerwing M, Sheppard C, et al. Ultrasonography for the diagnosis of diseases of the tendon and tendon sheath of the biceps brachii muscle. Vet Surg 2001;30(1):64–71.
7. Barella G, Lodi M, Faverzani S. Ultrasonographic findings of shoulder teno-muscular structures in symptomatic and asymptomatic dogs. J Ultrasound 2018;21(2):145–52.
8. Long CD, Nyland TG. Ultrasonographic evaluation of the canine shoulder. Vet Radiol Ultrasound 1999;40(4):372–9.
9. Zwingenberger A, Benigni L, Lamb CR. Small animal diagnostic ultrasound. In: Mattoon JS, Nyland TG, editors. Chapter 14 musculoskeletal system. 3rd edition. United Kingdom: Elsevier; 2015.
10. Lassaigne CC, Boyer C, Sautier L, et al. Ultrasound of the normal canine supraspinatus tendon: comparison with gross anatomy and histology. Vet Rec 2020; 186(17):e14.
11. Doyle, Claire Sigrid Aurora. Ultrasonographic features of the supraspinatus tendon in large breed dogs without forelimb lameness. 2020. Available at: http://www.dissertations.wsu.edu/Thesis/Summer2020/C_Doyle_051420.pdf.
12. Abbey R, Pettitt R. Prevalence of mineralisation of the tendon of the supraspinatus muscle in non-lame dogs. J Small Anim Pract 2021;62(6):450–4.
13. Canapp SO, Canapp DA, Carr BJ, et al. Supraspinatus Tendinopathy in 327 Dogs: A Retrospective Study. VE 2016;1(3). https://doi.org/10.18849/ve.v1i3.32.
14. Maddox TW, May C, Keeley BJ, et al. Comparison between shulder comptued tomography and clinical findings in 89 dogs presented for thoracic limb lameness. Vet Radiol Ultrasound 2013;54(4):358–64.
15. Devor M, Sørby R. Fibrotic contracture of the canine infraspinatus muscle: pathophysiology and prevention by early surgical intervention. Vet Comp Orthop Traumatol 2006;19(2):117–21.
16. Ballegeer EA. Computed tomography of the musculoskeletal system. Vet Clin North Am Small Anim Pract 2016;46(3):373–420.
17. von Pfeil DJF, Megliola S, Horstman C, et al. Comparison of classic and needle arthroscopy to diagnose canine medial shoulder instability: 31 cases. Can Vet J 2021;62(5):461–8.
18. Klein W, Kurze V. Arthroscopic arthropathy: Iatrogenic arthroscopic joint lesions in animals. Arthroscopy 1986;2(3):163–8.

19. Rogatko CP, Warnock JJ, Bobe G, et al. Comparison of iatrogenic articular cartilage injury in canine stifle arthroscopy versus medial parapatellar mini-arthrotomy in a cadaveric model. Vet Surg 2018;47(S1):O6–14.
20. Murphy SE, Ballegeer EA, Forrest LJ, et al. Magnetic resonance imaging findings in dogs with confirmed shoulder pathology. Vet Surg 2008;37(7):631–8.
21. Alves-Pimenta S, Ginja MM, Colaço B. Role of elbow incongruity in canine elbow dysplasia: advances in diagnostics and biomechanics. Vet Comp Orthop Traumatol 2019;32(2):87–96.
22. Van Ryssen B, de Bakker E, Beaumlin Y, et al. Primary flexor enthesopathy of the canine elbow: imaging and arthroscopic findings in eight dogs with discrete radiographic changes. Vet Comp Orthop Traumatol 2012;25(03):239–45.
23. de Bakker E, Gielen I, Saunders JH, et al. Primary and concomitant flexor enthesopathy of the canine elbow: A phantom study. Vet Comp Orthop Traumatol 2013;26(06):425–34.
24. Rau FC, Wigger A, Tellhelm B, et al. Observer variability and sensitivity of radiographic diagnosis of canine medial coronoid disease. Tierarztl Prax Ausg K Kleintiere Heimtiere 2011;39(5):313–22.
25. Villamonte-Chevalier AA, Soler M, Sarria R, et al. Ultrasonographic and Anatomic Study of the Canine Elbow Joint: Ultrasonographic and Anatomic Study of the Canine Elbow Joint. Vet Surg 2015;44(4):485–93.
26. Knox VW, Sehgal CM, Wood AKW. Correlation of ultrasonographic observations with anatomic features and radiography of the elbow joint in dogs. Am J Vet Res 2003;64(6):721–6.
27. Lamb CR, Wong K. Ultrasonographic anatomy of the canine elbow. Vet Radiol Ultrasound 2005;46(4):319–25.
28. Cook CR, Cook JL. Diagnostic imaging of canine elbow dysplasia: a review. Vet Surg 2009;38(2):144–53.
29. Kramer M, d'Anjou MA. Chapter 16 - Musculoskeletal system. In: Penninck D, D'Anjou M, editors. Chapter 16 - Musculoskeletal system, Atlas of small animal ultrasonography. 1st edition. Ames (IA): Blackwell Publishing; 2008. p. 465–510.
30. Seyrek-Intas D, Michele U, Tacke S, et al. Accuracy of ultrasonography in detecting fragmentation of the medial coronoid process in dogs. J Am Vet Med Assoc 2009;234(4):480–5.
31. Villamonte-Chevalier A, van Bree H, Broeckx B, et al. Assessment of medial coronoid disease in 180 canine lame elbow joints: a sensitivity and specificity comparison of radiographic, computed tomographic and arthroscopic findings. BMC Vet Res 2015;11(1):243.
32. Samoy Y, Van Vynckt D, Gielen I, et al. Arthroscopic findings in 32 joints affected by severe elbow incongruity with concomitant fragmented medial coronoid process: arthroscopic findings in severe elbow incongruity. Vet Surg 2012. https://doi.org/10.1111/j.1532-950X.2012.00949.x.
33. Zweifel RT, DiDonato P, Hartmann A, et al. Improved computed tomography accuracy with a 1-mm versus 2- or 3-mm slice thickness for the detection of medial coronoid disease in dogs. Vet Comp Orthop Traumatol 2020;33(01):045–50.
34. Hersh-Boyle RA, Chou P, Kapatkin AS, et al. Comparison of needle arthroscopy, traditional arthroscopy, and computed tomography for the evaluation of medial coronoid disease in the canine elbow. Vet Surg 2021;50(S1):O116–27.
35. Franklin SP, Burke EE, Holmes SP. Utility of MRI for Characterizing Articular Cartilage Pathology in Dogs with Medial Coronoid Process Disease. Front Vet Sci 2017;4:25.

36. Snaps FR, Balligand MH, Saunders JH, et al. Comparison of radiography, magnetic resonance imaging, and surgical findings in dogs with elbow dysplasia. Am J Vet Res 1997;58(12):1367–70.
37. Snaps FR, Park RD, Saunders JH, et al. Magnetic resonance arthrography of the cubital joint in dogs affected with fragmented medial coronoid processes. Am J Vet Res 1999;60(2):190–3.
38. Young AN, Amsellem P, Muirhead TL, et al. Ulnar ostectomy decreases the stability of canine cadaver carpi as assessed with stress radiography. Vet Radiol Ultrasound 2019;60(1):19–27.
39. Langley-Hobbs SJ, Hamilton MH, Pratt JNJ. Radiographic and clinical features of carpal varus associated with chronic sprain of the lateral collateral ligament complex in 10 dogs. Vet Comp Orthop Traumatol 2007;20(04):324–30.
40. Jaegger G, Marcellin-Little DJ, Levine D. Reliability of goniometry in Labrador Retrievers. Am J Vet Res 2002;63(7):979.
41. Milgram J, Slonim E, Kass PH, et al. A radiographic study of joint angles in standing dogs. Vet Comp Orthop Traumatol 2004;17(02):82–90.
42. González-Rellán S, Fdz-de-Trocóniz P, Barreiro A. Ultrasonographic anatomy of the dorsal region of the carpus of the dog. Vet Radiol Ultrasound 2021;62(5): 591–601.
43. Hittmair KM, Groessl V, Mayrhofer E. Radiographic and ultrasonographic diagnosis of stenosing tenosynovitis of the abductor longus muscle in dogs. Vet Radiol Ultrasound 2012;53(2):135–40.
44. Tobolska A, Adamiak Z, Głodek J. Clinical applications of imaging modalities of the carpal joint in dogs with particular reference to the carpal canal. J Vet Res 2020;64(1):169–74.
45. Castelli E, Pozzi A, Klisch K, et al. Comparison between high-field 3 Tesla MRI and computed tomography with and without arthrography for visualization of canine carpal ligaments: A cadaveric study. Vet Surg 2019;48(4):546–55.
46. Nordberg CC, Johnson KA. Magnetic resonance imaging of normal canine carpal ligaments. Vet Radiol Ultrasound 1999;40(2):128–36.
47. Prole JHB. A survey of racing injuries in the Greyhound. J Small Anim Pract 1976;17(4):207–18.
48. Cullen KL, Dickey JP, Bent LR, et al. Internet-based survey of the nature and perceived causes of injury to dogs participating in agility training and competition events. J Am Vet Med Assoc 2013;243(7):1010–8.
49. Levy I, Hall C, Trentacosta N, et al. A preliminary retrospective survey of injuries occurring in dogs participating in canine agility. Vet Comp Orthop Traumatol 2009;22(04):321–4.
50. Evans HE. Appendicular skeleton: bones of the thoracic limb. In: Miller ME, Evans HE, editors. MIller's anatomy of the dog. 3rd edition. United Kingdom: Saunders; 1993. p. 196.
51. Ober CP, Freeman LE. Computed tomographic, magnetic resonance imaging, and cross-sectional anatomic features of the manus in cadavers of dogs without forelimb disease. Am J Vet Res 2009;70(12):1450–8.
52. Cullen R, Canapp D, Dycus D, et al. Clinical Evaluation of Iliopsoas Strain with Findings from Diagnostic Musculoskeletal Ultrasound in Agility Performance Canines – 73 Cases. VE 2017;2(2). https://doi.org/10.18849/ve.v2i2.93.
53. Breur GJ, Blevins WE. Traumatic injury of the iliopsoas muscle in three dogs. J Am Vet Med Assoc 1997;210(11):1631–4.
54. Vidoni B, Henninger W, Lorinson D, et al. Traumatic avulsion fracture of the lesser trochanter in a dog. Vet Comp Orthop Traumatol 2005;18(2):105–9.

55. Butler JR, Gambino J. Canine hip dysplasia. Vet Clin North Am Small Anim Pract 2017;47(4):777–93.
56. Mayhew PD, McKelvie PJ, Biery DN, et al. Evaluation of a radiographic caudolateral curvilinear osteophyte on the femoral neck and its relationship to degenerative joint disease and distraction index in dogs. J Am Vet Med Assoc 2002; 220(4):472–6.
57. Smith GK, Gregor TP, Rhodes WH, et al. Coxofemoral joint laxity from distraction radiography and its contemporaneous and prospective correlation with laxity, subjective score, and evidence of degenerative joint disease from conventional hip-extended radiography in dogs. Am J Vet Res 1993;54(7):1021–42.
58. Powers MY, Karbe GT, Gregor TP, et al. Evaluation of the relationship between Orthopedic Foundation for Animals' hip joint scores and PennHIP distraction index values in dogs. J Am Vet Med Assoc 2010;237(5):532–41.
59. Cannon MS, Puchalski SM. Ultrasonographic evaluation of normal canine iliopsoas muscle. Vet Radiol Ultrasound 2008;49(4):378–82.
60. Tomlinson JE. Using therapeutic ultrasound to treat muscle injuries. In: Using therapeutic ultrasound to treat muscle injuries. Nashville (TN): American College of Veterinary Surgeons; 2015. p. 495–6.
61. Fischer A, Flöck A, Tellhelm B, et al. Static and dynamic ultrasonography for the early diagnosis of canine hip dysplasia. J Small Anim Pract 2010;51(11):582–8.
62. Bergamino C, Etienne AL, Busoni V. Developing a technique for ultrasound-guided injection of the adult canine hip: ultrasound-guided injection of the canine hip. Vet Radiol Ultrasound 2015;56(4):456–61.
63. Stepnik MW, Olby N, Thompson RR, et al. Femoral neuropathy in a dog with iliopsoas muscle injury. Vet Surg 2006;35(2):186–90.
64. Mahn MM, Cook JL, Cook CR, et al. Arthroscopic verification of ultrasonographic diagnosis of meniscal pathology in dogs. Vet Surg 2005;34(4):318–23.
65. Plesman R, Gilbert P, Campbell J. Detection of meniscal tears by arthroscopy and arthrotomy in dogs with cranial cruciate ligament rupture: a retrospective, cohort study. Vet Comp Orthop Traumatol 2013;26(01):42–6.
66. Fuller MC, Hayashi K, Bruecker KA, et al. Evaluation of the radiographic infrapatellar fat pad sign of the contralateral stifle joint as a risk factor for subsequent contralateral cranial cruciate ligament rupture in dogs with unilateral rupture: 96 cases (2006–2007). J Am Vet Med Assoc 2014;244(3):328–38.
67. Campbell CA, Horstman CL, Mason DR, et al. Severity of patellar luxation and frequency of concomitant cranial cruciate ligament rupture in dogs: 162 cases (2004–2007). J Am Vet Med Assoc 2010;236(8):887–91.
68. Arnault F, Cauvin E, Viguier E, et al. Diagnostic value of ultrasonography to assess stifle lesions in dogs after cranial cruciate ligament rupture : 13 cases. Vet Comp Orthop Traumatol 2009;22(06):479–85.
69. Gnudi G, Bertoni G. Echographic examination of teh stifle joint affected by cranial cruciate ligament rupture in the dog. Vet Radiol Ultrasound 2001;42(3): 266–70.
70. Franklin SP, Cook JL, Cook CR, et al. Comparison of ultrasonography and magnetic resonance imaging to arthroscopy for diagnosing medial meniscal lesions in dogs with cranial cruciate ligament deficiency. J Am Vet Med Assoc 2017; 251(1):71–9.
71. Coss P. The Use of Ultrasonography for Detection of Meniscal Damage in Dogs. VE 2019;4(2). https://doi.org/10.18849/ve.v4i2.207.

72. Frisbie DD, Barrett MF, McIlwraith CW, et al. Diagnostic stifle joint arthroscopy using a needle arthroscope in standing horses: Diagnostic Stifle Joint Arthroscopy. Vet Surg 2014;43(1):12–8.
73. Samii VF, Dyce J, Pozzi A, et al. Computed tomographic arthrography of the stifle for detection of cranial and caudal cruciate ligament and meniscal tears in dogs. Vet Radiol Ultrasound 2009;50(2):144–50.
74. Tivers MS, Mahoney PN, Baines EA, et al. Diagnostic accuracy of positive contrast computed tomography arthrography for the detection of injuries to the medial meniscus in dogs with naturally occurring cranial cruciate ligament insufficiency. J Small Anim Pract 2009;50(7):324–32.
75. Soler M, Murciano J, Latorre R, et al. Ultrasonographic, computed tomographic and magnetic resonance imaging anatomy of the normal canine stifle joint. Vet J 2007;174(2):351–61.
76. Baird DK, Hathcock JT, Rumph PF, et al. Low-field magnetic resonance imaging of the canine stifle joint: normal anatomy. Vet Radiol Ultrasound 1998;39(2): 87–97.
77. Blond L, Thrall DE, Roe SC, et al. Diagnostic accuracy of magnetic resonance imaging for meniscal tears in dogs affected with naturally occurring cranial cruciate ligament rupture. Vet Radiol Ultrasound 2008;49(5):425–31.
78. Barrett E, Barr F, Owen M, et al. A retrospective study of the MRI findings in 18 dogs with stifle injuries. J Small Anim Pract 2009;50(9):448–55.
79. Galindo-Zamora V, Dziallas P, Ludwig DC, et al. Diagnostic accuracy of a short-duration 3 Tesla magnetic resonance protocol for diagnosing stifle joint lesions in dogs with non-traumatic cranial cruciate ligament rupture. BMC Vet Res 2013; 9(1):40.
80. Böttcher P, Brühschwein A, Winkels P, et al. Value of low-field magnetic resonance imaging in diagnosing meniscal tears in the canine stifle: a prospective study evaluating sensitivity and specificity in naturally occurring cranial cruciate ligament deficiency with arthroscopy as the gold standard: low-field mri for diagnosis of meniscal tears. Vet Surg 2010;39(3):296–305.
81. D'Anjou MA, Moreau M, Troncy É, et al. Osteophytosis, subchondral bone sclerosis, joint effusion and soft tissue thickening in canine experimental stifle osteoarthritis: comparison between 1.5 T magnetic resonance imaging and computed radiography. Vet Surg 2008;37(2):166–77.
82. Widmer WR, Buckwalter KA, Braunstein EM, et al. Radiographic and magnetic resonance imaging of the stifle joint in experimental osteoarthritis of dogs. Vet Radiol Ultrasound 1994;35(5):371–84.
83. Olive J, d'Anjou MA, Cabassu J, et al. Fast presurgical magnetic resonance imaging of meniscal tears and concurrent subchondral bone marrow lesions: Study of dogs with naturally occurring cranial cruciate ligament rupture. Vet Comp Orthop Traumatol 2014;27(01):01–7.
84. Corr SA, Draffan D, Kulendra E, et al. Retrospective study of Achilles mechanism disruption in 45 dogs. Vet Rec 2010;167(11):407–11.
85. Gamble LJ, Canapp DA, Canapp SO. Evaluation of Achilles Tendon Injuries with Findings from Diagnostic Musculoskeletal Ultrasound in Canines – 43 Cases. VE 2017;2(3). https://doi.org/10.18849/ve.v2i3.92.
86. Gielen I, van Ryssen B, van Bree H. Computerized tomography compared with radiography in the diagnosis of lateral trochlear ridge talar osteochondritis dissecans in dogs. Vet Comp Orthop Traumatol 2005;18(02):77–81.

87. Carlisle CH, Robins GM, Reynolds KM. Radiographic signs of osteochondritis dissecans of the lateral ridge of the trochlea tali in the dog. J Small Anim Pract 1990;31(6):280–6.
88. Mauragis D, Berry CR. Small animal tarsus & pes radiography. Today's Vet Pract 2012;2(6):47–54.
89. Sjöström L, Håkanson N. Traumatic injuries associated with the short lateral collateral ligaments of the talocrural joint of the dog. J Small Anim Pract 1994; 35(3):163–8.
90. Caine A, Agthe P, Posch B, et al. Sonography of the soft tissue structures of the canine tarsus. Vet Radiol Ultrasound 2009;50(3):304–8.
91. Lamb CR, Duvernois A. Ultrasonographic anatomy of the normal canine calcaneal tendon. Vet Radiol Ultrasound 2005;46(4):326–30.
92. Evans HE. Muscles of the pelvic limb. In: Evans HE, Miller ME, editors. Miller's anatomy of the dog. United Kingdom: Third; 1993. p. 349–83.
93. Baltzer WI, Rist P. Achilles tendon repair in dogs using the semitendinosus muscle: surgical technique and short-term outcome in five dogs. Vet Surg 2009; 38(6):770–9.
94. Case JB, Palmer R, Valdes-Martinez A, et al. Gastrocnemius Tendon strain in a dog treated with autologous mesenchymal stem cells and a custom orthosis. Vet Surg 2013;42(4):355–60.
95. Gielen I, van Bree H, Van Ryssen B, et al. Radiographic, computed tomographic and arthroscopic findings in 23 dogs with osteochondrosis of the tarsocrural joint. Vet Rec 2002;150(14):442–7.
96. Gielen I, Van Ryssen B, Coopman F, et al. Comparison of subchondral lesion size between clinical and non-clinical medial trochlear ridge talar osteochondritis dissecans in dogs. Vet Comp Orthop Traumatol 2007;20(01):08–11.
97. Hercock CA, Innes JF, McConnell F, et al. Observer variation in the evaluation and classification of severe central tarsal bone fractures in racing Greyhounds. Vet Comp Orthop Traumatol 2011;24(03):215–22.
98. Rutherford S, Ness MG. Dorsal Slab Fracture of the Fourth Carpal Bone in a Racing Greyhound: Dorsal Slab Fracture of the Fourth Carpal Bone. Vet Surg 2012;41(8):944–7.
99. Lin M, Glass EN, Kent M. Utility of MRI for Evaluation of a Common Calcaneal Tendon Rupture in a Dog: Case Report. Front Vet Sci 2020;7:602.
100. Deruddere KJ, Milne ME, Wilson KM, et al. Magnetic resonance imaging, computed tomography, and gross anatomy of the canine tarsus: mri, ct, and gross anatomy of the canine tarsus. Vet Surg 2014;43(8):912–9.

Canine Mobility Maintenance and Promotion of a Healthy Lifestyle

Meghan T. Ramos, VMD*, Cynthia M. Otto, DVM, PhD

KEYWORDS

• Musculoskeletal • Sports medicine • Physical fitness • Injury prevention

KEY POINTS

- A healthy lifestyle emphasizes appropriate body composition, maintenance of mobility, and early identification and intervention of degenerative disorders.
- Weight management and physical fitness are essential to preventing or delaying the onset of musculoskeletal disorders.
- The veterinary profession is evolving towards prevention of musculoskeletal disease through redefining acceptable BCS, MCS, and establishment of life stage appropriate exercise programs.

INTRODUCTION

Mobility is defined as the ability to move without restriction or pain. This article highlights the considerations of mobility throughout a dog's life. The beginning of the article discusses general features of mobility as it applies to dogs across all life stages (structurally immature puppy to senior dog). The remainder of the article focuses on specific considerations and interventions at each life stage of a dog. Mobility is influenced by a dog's structure, posture, proprioception, muscle condition, body condition, and function. A dog's mobility directly impacts their quality of life and longevity. The role of targeted physical exercise in maintaining mobility throughout a dog's lifetime is highlighted. The importance of implementing mobility plans, recognizing altered mobility, and addressing quality-of-life concerns resulting from decreased mobility is a consistent theme.

Structure and Posture of Mobility

Mobility is the product of the interplay between bones, nerves, muscles, fascia, and other soft tissue structures. Functional neuromuscular exercise incorporates motor

Penn Vet Working Dog Center, Clinical Sciences and Advanced Medicine, School of Veterinary Medicine, University of Pennsylvania, 3401 Grays Ferry Avenue, Philadelphia, PA 19146, USA
* Corresponding author.
E-mail address: megramos@upenn.edu

Vet Clin Small Anim 52 (2022) 907–924
https://doi.org/10.1016/j.cvsm.2022.03.001
0195-5616/22/

skills such as balance, coordination, gait, and proprioception.[1] A dog's mobility is determined by its ability to move and transition from positions such as a sit, down, stand, walk, jump, and run without pain. The coordination of movement is dictated by the dog's anatomic structure, neuromuscular function, and presence of pain, or discomfort.

Anatomic structure can affect mobility through breed predispositions for developmental and/or hereditary conditions such as hip or elbow dysplasia, lumbosacral disorders, and chondrodystrophic conformation. Understanding the normal anatomic structure of distinct breeds enables veterinarians to conceptualize the functional anatomy and anticipate risks. The angulation of pelvic limbs is studied in several dog breeds. The angulation is determined by structure of the axial and long bones and influenced by the interplay of the skeletal muscles, tendons, ligaments, and nerves.[2,3] A recent study classified the pelvic limbs of medium-sized dogs into 3 distinct groups: most angulated (German shepherd), least angulated or most straight (Doberman pinscher), and moderately angulated (Labrador retriever) (**Fig. 1**).[4] These findings may provide insight into understanding the association of pelvic limb structure with some orthopedic disorders.[4–6] For example, a pelvic limb with little angulation (straight) has been proposed as a risk factor in the development of stifle disorders.[4,7] These predispositions may be at least partially mitigated by responsible breeding and early implementation of mobility training. For optimal quality of life and development of a healthy human-animal bond, mobility training should start when the puppy is acquired and continue throughout its life.

Similar to humans, in companion animals, correct posture is an often-overlooked component of a healthy lifestyle. Human studies have demonstrated the important regulatory role of postural stability and balance play in initiating and executing daily movements.[8–10] Translating and applying these findings to dogs suggests that a cornerstone of mobility maintenance and training may be the consistent implementation of proper canine posture (**Figs. 2–4**). Posture relies on the interaction between the nervous and musculoskeletal systems to hold the body in position and carry the body through space.[11,12] In humans posture is evaluated across the spectrum of age, from babies to geriatric patients, during both static and dynamic movements.[12,13] Therefore

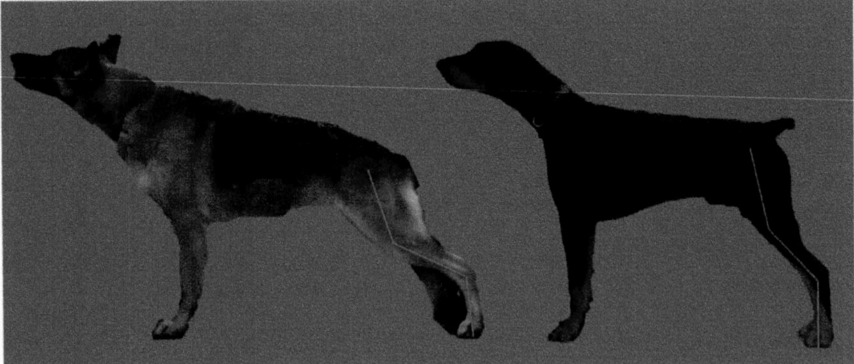

Fig. 1. Hind limb angulations of medium to large breeds. Left side of the image represents the most angulated German shepherd. and the right image represents the least angulated or most straight Doberman pinscher. The orange lines highlight the angles of the hind limb. The photograph is an original image taken by Dr. Meghan Ramos at the Penn Vet Working Dog Center.

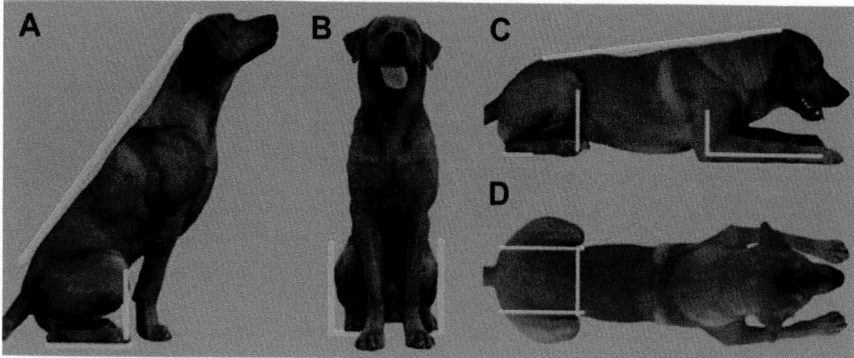

Fig. 2. The proper posture in the sit and down positions. (*A*) The proper sit position. Note the straight line from the head to the base of the tail. The stifle is dorsal to or just cranial to the digits. (*B*) A square sit in which the hips, stifle, and digits are within the same sagittal plane. (*C*) The proper posture down position. Note the straight line from the head to the base of the tail. The forelimb is flexed at the elbow and shoulder. The stifle is dorsal to or just cranial to the digits. (*D*) The dorsal view of a proper posture down. Ipsilateral limbs are aligned in the sagittal plane, and the hind limb digits are obscured by the stifles. All photographs are original images taken by Kasey Seizova at the Penn Vet Working Dog Center and previously published in the Vet Clin Small Anim 51 (2021) 859–876. https://doi.org/10.1016/j.cvsm.2021.04.005 vetsmall.theclinics.com 0195-5616/21/ª 2021 Elsevier Inc.

dog posture should be evaluated and trained during all life stages in both static positions (sit, stand, down) and dynamic movements (walking, running, jumping). As veterinarians, there is a need to educate oneself and owners on how to critically evaluate normal posture. Subtle changes in posture such as lateral deviation of a forepaw or a kyphotic spine during a sit may signal an injury or underlying musculoskeletal problem. Promoting and monitoring proper posture (**Fig. 5**) in a puppy may make the difference between writing off an awkward gait as "puppy" and identifying spinal stenosis or dysplastic disorders.[3,7,14] Studies in human sports medicine demonstrate that correct

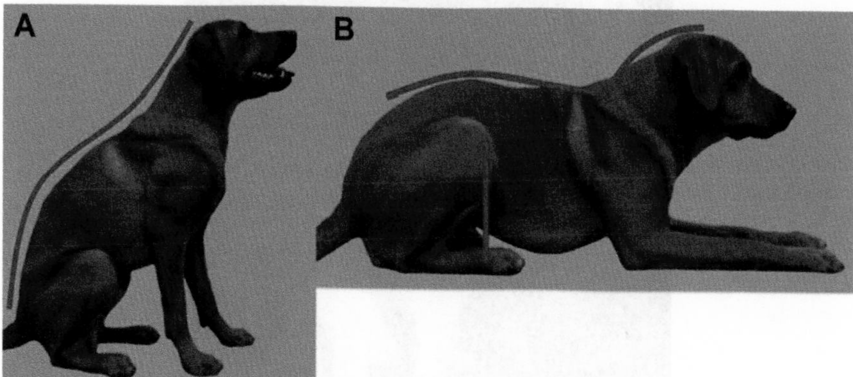

Fig. 3. Kyphosis in the sit and down positions. (*A*) Kyphosis in a sit as highlighted by the red line. (*B*) Kyphotic spine in a down position. Note the stifles are not over the hind limb digits in both images. All photographs are original images taken by Kasey Seizova at the Penn Vet Working Dog Center and previously published in the Vet Clin Small Anim 51 (2021) 859–876. https://doi.org/10.1016/j.cvsm.2021.04.005 vetsmall.theclinics.com 0195-5616/21/ª 2021 Elsevier Inc.

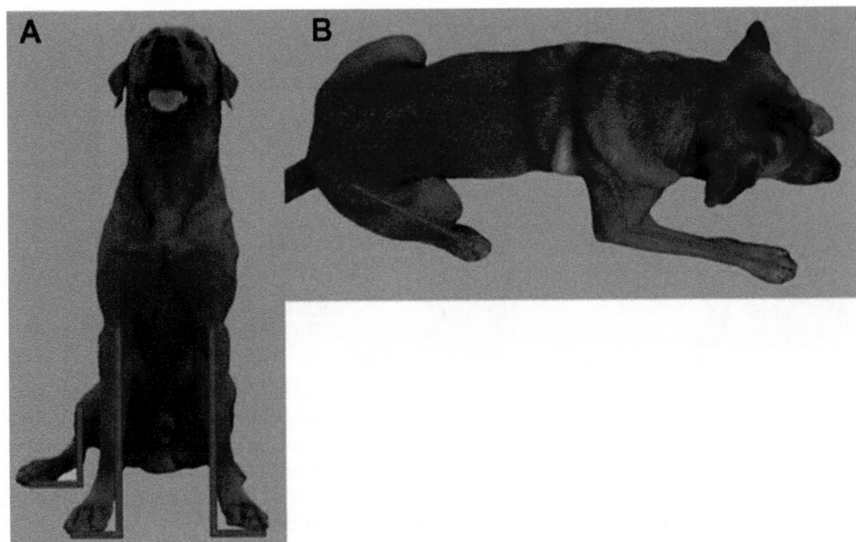

Fig. 4. The improper posture in the sit and down positions. (*A*) The abduction of the right hind limb paw and stifle. The image demonstrates the lateral deviation of the forelimbs as seen by the forepaws. (*B*) The abduction of the forelimb and hind limb in a down position. All photographs are original images taken by Kasey Seizova at the Penn Vet Working Dog Center and previously published in the Vet Clin Small Anim 51 (2021) 859–876. https://doi.org/10.1016/j.cvsm.2021.04.005 vetsmall.theclinics.com 0195-5616/21/ª 2021 Elsevier Inc.

posture during athletic movement and static positioning has positive effects on overall health.[11–13] In a senior dog, maintaining proper posture may decrease the risk of injury, heighten the owner's ability to observe postural changes, and lead to earlier intervention. The practice of having clients take photographs or videos of their dogs every 6 to

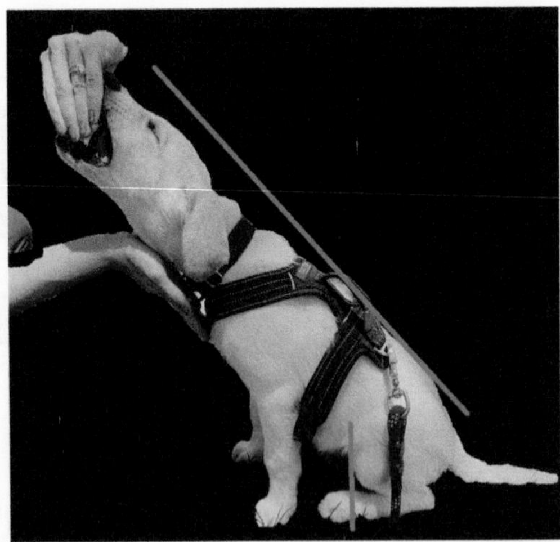

Fig. 5. An 8-week-old Labrador retriever puppy performing an acceptable posture sit for his age. The puppy does not complete the extension of his spine or stifles over toes in the photograph. The dog would be expected to improve its posture with age. The photograph is an original image taken by Dr Meghan Ramos at the Penn Vet Working Dog Center.

12 months in a sit, down, and stand position establishes a tangible and trackable screening tool of posture and lifelong mobility.

Neuromuscular and Musculoskeletal Mobility

Following structure and posture, mobility maintenance and training is focused on function neuromuscular exercises. These exercises incorporate motor skills such as balance, coordination, gait, and proprioception. Motor skills are important throughout life, but they are especially critical in puppy and senior life stages. Exercises to engage motor skills at different life stages are highlighted in the following discussion. In a puppy, a dog's neuroplasticity is at the highest capacity lending them to quickly learn and develop preferential gait patterns, balance, and coordination. Similar to humans, dogs in the senior life stage begin to experience cognitive decline as seen by decreasing neuroplasticity. During this time, it is important to maintain motor skills training to keep the neurologic pathways active aiming to prevent demyelination or inefficient transmission at neuromuscular junction.[11,15] A decrease in either aspect will contribute to decrease in both mobility and quality of life.

From puppy to end of life, maintaining an appropriate or low body fat composition may be the single most important factor in overall health and mobility. Appropriate levels of body fat are highly correlated with health and longevity in dogs[16–18]; this is one area in which the human-animal bond is often perceived to be at odds with the overall health of the dog. Many owners equate providing food, including high-calorie treats, with love for their pet. Strategies to help fight the obesity crisis can be directed at the dog (diet, exercise) or at the owner (education, reinforcement). Some tips include encouraging healthy low-calorie treats (eg, green beans, carrots) as replacement for human foods or high-calorie treats and praising owners for keeping their dogs lean or for accomplishing small steps toward achieving ideal weight for their overweight dog. One educational approach may be to help owners understand that excessive body condition (eg, 7/9 vs 5/9) will shorten their pets' life by as much as 2 years.[19,20] Obesity, its impacts on mobility as well, and suggested intervention are discussed in more detail in Barbara Esteve Ratsch and colleagues' article, "Clinical Guide to Obesity and Non-Herbal Nutraceuticals in Canine Orthopedic Conditions," in this issue. Second in importance to body fat composition is muscle mass development and retention with age. Muscular development is positively associated with health and inversely with injury.[21–23] The World Small Animal Veterinary Association Global Nutrition Committee muscle condition scoring (MCS) system was developed for evaluation of illness and sarcopenia (**Table 1**) and focuses on loss of muscle compared with a normal sedentary pet.[23] Considering the importance of mobility and assessment of canine athletes, the muscle condition score needs to be expanded beyond "normal" to include optimal muscle mass and tone (a score of 4/5) and excessive hypertrophy, which could result from overtraining (similar to what might be seen in a human power lifter), inappropriate weight distribution secondary to a primary musculoskeletal pathology (ie, should muscle hypertrophy in bilaterally hind limb lame dogs), or genetic variations (eg, mutations in the myostatin gene, commonly called double muscling).[24] Application of this scoring system clinically during palpation can be achieved by comparing tactile feel of both muscle volume and tone to an IV fluids. An MCS of 3/5 would have a tactile resistance to depression like an IV bag that had a small amount of fluid removed (or uncooked chicken breast), whereas an MCS of 4/5 would have a resistance to depression like an IV bag that had slightly increased amount of colloidal fluid (or a plump cooked chicken breast) and a 5/5 resistance to depression would be similar to an IV fluid bag that is overfilled and taut (or a cooked stuffed chicken breast).

Table 1
Muscle condition score

Muscle Condition Score	WSAVA (Current Method)[20]	Proposed
1	Moderate atrophy	Moderate atrophy
2	Mild atrophy	Mild atrophy
3	Normal muscle	Adequate muscle mass and tone (able to depress muscle on palpation)
4	NA	Increased muscle mass and firm tone (resistant to depression on palpation)
5	NA	Overdeveloped muscle mass increased tone (hypertrophy)

The table provides a proposed muscle condition scoring system.
Abbreviation: WSAVA, World Small Animal Veterinary Association.

Highlighted in the following discussion are the ideal muscle characteristics by life stage and recommendations to engage and maintain muscle mass.

Most adolescent and adult dogs inherently develop muscle with an active lifestyle. However, dogs naturally bear approximately two-thirds of their weight on their forelimbs during normal physical activity, therefore disproportionate muscle development occurs.[2] The loss of mobility with aging disproportionately affects the hind limbs and core. In the authors' opinion, all dogs should perform a targeted or foundational fitness program to balance muscle mass and maintain mobility. The goal of the program is to focus on muscle groups that contribute to common physical tasks such as running, jumping (up and down), and quickly or abruptly changing direction (ball retrieve). These tasks require the use of muscles of the core (spine and abdominals), hind limbs, and supporting soft tissue structures, which are minimally or briefly engaged with routine activities such as walking or obedience.[6,7,25–27] The lack of muscle

Table 2
Fitness focus areas[45,61]

Term	Definition	Activities Requiring This Focus Area
Balance	The ability to maintain equilibrium while stationary or moving	Navigating uneven terrain or obstacles, turning, landing from jumping stairs
Stability	The ability to maintain control through balance and coordination throughout a movement and return to original position or stabilize ones position	Jumping, sprinting, braking, turning, stairs, navigating uneven terrain or obstacles
Strength	The ability of muscle(s) to exert force	Pulling, sprinting, jumping, or rough socializing.
Endurance a. Cardiorespiratory b. Muscular	a. The ability of the circulatory and respiratory system to supply oxygen during sustained physical activity b. The ability of muscle to continue to perform without fatigue	a. Walking, trotting, sprinting, swimming, pulling of an object. b. Body weight exercise, ladder climbing, jumping, tugging

The table provides definitions and common activities that use the fitness focus areas.

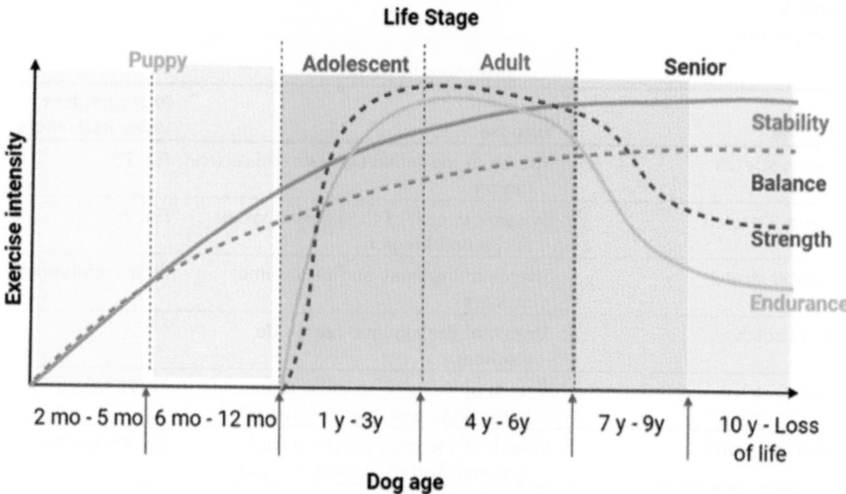

Fig. 6. A summary image of the intensity and types of exercise for each life stage. This summary is applicable for an aging healthy pet dog. Adjustments must be made to the intensity and exercise type for any dog with a musculoskeletal disorder beyond normal age-related degenerative changes. Active working or sporting dogs have a more advanced timeline and higher exercise intensity requirements due to the physical demands of their work or sport. The figure is an original image created by Dr Meghan Ramos at the Penn Vet Working Dog Center.

development without consistent and targeted exercises predisposes these areas to musculoskeletal injuries (ligament injuries, sprains, strains, spinal instability).

Age Considerations for Healthy Mobility

The remainder of this article highlights considerations for healthy lifestyle choices and mobility maintenance for specific life stages. The mobility maintenance in each life stage consists of a combination of fitness focus areas. The focus areas are stability, balance, strength, and endurance (definitions see **Table 2**). Although present at each life stage, the expectations, intensity, and duration vary for each focus area depending on the dog's age. **Fig. 6** illustrates a summary image of the intensity of the focus areas throughout the life stages. **Table 3** highlights specific exercises and their focus areas. **Table 4** summarizes the priority of each exercise for each life stage.

Puppy: Young Puppy—8 Weeks to 5 Months, Older Puppy—5 Months to 12 Months or Skeletal Maturity

Mobility and healthy lifestyle recommendations for a puppy can be divided into 2 age groups based on bone maturity. A puppy between 8 weeks and 5 months is considered a "young puppy" and between 5 months and 12 months or skeletal maturity is considered an "older puppy."[28,29] These age categories are somewhat dynamic, because skeletal maturation in smaller breeds will be faster and that in large/giant breeds will be slower. Current understanding of safe and effective strength and stability exercises for puppies is limited, and what is published is controversial.[30,31] It is accepted that young puppies should be physically active because inactivity can lead to musculoskeletal deformities,[32] although which activities should be included are subject to debate. One paper reported that puppies engaged in climbing stairs

Table 3
Exercise list

Exercise	Purpose	Photograph or Video References
Stretching Exercises		
Cookie stretch	Stretch of the spinal/epaxials and cervical region	**Fig. 7**B
Figure-8 stretch	Dynamic stretch of the spinal/epaxials and cervical region	**Fig. 7**C
Counter stretch	Stretch of inguinal, and pelvic limb muscles	Photo reference[51]
Frog stretch	Stretch of the inguinal region (ie, iliopsoas)	[2,5]
Bow stretch	Stretch of the core, spinal/epaxial, hamstrings, and gracilis muscles.	Photo reference[51]
Paws-up stretch	Stretch of the core, spinal/epaxial, inguinal, and pelvic limb muscles	**Fig. 7**A and Ref.[51]
Posture Exercises		
Posture-sit	Stability of the core and back muscles	**Fig. 2**
Posture-down	Stability of the core and back muscles	**Fig. 2**
Strength, Stability, Balance Exercises		
Down to stand	Whole-body stability and strength	[2,5]
Squat or sit to stand	Strength of the hind limbs	[40]
Back-up	Stability and strength of forelimbs and hind limbs	[40]
Plank	Stability and strength of the core and spinal/epaxials	[40]
Pivot	Strength of the medial and lateral muscles of the hind limbs	[40]
Cavaletti	Stability and balance of the forelimbs and hind limbs	[2,5]
Chipmunk or beg	Stability and strength of the core and spinal/epaxials	[40]
Unstable surfaces	Whole-body stability and balance	[2,5]
High fives	Strength and stability of the forelimbs	[2,5]
Diagonal stand	Stability of the forelimbs and hind limbs	[2,5]
Ladder	Whole-body stability, strength, and balance	[2,5]
Stairs	Whole-body stability, strength, and balance	[2,5]
Side stepping	Strength and stability of the medial and lateral muscles of the forelimb and hind limb	[2,5]
Endurance Exercises		
Treadmill (land or underwater)	Cardiorespiratory endurance	[2,5]
Sled pulling	Cardiorespiratory and muscular endurance	
Parachute running	Cardiorespiratory endurance	
Swimming	Cardiorespiratory endurance	[2,5]

The table provides the list of exercises, the targeted musculoskeletal groups, and resources to find the exercises.

Table 4
Exercises by life stage

		Young Puppy	Older Puppy	Adolescent	Adult	Senior
Posture	Posture-sit	H	H	H	H	H
	Posture-down	H	H	H	H	H
Stretches	Cookie	H	H	M	M	H
	Fig. 8	M	H	H	H	M
	Paws-up	L	M	H	H	H
	Bow	N	M	H	H	H
	Counter	N	M	M	M	H
	Frog	N	N	M	H	M
Strength, Stability, Balance	Down to stand	L	H	H	H	H
	Squat or sit to stand	L	M	H	H	M
	Back-up	M	M	M	H	H
	Plank	L	H	H	H	H
	Pivot	L	M	H	H	M
	Cavaletti	M	H	L	L	H
	Chipmunk or beg	N	N	L	M	L
	Unstable surfaces	M	H	H	M	H
	High fives	L	L	M	M	M
	Diagonal Stand	N	L	L	L	H
	Ladder	N	N	M	M	L
	Stairs	N	M	M	H	H
	Side stepping	M	M	L	L	H
End ura	Treadmill	N	N	H	H	M
	Sled pulling	N	N	M	H	N
	Parachute running	N	N	H	H	N
	Swimming	N	L	M	M	H

The table provides the recommendations and priorities of the exercises at each life stage.
Abbreviations: H, high priority; L, low priority; M, medium priority; N, not recommended.

had a higher incidence of hip dysplasia than those that did not climb stairs[30]; however, dogs kept indoors had a higher incidence than dogs with access to the outdoors.[33] In a series of studies evaluating young beagle puppies undergoing treadmill exercise, adverse effects were minimal and benefits including enhanced cartilage development were reported.[34–36] In any exercise program, the health and welfare of the puppy should be foremost and the enhancement of the human animal bond a clear goal. Owners should be educated to recognize signs of stress or discomfort in any dog participating in physical and behavioral training. Owners should be encouraged to use positive reinforcement training methods to create a positive learning environment and enhance the bond with the dog. For young puppies, it is important to develop and reinforce the neuromuscular connections associated with good posture and gait. As part of a complete physical examination of a young puppy, the musculoskeletal system should be thoroughly evaluated. One approach is to begin the examination from a distance and watch the puppy as it walks, trots, and transitions between a sit and a stand or a down position, being sure to have nonslip flooring for the examination. The next step is to observe their posture in a sit and in a down. Can the puppy hold itself in a proper posture position? If it can hold itself, for what duration and how does it transition out of the position does it collapse or gently settle? In addition, the soft tissues, bones, and joints should be palpated for muscle mass, tone, asymmetry, and pain. The owner should be asked how the puppy navigates obstacles and provide video; otherwise during an examination the dog can be evaluated over a low set of objects on the ground.

Healthy lifestyle choices for a young puppy include engagement and focused mobility exercises. Engagement occurs through interaction with and exposure to new and varied environments, mental stimulation with toys, and positive interaction with the owner. Mobility exercises at this stage are highlighted in **Table 4**. Toy play and running should be limited to short distances on good footing without potential hazards like colliding into fixed obstacle or older or larger dogs. A potentially safer way to engage in retrieval activities is to lightly restrain the dog at the shoulders, throw the object, and allow it to settle before releasing the puppy. This "dead ball" retrieving style promotes running in a straight-line versus unexpected twists or turns, which can result in soft tissue injuries. Alternatively, throwing into or hiding the object in high grass, where the puppy must search for it, will minimize "crashing" into the object and engage their brain and their nose (a valuable way to tire them out). Activities to avoid with young puppies are prolonged training sessions of more than 15 minutes, structured running particularly on pavement, interaction with rough or large breeds for social play, and jumping up or down from heights higher than the puppy's carpus.[14,28,30]

An older puppy should build on the engagement and focused mobility exercises introduced as a young puppy. Mobility exercises introduced at this stage are outlined in **Table 4**. Goals for an older puppy are more extensive environmental exposure and the development of muscle memory through increased repetitions of short duration while avoiding repetitive motion injury. If the puppy is reluctant to perform an exercise or cannot appropriately perform the exercise, this might be a challenge with the training, or it could be a physical limitation. A puppy that had been previously capable of performing an exercise may have a decrease in performance during a growth spurt or could be manifesting a subtle musculoskeletal injury or metabolic bone disease. Owners are quick to attribute difficulties in performing the exercises as the dog "being stubborn"; however, this is rarely the case. A complete sports medicine evaluation, potentially a behavioral/training consult or diagnostic imaging, may be indicated. One example is for puppies that are reluctant or unable to establish or maintain a "posture sit" and/or "posture down" position, pelvic and coxofemoral radiographs are recommended. In addition to the young puppy restrictions, an older puppy should not perform repetitive high-impact activities such as long-distance running, weave poles, or repeated jumping up and down at a height above the elbow.[14,29,30]

Adolescent: 1 to 3 Years

Evaluation methods and healthy lifestyle activities in an adolescent dog can vary widely depending on the exercise requirements and trainability of the breed and more specifically, the individual dog. Recommendations to a client should be made with the needs of the dog and expectations of the client in mind. The following outline provides healthy habits and mobility exercises for most adolescent dogs. The early diagnosis of musculoskeletal conditions, like hip or elbow dysplasia, that increase the risk of impaired mobility may allow interventions that slow the disease progression and enhance the quality of life. To safely embark on a mobility plan, adolescent dogs should have a complete physical examination, body condition scoring, nutritional recommendations, and ideally imaging of coxofemoral and elbow joints through Orthopedic Foundation of Animals or PennHIP radiographs.[37,38] For breeds predisposed to transitional vertebrae, such as French bulldogs (thoracolumbar) and German shepherds (lumbosacral), additional imaging of the spine may be warranted before vigorous activities such as agility, apprehension sports, or training as a working dog.[39–43] Instability in these areas may increase risk of degenerative joint changes, debilitating pain, and/or neurologic impairment.[43] The radiographs act as both a screening tool and a baseline for comparison to future diagnostic imaging.

Following radiographic assessment of musculoskeletal disorders, the mobility exercises highlighted in the Puppy section should continue and physical conditioning with a focus on muscular strength development and cardiovascular endurance should begin. Details on conditioning programs are highlighted in Juliette Hart's article, "Economic and Clinical Benefits of Orthopedic/Sports Medicine and Rehabilitation," in this issue. An important recommendation for the client is that the exercises must be consistent, controlled, and safe. Before and immediately following exercise, the

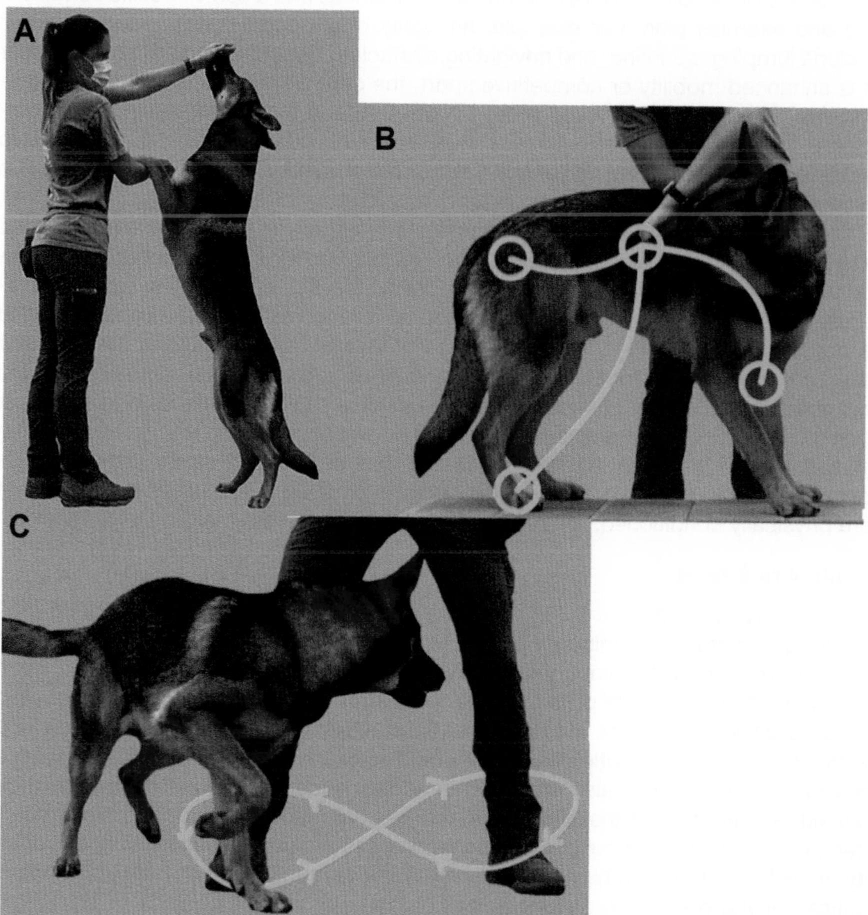

Fig. 7. The paws-up (*A*), cookie (*B*), and figure-8 (*C*) stretches. All stretches are to be performed after a minute of consistent walking. The paws-up stretch targets hip and abdominal tissues for extension. The cookie stretches target the neck and trunk in the lateral directions. The figure-8 is a dynamic stretch that targets whole-body lateral flexion and extension. The blue arrows and lines represent the motion of the dog's head in (*B*) and the whole-body movement in (*C*). All photographs are original images taken by Kasey Seizova at the Penn Vet Working Dog Center.

dog should have a simple warm up and cool down routine starting with a light walk and trot and followed with active stretches as highlighted in **Fig. 7**. Often, weekends for dogs and humans are the opportunity for intensive activity; although these can be enjoyable, a more consistent exercise regime is ideal to avoid injury/setbacks of the weekend warrior.[44] To maximize enjoyment and minimize the risk of injury, it is critical that the dog, and the human, be conditioned for the activity. Dogs should start a daily exercise program with mild activity such as walking or light trotting and active stretches followed by moderate activities such as controlled ball play, swimming, or exercise programs such as the Penn Vet Working Dog Center Fit to Work Foundational Fitness Program.[45] In general, flexibility and general cardiovascular exercises should be done daily; strength training should be included 2 to 3 times a week and might involve sport-specific exercises. For example, dog competing in sports like agility or apprehension should implement a foundational fitness and a sport-specific conditioning and exercise plan. For example, an agility dog's sport-specific training would include jumping, sprinting, and navigating obstacles. Regardless of the goal, whether it is enhanced mobility or competitive sport, the conditioning should advance incrementally, recognizing that it requires both physical and behavioral training to accomplish the exercises. The time spent training with the dog also enhances the relationship and the bond between the dog and the owner, if the training is conducted with positive reinforcement.

Adolescent dogs are eager to be active and engage with their owners in explosive activities (free-ball chasing, jumping, running, playdates) with or without the appropriate warm-up, muscle strength, or stability for the activity. The lack of self-preservation, inadequate muscular development, and weekend warrior approach to exercise makes this life stage the highest risk for musculoskeletal and primarily soft tissue injuries. The combination can lend itself to subtle or acute lameness, which result in compensatory changes in gait or exercise that summate to longer-term or chronic conditions of decreased mobility. The attentive owner who is participating in a fitness program may identify these changes before they cause disability, thus benefiting the long-term mobility of their dog. In addition, it is thought that dogs that are physically conditioned, are more resilient to injury, or are more rapid to recover.

Adult: 4 to 6 Years

The mobility of adult dogs is highly influenced by their younger years. If the healthy habits of maintaining canine mobility and health outline in previous sections have been implemented, the adult years may be the most rewarding for both the client and dog. The dog is in its physical and mental prime, and the clients have cultivated an unparalleled bond with the dog. This bond facilitates continued compliance and early identification of subtle changes. Adult dog exercise programs should advance beyond the beginner levels introduced in adolescence. Special attention should be placed on targeting of the abdominal and epaxial musculature during these years because lower back and hip pain are common causes of decreased mobility and quality of life.[46,47] Studies in human sports medicine demonstrate that core activation is critical for the prevention and treatment of lower back or hip pain.[48–50] The target for lower back or hip pain in human sports medicine and physical therapy is muscle development and neuromuscular training of the abdominal, epaxial, and hip musculature. A common and effective exercise to target these muscles in humans is the plank (supine or prone bridge, **Fig. 8**), and although extensive data are lacking, this seems to be a low-impact and beneficial exercise for dogs.[48–50]

Adult dogs that were inadequately exercised or experienced repetitive motion or mild soft tissue injuries during adolescence may begin to demonstrate subtle clinical

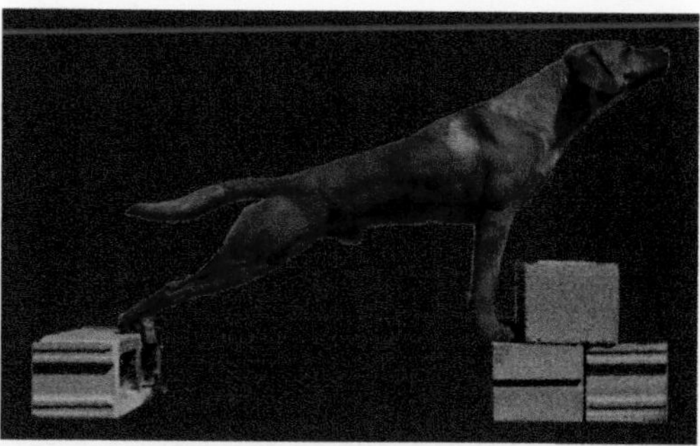

Fig. 8. The plank exercise. The plank exercise often referred to as the prone or supine bridge builds strength and stability of the core. The photograph is an original image taken by Dr Meghan Ramos at the Penn Vet Working Dog Center.

signs of overuse, compensatory, or repetitive injuries. Communication with the client about the dog's ability to perform specific movements, changes in repetitions of exercise, and any reluctance or slowing down during exercise will highlight these subtle changes. Examples may include the dog moving slower from a stand to a sitting position or holding a hind paw out to the side rather than tucked under them during a down or a sit. Management of these mild cases should be evaluated to identify underlying conditions, control pain, and start interventions to prevent progression of disease and decrease in mobility. Common therapeutic options include nonsteroidal anti-inflammatory drugs and nutraceutical supplementation. Although lacking robust scientific evidence, other options for this time are chiropractic adjustments, acupuncture, and laser therapy. Activity modifications for postural changes primarily focus on promoting stability within the axial or abaxial musculature and strengthening the supporting muscles that are compensating for the injury. For elaborate details on mobility assessments and supplementation see Christina Montalbano's article, "Comprehensive Mobility Assessment"; and Barbara Esteve Ratsch and colleagues' article, "Clinical Guide to Obesity and Non-Herbal Nutraceuticals in Canine Orthopedic Conditions," in this issue, respectively.

Senior Dogs: 7 Years and Older

Despite the best health practices and therapeutic interventions, the normal aging process inevitably leads to a decrease in mobility; however, aging is not stochastic, in that some dogs will reach senior status before 7 years and others may continue to function as active adults through their early teens. The decline is commonly a vicious cycle of pain, often caused by osteoarthritis or nerve pain, followed by reduced activity, which leads to muscle atrophy, which leads to more pain and further reduction in activity. Muscle atrophy particularly of the epaxials, abdominals (manifest as kyphosis or lordosis), and pelvic limbs may contribute to instability of the hips and spine and the progressive inability to rise (**Fig. 9**).[51–56] The progression and severity of these changes are more pronounced in dogs with a high body condition score and decreased muscle tone.[15,16,18,21] Therefore, the goals for a senior dog are to maintain a lean body condition score while retaining muscle mass through functional neuromuscular exercises. The plan to achieve these goals will vary depending on the individual client expectations and the dog's comorbidities, body condition, and lifestyle. Establishing the client's expectations for the dog is the first step in mobility management because loss of mobility is a major factor in end-of-life decisions. Most owners will adjust their expectations of their dog as it ages, although some may still want to engage in intensive physical activity. Some owners may consider mobility changes

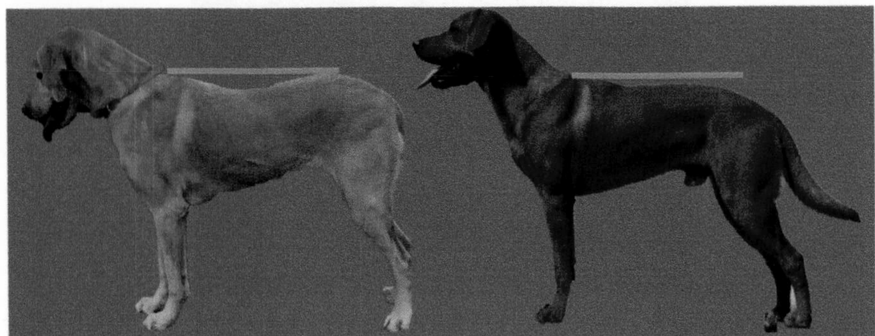

Fig. 9. A senior dog on the left and an adolescent dog on the right. Note the diffuse muscle atrophy and resulting lordosis of the senior dog. The photograph is an original image taken by Dr Meghan Ramos at the Penn Vet Working Dog Center.

as an inevitable sign of aging, but the astute veterinarian may be able to provide owners with tools to slow or even reverse some of these changes extending the quality of life for the dog. To support the bond between the dog and the owner, it is important to establish realistic expectations and ensure the comfort and welfare of the dog. Common expectations of senior dogs are to be able to interact with family members, walk, eat, defecate, and urinate without discomfort.

Healthy lifestyle choices for most senior dogs include mental stimulation and focused stability exercises.[31] Mental stimulation can be provided through enrichment puzzles or walks in new environments. Stability exercises at this stage are often focused on low-impact activities. Engagement of the fascial planes through active stretching is important in preventing fibrosis and muscle contracture.[57–60] Nonslip footing is especially important in the senior dog as proprioception may be reduced and healing mechanisms are delayed with age.[31] As with puppies, senior dogs should be active with controlled activity and education of clients on signs of stress or discomfort to ensure the dog is safe and comfortable.

SUMMARY

Promotion of a healthy canine lifestyle and mobility maintenance is a lifelong commitment and an opportunity to enhance the welfare, longevity of the dog, as well as the human-animal bond. The journey begins by setting expectations and focusing on simple and effective lifestyle changes. Understanding the structure of a dog breed and therefore its predispositions to abnormal mobility are the first key steps to successful intervention. Education and implementation of correct posture and motor skills training at a young age and throughout a dog's life are essential for maintaining mobility long term. This article highlights healthy habits and current knowledge of mobility at all life stages. Future development and validation of an expanded muscle condition score and scientifically valid, progressive, and safe exercise programs for all life stages are warranted.

CLINICS CARE POINTS

- A healthy lifestyle emphasizes appropriate body composition, maintenance of mobility, and early identification and intervention of degenerative disorders.

- Weight management and physical fitness are essential to preventing or delaying the onset of musculoskeletal disorders.
- The veterinary profession is evolving toward prevention of musculoskeletal disease through redefining acceptable BCS, MCS, and establishment of life stage-appropriate exercise programs.

DISCLOSURE

The authors do not have any commercial or financial conflicts of interest regarding the material presented in this article. The authors are employed with the Penn Vet Working Dog Center (PVWDC). The PVWDC currently receives funding from Pennsylvania Emergency Management $A_{genc}y$, Pennsylvania Game Commission, National Institutes of Health, Department of Homeland Security, United States Department of Agriculture, Kleberg Foundation, and Zoetis. The sports medicine and rehabilitation residency at the PVWDC at the time of publication is sponsored by Dechra. Donors to the PVWDC are Dechra, Nestle-Purina, Royal Canin, Nutramax, Boehringer-Ingelheim, Merial, Merck, and Respond Systems. The PVWDC was previously funded by Nestle-Purina, Virox, and Red Arch Cultural Heritage Law & Policy Research Foundation.

REFERENCES

1. Proceedings of the 10th International Symposium on Veterinary Rehabilitation and Physical Therapy; and the Summit of the American Association of Rehabilitation Veterinarians; and the American College of Veterinary Sports Medicine and Rehabilitation. Acta Vet Scand 2019;61(1):1–29.
2. Zink CM, Dyke JBVan. Canine Sports Medicine and Rehabilitation. Vol 1.
3. Brown CM, Bonnie Dalzell. Dog locomotion and gait analysis. 1986. Available at: http://books.google.com/books?id=aC9WAAAAYAAJ.
4. Sabanci SS, Ocal MK. Categorization of the pelvic limb standing posture in nine breeds of dogs. Anat Histol Embryol 2018;47(1):58–63.
5. Millis DL, Levine D. Canine rehabilitation and physical therapy. 2nd Edition 2013. https://doi.org/10.1016/C2009-0-52108-3.
6. Adrian CP, Haussler KK, Kawcak C, et al. The role of muscle activation in cruciate disease. Vet Surg 2013;42(7):765–73.
7. Adrian CP, Haussler KK, Kawcak CE, et al. Gait and electromyographic alterations due to early onset of injury and eventual rupture of the cranial cruciate ligament in dogs: A pilot study. Vet Surg 2019;48(3):388–400.
8. Sousa ASP, Silva A, Tavares JMRS. Biomechanical and neurophysiological mechanisms related to postural control and efficiency of movement: A review. Somatosensory Mot Res 2012;29(4):131–43.
9. Błaszczyk JW, Fredyk A, Błaszczyk PM, et al. Step Response of Human Motor System as a Measure of Postural Stability in Children. IEEE Trans Neural Syst Rehabil Eng 2020;28(4):895–903.
10. Ganz DA, Bao Y, Shekelle PG, et al. Will my patient fall? JAMA 2007;297(1):77–86.
11. Ludwig O, Kelm J, Hammes A, et al. Neuromuscular performance of balance and posture control in childhood and adolescence. Heliyon 2020;6(7):e04541.
12. Viton JM, Mesure S, Bensoussan L, et al. Analyse de la posture et du mouvement et médecine du sport. Ann de Réadaptation de Médecine Physique 2004;47(6):258–62.

13. Howell DR, Hanson E, Sugimoto D, et al. Assessment of the Postural Stability of Female and Male Athletes. Clin J Sport Med 2017;27(5):444–9.
14. Lopez MJ, Quinn MM, Markel MD. Evaluation of gait kinetics in puppies with coxofemoral joint laxity. Am J Vet Res 2006;67(2):236–41.
15. Hill M. The Neuromuscular Junction Disorders. J Neurol Neurosurg Psychiatr 2003;74(90002):32ii–37.
16. Salt C, Morris PJ, Wilson D, et al. Association between life span and body condition in neutered client-owned dogs. J Vet Intern Med 2019;33(1):89–99.
17. German AJ, Blackwell E, Evans M, et al. Overweight dogs exercise less frequently and for shorter periods: results of a large online survey of dog owners from the UK. J Nutr Sci 2017;6:e11.
18. Adams VJ, Watson P, Carmichael S, et al. Exceptional longevity and potential determinants of successful ageing in a cohort of 39 Labrador retrievers: results of a prospective longitudinal study. Acta Vet Scand 2016;58(1):29.
19. Kealy RD, Lawler DF, Ballam JM, et al. Effects of diet restriction on life span and age-related changes in dogs. J Am Vet Med Assoc 2002;220(9):1315–20.
20. Kealy RD, Olsson SE, Monti KL, et al. Effects of limited food consumption on the incidence of hip dysplasia in growing dogs. J Am Vet Med Assoc 1992;201(6):857–63.
21. McLeod M, Breen L, Hamilton DL, et al. Live strong and prosper: the importance of skeletal muscle strength for healthy ageing. Biogerontology 2016;17:497–510.
22. Yang NP, Hsu NW, Lin CH, et al. Relationship between muscle strength and fall episodes among the elderly: the Yilan study, Taiwan. BMC Geriatr 2018;18. https://doi.org/10.1186/s12877-018-0779-2.
23. Freeman LM, Michel KE, Zanghi BM, et al. Evaluation of the use of muscle condition score and ultrasonographic measurements for assessment of muscle mass in dogs. Am J Vet Res 2019;80(6):595–600.
24. Mosher DS, Quignon P, Bustamante CD, et al. A Mutation in the Myostatin Gene Increases Muscle Mass and Enhances Racing Performance in Heterozygote Dogs. Takahashi JS. Plos Genet 2007;3(5):e79.
25. Otto CM, Cobb ML, Wilsson E. Editorial: Working Dogs: Form and Function. Front Vet Sci 2019;6:351. https://doi.org/10.3389/fvets.2019.00351.
26. Worth AJ, Cave NJ. A veterinary perspective on preventing injuries and other problems that shorten the life of working dogs. Revue scientifique Tech (International Off Epizootics) 2018;37(1):161–9.
27. Gamble KB, Jones JC, Biddlecome A, et al. Qualitative and quantitative computed tomographic characteristics of the lumbosacral spine in German shepherd military working dogs with versus without lumbosacral pain. J Vet Behav 2020;38:38–55.
28. Torzilli PA, Takebe K, Burstein AH, et al. Structural Properties of Immature Canine Bone. J Biomechanical Eng 1981;103(4):232–8.
29. O'brien TR, Morgan JP, Suter PF. Epiphyseal plate injury in the dog: a radiographic study of growth disturbance in the forelimb. J Small Anim Pract 1971;12(1):19–36.
30. Krontveit RI, Nødtvedt A, Sævik BK, et al. Housing- and exercise-related risk factors associated with the development of hip dysplasia as determined by radiographic evaluation in a prospective cohort of Newfoundlands, Labrador Retrievers, Leonbergers, and Irish Wolfhounds in Norway. Am J Vet Res 2012;73(6):838–46.
31. Bellows J, Colitz CMH, Daristotle L, et al. Common physical and functional changes associated with aging in dogs. J Am Vet Med Assoc 2015;246(1):67–75.

32. Cetinkaya MA, Yardimci C, Sağlam M. Carpal laxity syndrome in forty-three puppies. Vet Comp Orthop Traumatol 2007;20(2):126–30.
33. Krontveit RI, Sævik BK. Challenges in tackling inherited skeletal disorders in the dog. Vet J 2013;196(1):8–9.
34. Kiviranta I, Tammi M, Jurvelin J, et al. Articular cartilage thickness and glycosaminoglycan distribution in the canine knee joint after strenuous running exercise. Clin Orthopaedics Relat Res 1992;(283):302–8.
35. Kiviranta I, Tammi M, Jurvelin J, et al. Moderate running exercise augments glycosaminoglycans and thickness of articular cartilage in the knee joint of young beagle dogs: Running exercise and cartilage glycosaminoglycans. J Orthop Res 1988;6(2):188–95.
36. Arokoski J, Kiviranta I, Jurvelin J, et al. Long-distance running causes site-dependent decrease of cartilage glycosaminoglycan content in the knee joints of beagle dogs. Arthritis Rheum 1993;36(10):1451–9.
37. Haney PS, Lazarowski L, Wang X, et al. Effectiveness of PennHIP and orthopedic foundation for animals measurements of hip joint quality for breeding selection to reduce hip dysplasia in a population of purpose-bred detection dogs. J Am Vet Med Assoc 2020;257(3):299–304.
38. Leighton EA, Holle D, Biery DN, et al. Genetic improvement of hip-extended scores in 3 breeds of guide dogs using estimated breeding values: Notable progress but more improvement is needed. PLoS ONE 2019;14(2):1–33.
39. Flückiger M, Steffen F, Hässig M, et al. Asymmetrical lumbosacral transitional vertebrae in dogs may promote asymmetrical hip joint development. Vet Comp Orthop Traumatol 2017;30(02):137–42.
40. Bertram S, ter Haar G, De Decker S. Congenital malformations of the lumbosacral vertebral column are common in neurologically normal French Bulldogs, English Bulldogs, and Pugs, with breed-specific differences. Vet Radiol Ultrasound 2019; 60(4):400–8.
41. Gluding D, Stock KF, Tellhelm B, et al. Genetic background of lumbosacral transitional vertebrae in German shepherd dogs. J Small Anim Pract 2021;62(11): 967–72.
42. Komsta R, Łojszczyk-Szczepaniak A, Dębiak P. Lumbosacral Transitional Vertebrae, Canine Hip Dysplasia, and Sacroiliac Joint Degenerative Changes on Ventrodorsal Radiographs of the Pelvis in Police Working German Shepherd Dogs. Top Companion Anim Med 2015;30(1):10–5.
43. Worth A, Thompson D, Hartman A. Degenerative lumbosacral stenosis in working dogs: Current concepts and review. N Zealand Vet J 2009;57(6):319–30.
44. Beraud R, Moreau M, Lussier B. Effect of exercise on kinetic gait analysis of dogs afflicted by osteoarthritis. Vet Comp Orthop Traumatol 2010;23(2):87–92.
45. Farr BD, Ramos MT, Otto CM. The Penn Vet Working Dog Center Fit to Work Program: A Formalized Method for Assessing and Developing Foundational Canine Physical Fitness. Front Vet Sci 2020;7. https://doi.org/10.3389/fvets.2020.00470.
46. Bockstahler B, Tichy A, Aigner P. Compensatory load redistribution in Labrador retrievers when carrying different weights – a non-randomized prospective trial. BMC Vet Res 2016;12(1):92.
47. Carnevale M, Jones J, Li G, et al. Computed Tomographic Evaluation of the Sacroiliac Joints of Young Working Labrador Retrievers of Various Work Status Groups: Detected Lesions Vary Among the Different Groups and Finite Element Analyses of the Static Pelvis Yields Repeatable Measures of Sacroiliac Ligament Joint Strain. Front Vet Sci 2020;7:528. https://doi.org/10.3389/fvets.2020.00528.

48. Jeon I-C, Kwon O-Y, Weon J-H, et al. Comparison of Hip- and Back-Muscle Activity and Pelvic Compensation in Healthy Subjects During 3 Different Prone Table Hip-Extension Exercises. J Sport Rehabil 2017;26(4):216–22.
49. Youdas JW, Boor MMP, Darfler AL, et al. Surface Electromyographic Analysis of Core Trunk and Hip Muscles During Selected Rehabilitation Exercises in the Side-Bridge to Neutral Spine Position. Sports Health 2014;6(5):416–21.
50. Bockstahler B, Kräutler C, Holler P, et al. Pelvic Limb Kinematics and Surface Electromyography of the Vastus Lateralis, Biceps Femoris, and Gluteus Medius Muscle in Dogs with Hip Osteoarthritis. Vet Surg 2012;41(1):54–62.
51. Zotti MGT, Boas FV, Clifton T, et al. Does pre-operative magnetic resonance imaging of the lumbar multifidus muscle predict clinical outcomes following lumbar spinal decompression for symptomatic spinal stenosis? Eur Spine J 2017;26(10):2589–97.
52. Shafaq N, Suzuki A, Matsumura A, et al. Asymmetric Degeneration of Paravertebral Muscles in Patients With Degenerative Lumbar Scoliosis. Spine 2012;37(16):1398–406.
53. Sun D, Liu P, Cheng J, et al. Correlation between intervertebral disc degeneration, paraspinal muscle atrophy, and lumbar facet joints degeneration in patients with lumbar disc herniation. BMC Musculoskelet Disord 2017;18(1):167.
54. Boström A, Channon S, Jokinen T, et al. Structural characteristics and predicted functional capacities of epaxial muscles in chondrodystrophic and non-chondrodystrophic dogs with and without suspected intervertebral disc herniation- a preliminary study. Res Vet Sci 2019;123:204–15.
55. Schaub KI, Kelleners N, Schmidt MJ, et al. Three-Dimensional Kinematics of the Pelvis and Caudal Lumbar Spine in German Shepherd Dogs. Front Vet Sci 2021;8. Available at: https://www.frontiersin.org/article/10.3389/fvets.2021.709966. Accessed February 4, 2022.
56. Schilling N, Carrier DR. Function of the epaxial muscles in walking, trotting and galloping dogs: implications for the evolution of epaxial muscle function in tetrapods. J Exp Biol 2010;213(9):1490–502.
57. Wall R. Introduction to Myofascial Trigger Points in Dogs. Top Companion Anim Med 2014;29(2):43–8.
58. Bilzer T, Faissler D, Neumann J, et al. Myopathie der Labrador Retriever: neuromuskuläre Veränderungen bei kranken und klinisch gesunden Hunden. Tierarztl Prax Ausg K 2004;32(03):130–9.
59. Formenton MR, Pereira MAA, Fantoni DT. Small Animal Massage Therapy: A Brief Review and Relevant Observations. Top Companion Anim Med 2017;32(4):139–45.
60. Corti L. Massage Therapy for Dogs and Cats. Top Companion Anim Med 2014;29(2):54–7.
61. Ramos MT, Farr BD, Otto CM. Sports Medicine and Rehabilitation in Working Dogs. Vet Clin North America: Small Anim Pract 2021;51(4):859–76.

Evidence-Based Complementary and Alternative Canine Orthopedic Medicine

Erin Miscioscia, DVM, CVA*, Jennifer Repac, DVM, CCRT, CVA, CVCH

KEYWORDS

- Canine • Orthopedic • Complementary and alternative veterinary medicine
- Acupuncture • Chiropractic • Manual therapy
- Traditional Chinese veterinary medicine • Herbal

KEY POINTS

- Complementary therapies can serve as useful adjuncts to traditional orthopedic veterinary treatments, especially for chronic pain management.
- There is more evidence in human medicine validating complementary orthopedic therapies such as acupuncture, chiropractic, and herbal supplements. Further high-quality studies are generally needed in veterinary medicine.
- There is growing evidence for acupuncture therapy as part of the multimodal analgesic management of small animal patients with chronic musculoskeletal pain.
- Growing research demonstrates the potential utility of some herbal supplements for canine osteoarthritis management; however, herbal supplements should not supplant pharmaceutical intervention when necessary (eg, nonsteroidal anti-inflammatory drugs).

INTRODUCTION

Complementary and alternative veterinary medicine (CAVM) describes therapies that are not typical components of traditional veterinary education. Although CAVM is becoming popular in veterinary postgraduate education, it is generally viewed as complementary to traditional medicine.[1] Demand for CAVM in the treatment of musculoskeletal conditions continues to grow. Recent studies in sporting dogs have

Department of Comparative, Diagnostic and Population Medicine, College of Veterinary Medicine, University of Florida, 2015 Southwest 16th Avenue, Gainesville, FL 32608, USA
* Corresponding author.
E-mail address: emiscioscia@ufl.edu

Vet Clin Small Anim 52 (2022) 925–938
https://doi.org/10.1016/j.cvsm.2022.02.003
0195-5616/22/Published by Elsevier Inc.

reported that 18% of owners use herbal supplements, and 73% and 12% use chiropractic and acupuncture, respectively.[2,3] While CAVM encompasses an ever-expanding list of unconventional therapies, this review focuses on those that are more commonly used and researched.

ACUPUNCTURE

Background

Acupuncture is a 3000-year-old therapy in which small gauge needles are placed at specific locations, or acupoints, in the body for a therapeutic effect. Acupoints, often located along meridians or channels, are characterized by low electrical impedance and high electrical skin conductance.[4,5] These points often overlay fascial planes, motor points, nerve branches, and/or regions of increased free nerve endings and mast cells.[5–8] There are several techniques used to stimulate acupoints, described in **Table 1**.[5,9–11]

Mechanism of action

Acupuncture alters the pain pathway through the release of neurochemicals including: enkephalins, endorphins, dynorphins, serotonin, norepinephrine, glutamate, neurokinin, and cannabinoids.[5,9,12] In addition, interplay between connective tissue and the neuro-immune microenvironment of acupoints, as well as the modulation of inflammatory mediators, likely contribute to the effects of acupuncture.[6,7,9,13] Several studies have evaluated the effect of acupuncture on osteoarthritis, demonstrating reduced expression of matrix metalloproteinases (MMPs), interleukin (IL) IL-1β, IL-6, and tumor necrosis factor (TNF)-α, as well as reduced cartilage matrix degradation.[14–18]

Acupuncture research shortcomings

A review of the efficacy of acupuncture in companion animals concluded that high-quality, randomized controlled trials (RCTs) with consistent and clinically relevant outcome measures (OMs) are needed to confirm conclusions of efficacy.[19] Similarly, a recent evaluation of systematic reviews of acupuncture for chronic pain in humans described the shortcomings of many of the included RCTs, contributing to downgraded evidence and uncertain conclusions.[20] These shortcomings included inadequate sample size, inappropriate controls and the challenge of dosing adequacy. In human studies where controls received no acupuncture, the placebo effect is a confounding factor. Alternatively, 'sham' acupuncture may be used, in which needles are

Table 1
Common techniques used to stimulate acupoints

Technique	Description
Dry needle acupuncture (DN AP)	Placement of small gauge needle into acupoints
Electroacupuncture (EAP)	Electric leads applied to needles placed into acupoints
Moxibustion	Heat applied to needles placed into acupoints (commonly by burning *Artemisia vulgaris*)
LASER acupuncture (LAP)	Application of therapeutic laser directly to an acupoint
Aquapuncture	Injection of a sterile liquid into an acupoint (eg: vitamin B12)
Implantation	Implantation of a substance into an acupoint (eg: gold bead or wire)
Acupressure	Manual pressure at an acupoint

either inserted at nonacupoints or superficially touch the skin. Unfortunately, both of these 'sham' techniques have the potential of contributing to physiologic effects. Further, dosing and acupoint protocols are typically individualized in clinical practice, presenting a challenge when standardizing acupuncture for RCTs. Utilizing dogs as models to study acupuncture offers a unique advantage over human trials given the ease of blinding owners to patient treatment groups.

Acupuncture for orthopedic medicine

Human Evidence

Meta-analysis of acupuncture for chronic pain in people showed that acupuncture was superior to sham or no acupuncture control groups for all conditions.[21] Similarly, another meta-analysis found acupuncture to be more effective than sham for chronic neck and shoulder pain (high evidence), low-back and myofascial pain (moderate evidence), and osteoarthritis (low evidence), but not chronic arm pain, rheumatoid arthritis, or acute neck and back pain.[22] While promising, it is important to recognize the limitations, as well as the varied outcomes across these trials.

Systematic reviews of acupuncture therapy for human peripheral joint osteoarthritis (OA) commonly showed minimal to no adverse effects, and statistically significant, though questionably clinically relevant, benefit when compared to sham acupuncture. Conversely, significant and likely clinically relevant benefit was observed when compared to no acupuncture, though placebo effect may have contributed.[23–27] A review of RCTs of acupuncture for human knee OA described the overall high risk of bias of published trials due to methodological limitations in study designs, conduct, and analyses.[28] Meta-analysis of 33 RCTs evaluating acupuncture for human myofascial pain syndrome concluded that most acupuncture therapies were effective in reducing pain and improving function.[29] Injection of myofascial trigger points (MTrPs) with bupivacaine was associated with a higher risk of adverse events.

Canine Evidence

Several controlled trials have evaluated acupuncture for various indications in canine orthopedic medicine, inclusive of general musculoskeletal pain, peripheral joint OA/dysplasia, postoperative management, and tissue healing (bone, tendon) (**Table 2**). Of the 9 trials described, 8 were RCTs and sample sizes ranged from 9 to 73 dogs. Interventions varied, with 2 studies utilizing dry needle acupuncture (DN AP), 4 electroacupuncture (EAP), 2 gold implant, and 1 did not specify the technique. OMs also varied, with 5 studies utilizing at least one objective OM. The most common OMs used were client-completed clinical metrology instruments (CMIs, 5/9), ground reaction forces (GRFs, 4/9), and subjective orthopedic scores (SOS, 4/9).

Five out of 9 evaluated trials detected significant improvements in at least one OM compared to controls, the majority of which were subjective (CMIs) and therefore subject to potential bias.[30–34] Most of these trials evaluated acupuncture for improving pain and function in dogs with peripheral joint OA/dysplasia. Of the trials that detected no significant differences between acupuncture and control groups, 3/4 had a sample size less than 20.[11,35–37] None of the studies evaluating objective gait analysis detected significant differences between groups.[31,32,35,36] Similar to the findings of Rose *and colleagues*[19] this supports the need for larger, higher quality RCTs with consistent OMs to further evaluate the use of acupuncture in small animal orthopedic medicine. Currently, the literature supports the safety and potential benefit of acupuncture (DN AP, EAP, gold bead implant) in some dogs with musculoskeletal pain, especially associated with OA.[30–34]

Table 2
Controlled trials evaluating the efficacy of acupuncture for canine orthopedic medicine

Author, Year	n	Study Design, Control (C)	Indication	Intervention	Outcome Measure(s)	Outcome(s) (vs. Control unless Specified)
Lane 2016	47	Controlled crossover, C: no treatment	Musculoskeletal pain	AP & manual therapy weekly X2	CMI with VAS	Sign.: CMI (pain, function)
Baker-Meuten 2020	32	RCT crossover	Peripheral joint OA	DN AP weekly X4	GRF, AC, SOS, CMI	Sign.: CMI (CSOM); NSD: GRF, AC, SOS, CMI (CBPI)
Teixeira 2016	70	RCT C: no treatment OR carprofen	Hip dysplasia	DN AP weekly X5	GRF, CMI with VAS	Sign.: CMI (AP vs no treatment); NSD: GRF (all groups), CMI (carprofen vs other groups)
Jaeger 2007	73	RCT C: no treatment	Hip dysplasia	Gold bead AP implant in place 18–24 mo	SOS, CMI	Sign.: SOS & CMI (pain, function); NSD: CMI (QOL, lameness)
Hielm-Bjorkman	38	RCT C: sham skin piercing	Hip dysplasia	Gold wire AP implant in place 6 mo	SOS, CMI	NSD
Kapatkin 2006	9	RCT crossover C: sham AP	Elbow OA	EAP weekly X3	GRF, SOS (VAS pain)	NSD
Shmalberg 2014	18	RCT C: no treatment	1-mo postop TPLO or CCWO	EAP once, immediate posttreatment	GRF, ROM	NSD
Naddaf 2014	12	RCT C: no treatment	Ulna fracture healing	EAP daily X10 Duration: 45–90 d	Radiographic score, histology score	NSD
Sharifi 2009	10	RCT C: no treatment	Calcaneal tendon healing	EAP daily X15, Duration: 60 d	Histologic healing	Sign.: histologic healing

Abbreviations: AC, activity count; AP, acupuncture; CBPI, canine brief pain inventory; CCWO, cranial closing wedge osteotomy; CMI, client metrology instrument (client completed); CSOM, client specific outcome measures; DN, dry needle; EAP, electroacupuncture; GRF, ground reaction forces; n, number of dogs in trial; NSD, no significant difference in all or specified OM between groups; OA, osteoarthritis; QOL, quality of life; RCT, randomized controlled trial; ROM, range of motion; Sign, statistically significant improvement in specified OM for the intervention group versus control; SOS, subjective orthopedic score; TPLO, tibial plateau leveling osteotomy; VAS, visual analog scale.

CLINICS CARE POINTS

- Acupuncture is safe and shows promise as part of the multimodal analgesic management of small animals with chronic musculoskeletal pain.[38,39] Higher quality studies with low risk of bias are indicated.
- Most canine osteoarthritis trials utilized weekly acupuncture sessions, which is a practical initial frequency (see **Table 2**).

CHIROPRACTIC

Ancient Manipulative Therapies

The practice of joint manipulation dates back to ancient Chinese medicine as early as 3 B.C E.[40] Writings of Pein Chiao from the 5th century B.C.E. reported the use of spinal manipulation for the treatment of insomnia, paralysis, lumbago, fatigue, rheumatism, and neurologic disorders. Various forms of joint and bone manipulation have also been recorded as part of Indian, Native American, Persian, and South American cultures.

Modern Chiropractic

D.D. Palmer founded chiropractic in the late 19th century.[41] His theory asserted that structural abnormalities of the spine (vertebral subluxation complexes) alter the body's neurologic coping ability, leading to decreased healing capacity and subsequent disease. However, the causal link between vertebral subluxation complexes and disease has yet to be scientifically elucidated.

Mechanism of Action

In contrast to conventional medicine's definition of subluxation, which refers to joint dislocation, a chiropractic subluxation is broadly described as a spinal biomechanical dysfunction or hypomobility. Chiropractic theory describes the dysfunction caused by a vertebral subluxation complex that results in changes in alignment, movement quality, and function. These changes subsequently affect joint motion, connective tissue, muscle, circulation, and neural integrity.

Chiropractic therapy aims to remedy vertebral subluxation complexes through a variety of motion-restoring manual therapies including joint traction, joint mobilization, and adjustments. Often the terms "spinal manipulation" and "adjustment" are used interchangeably; however, some disciplines emphasize that adjustments specifically refer to maneuvers performed on a boney contact point with a short lever arm.[42] For simplicity, "chiropractic" will be used in this review to include both adjustments and spinal manipulation therapy. Both terms refer to high-velocity, low-amplitude thrusts applied to a motion segment, pushing slightly beyond the end of the passive range of motion (into the paraphysiological space). Motion segments are most commonly vertebral segments, although the manipulation of peripheral joints may also be performed. This force is most commonly applied manually, along the "line of correction" which corresponds with the angle of the joint interface. These maneuvers are typically applied manually; however, some practitioners are trained using a mechanical spring-loaded "activator," which delivers an adjustable amount of focal pressure. Adjustments are only delivered to motion segments that were previously assessed as hypomobile through motion and palpation examination. A chiropractic adjustment provides therapeutic effect through several proposed mechanisms: reduction of nerve compression, restoration of intrinsic spinal reflex activity, and alleviation of fibrotic tissue stiffness.[42] Chiropractic is also thought to act by the stimulation of Aβ, Aδ, and C afferent nerve fibers similar to how acupuncture and transcutaneous electrical nerve stimulation (TENS) are used to block nociception.

Human Evidence

The majority of chiropractic research in human medicine focuses on the treatment of back pain. A systematic review on chronic low back pain showed greater decreases in pain and disability scores in patients receiving spinal manipulation compared with those in combined physical therapy and exercise programs.[43] Another systematic review on acute low back pain demonstrated moderate evidence of improved pain and function without serious adverse events.[44] According to the Annals of Internal Medicine's 2017 clinical guidelines, spinal manipulation, and acupuncture were both recommended over pharmacologic intervention for the treatment of chronic and acute low back pain.[45] There have also been studies demonstrating improved proprioception and coordination post cervical, and sacroiliac adjustment, respectively.[46,47]

Veterinary Evidence

Several equine studies, using a variety of OMs, support chiropractic therapy. One study showed decreased electromyographic (EMG) activity of splenius musculature 30 minutes post-treatment.[48] Another study measuring bioimpedance demonstrated increased contraction of trapezius musculature and increased use of the gluteus muscles post-treatment.[49] Chiropractic adjustment has also been demonstrated to increase spinal dorsoventral displacement, applied force, spinal range of motion, and axial pelvic rotation.[50,51] In one study, chiropractic increased mechanical nociceptive thresholds of patients post-treatment; however, a more recent RCT failed to show improvements in pain thresholds and pain and stiffness scoring.[52,53]

There is one canine study supporting the use of chiropractic performed in Boxer puppies.[54] Dogs in the treated group had a significantly lower incidence of radiographic spondylosis deformans at 1 year of age compared to the control group. However, this study was unblinded and thus subject to bias.

As with many veterinary studies, the existing veterinary chiropractic research is often underpowered and with fundamental study design flaws, such as lack of a control group. Additionally, the large variation in treatment protocols and OMs makes it difficult to draw conclusions.[55]

Clinical Application

Chiropractic examinations and treatments are typically recommended on a monthly basis. However, more gentle joint mobilization (low velocity) may be performed more frequently. Traction therapies can be taught to owners for home therapy use. Spinal pain is the most common indication; however, chiropractic can be used to address the indirect compensatory effects of any musculoskeletal condition. The most extreme example of this would be an amputee with the resultant rotation of the spine locally and altered positioning distally in the kinetic chain. Chiropractic is not recommended for patients with hypermobility, spinal instability, fracture, infection, neoplasia, or recent surgery. Extreme caution should be exercised in cases of suspected intervertebral disc extrusion and adjustments should not be applied directly at the lesion. Despite historical safety concerns regarding cervical adjustments, a human systematic review did not find a causal relationship between cervical arterial dissection and chiropractic.[56] However, this finding does not translate to the potential risk of adverse events in small animals receiving chiropractic therapy, which has yet to be fully investigated.

Herbal Medicine

Cannabis

There continues to be rapidly growing interest in the veterinary use of cannabis products. While marijuana is classified as a Schedule I drug, products containing less than 0.3% tetrahydrocannabinol (THC) are considered hemp according to the Agriculture Improvement Act.[57] The regulation of cannabidiol (CBD) products varies by state. Cannabis products can contain at least 480 different compounds including cannabinoids, terpenes, and phenylpropanoids.[58] These compounds bind to a variety of endogenous receptors throughout the body.[59] CB1 receptors are found primarily in the CNS, muscle, lung, gastrointestinal tract, vascular system, and reproductive organs. CB2 receptors are found in immune cells, glial cells, spleen, bone, and skin.

Several prospective clinical trials have demonstrated the efficacy of CBD for canine OA.[60–62] In contrast, 1 RCT showed no significant differences in supplemented osteoarthritic dogs.[63] The most commonly reported side effects include: elevation in alkaline phosphatase (ALP), gastrointestinal effects, lethargy, and ataxia, with a higher incidence in proportion to increased THC content.[60,64,65] Ingestion with a fatty meal and lecithin-containing preparations have been shown to improve absorption and delay time to $C_{max.}$[66] As with other herbal supplements, CBD products have highly variable active ingredient contents, such as cannabinoids and terpenes, and inactive ingredient contents. In a recent analysis of 29 CBD products, 4 were found to contain heavy metals and only 18 were labeled appropriately according to FDA guidelines.[67] This ingredient variability presents challenges in comparing CBD supplements and highlights the need for analysis and efficacy trials for individual products.

Curcumin

Curcumin is the active constituent of turmeric, which is derived from the rhizomes of *Curcuma longa.*[68] *In vitro*, curcumin has anti-inflammatory properties including the ability to decrease prostaglandin (PG) E_2, nitric oxide (NO), IL-6, cyclooxygenase-2 (COX-2), and MMPs.[68,69] Curcumin has also been shown to downregulate IL-18 and inhibit macrophage proliferation with subsequent downregulation of TNFα.[70] In a rat OA model, curcumin combined with glucosamine prevented cartilage degradation, improved locomotor function, and reduced neuropathic pain.[71] Bioavailability of curcumin is extremely low unless the product is formulated as chylomicrons or coadministered with piperine, limiting therapeutic dosing to these specific formulations.[68]

A 2016 meta-analysis containing 8 human RCTs supported the use of curcumin for OA; however, more trials are needed to solidify a firm conclusion.[72] Canine evidence remains inconsistent, and few studies have tested curcumin as a sole agent. A RCT showed improvements in pain scores, but not objective GRFs, of osteoarthritic dogs compared to controls when fed a diet supplemented with curcumin, hydrolyzed collagen, and green tea extract for 3 months.[73] Another RCT compared the use of a base nutraceutical (glucosamine-chondroitin, fish oil, vitamin C and E, saccharomyces) with and without a Boswellia-curcumin additive.[74] The group supplemented with Boswellia-curcumin demonstrated an increase in GRF, whereas the group on the base nutraceutical did not. In contrast, an earlier study evaluating curcumin alone failed to demonstrate differences in GRFs and CMIs, between treatment and control groups.[75] Unlike the 2 studies using combination products,[73,74] the supplement in this study[75] was not specifically formulated to enhance bioavailability.

Boswellia Serrata

Oleogum resin obtained from the bark of the *Boswellia serrata* tree (commonly known as frankincense) has been used medicinally in ancient cultures for thousands of years.[76]

AKBA (3-acetyl-11-keto-β-boswellic acid) and KBA (11-keto-β-boswellic acid) are the primary active boswellic acids in *Boswellia serrata* extract (BSE). Research has demonstrated the efficacy of BSE for the treatment of human colitis, bronchial asthma, neoplasia, and arthritis.[76–78] BSE's healing properties are attributed to anti-inflammatory inhibition of 5-lipoxygenase, TNF-α, and free oxygen radical formation.[76]

A meta-analysis of 7 human RCTs evaluating BSE supplementation for OA showed improvements in pain, stiffness, and function scores.[79] One uncontrolled canine clinical trial similarly demonstrated improved gait, pain, stiffness after 6 weeks of BSE supplementation.[80] BSE was generally well-tolerated with minor, infrequent adverse effects (diarrhea, flatulence). However, strong conclusions cannot be drawn due to the lack of a control group. Remaining canine studies used BSE in combination with other nutraceuticals, limiting the ability to determine efficacy as a sole agent.[74,81] Similar to CBD and other herbs, a study evaluating 13 BSE products demonstrated highly variable AKBA and KBA concentrations, as well as variations from label claims.[82]

Elk Antler Velvet

Elk antler velvet (EAV) was originally used in Chinese medicine for invigorating Kidney Yang and strengthening bone function.[83] EAV extract has been shown to decrease the level of intra-articular inflammatory mediators and plasma levels of IgG.[84] A study in mice showed velvet antler polypeptide partially reversed osteophyte formation and can modulate extracellular matrix through the inhibition of MMPs, ADAMTS4, and ADAMTS5.[85]

Canine studies on EAV are limited and results from the human literature remain inconclusive.[86] A canine RCT demonstrated improvements in GRFs, performance of activities of daily life, and vitality after 60 days of treatment.[87] No adverse effects were noted; however, 3/25 dogs in this study died (2 from adrenocortical insufficiency and 1 from hemangiosarcoma). Another canine RCT using a combination product (EAV, green-lipped mussel, shark cartilage, and enzogenol) showed improvements in CMIs.[88]

CLINICS CARE POINTS

- CBD supplementation has shown promise in the management of canine OA in several RCTs.[60–62]
- Curcumin, BSE and EAV supplementation require higher quality RCTs to support efficacy for canine OA; human studies support the use of curcumin and BSE.
- Herbal supplements must be critically evaluated for active ingredient content and bioavailability.[67,68,82]

SUMMARY

Owner and veterinary use of complementary therapies continue to become more widespread, especially for the management of chronic pain conditions such as OA. Many patients have comorbidities that preclude traditional medical options or have inadequate responses to conventional therapies. Evidence-based CAVM can serve as a safe and effective adjunct to help manage chronic pain conditions commonly seen in small animal orthopedic medicine. Veterinary scientific literature supports the use of acupuncture and some herbal supplements in the multimodal management of canine osteoarthritis. Most of the evidence supporting chiropractic is limited to equine and human literature.

DISCLOSURE

The authors have nothing to disclose.

REFERENCES

1. Gyles C. Complementary and alternative veterinary medicine. Can Vet J 2020;61(4):345–6.
2. Koh R, Montalbano C, Gamble LJ, et al. Internet survey of feeding, dietary supplement, and rehabilitative medical management use in flyball dogs. Can Vet J 2020;61(4):375–81.
3. Dinallo GK, Poplarski JA, Van Deventer GM, et al. A survey of feeding, activity, supplement use and energy consumption in North American agility dogs. J Nutr Sci 2017;6:e45. https://doi.org/10.1017/jns.2017.44.
4. Ahn AC, Colbert AP, Anderson BJ, et al. Electrical properties of acupuncture points and meridians: A systematic review. Bioelectromagnetics 2008;29(4):245–56.
5. Dewey C, Xie H. The scientific basis of acupuncture for veterinary pain management: a review based on relevant literature from the last two decades. Open Vet J 2021;11(2):203.
6. Langevin HM, Yandow JA. Relationship of acupuncture points and meridians to connective tissue planes. Anat Rec 2002;269(6):257–65.
7. Gong Y, Li N, Lv Z, et al. The neuro-immune microenvironment of acupoints—initiation of acupuncture effectiveness. J Leukoc Biol 2020;108(1):189–98.
8. Li A-H, Zhang J-M, Xie Y-K. Human acupuncture points mapped in rats are associated with excitable muscle/skin–nerve complexes with enriched nerve endings. Brain Res 2004;1012(1–2):154–9.
9. Zhang R, Lao L, Ren K, et al. Mechanisms of acupuncture–electroacupuncture on persistent pain. Anesthesiology 2014;120(2):482–503.
10. Yang J, Mallory MJ, Wu Q, et al. The safety of laser acupuncture: a systematic review. Med Acupunct 2020;32(4):209–17.
11. Hielm-Bjorkman A, Raekallio M, Kuusela E, et al. Double-blind evaluation of implants of gold wire at acupuncture points in the dog as a treatment for osteoarthritis induced by hip dysplasia. Vet Rec 2001;149(15):452–6.
12. Chen T, Zhang WW, Chu Y-X, et al. Acupuncture for pain management: molecular mechanisms of action. Am J Chin Med 2020;48(04):793–811.
13. Zhao Z-Q. Neural mechanism underlying acupuncture analgesia. Prog Neurobiol 2008;85(4):355–75.
14. Guan J, Geng W-Q, Li Y, et al. Decreased synovial fluid biomarkers levels are associated with rehabilitation of function and pain in rotator cuff tear patients following electroacupuncture therapy. Med Sci Monit 2020;26. https://doi.org/10.12659/msm.923240.
15. Xie L-L, Zhao Y-L, Yang J, et al. Electroacupuncture prevents osteoarthritis of high-fat diet-induced obese rats. Biomed Res Int 2020;2020:1–16. https://doi.org/10.1155/2020/9380965.
16. Zhang Y, Bao F, Wang Y, et al. Influence of acupuncture in treatment of knee osteoarthritis and cartilage repairing. Am J Transl Res 2016;8(9):3995–4002.
17. Bao F, Sun H, Wu Z-H, et al. Effect of acupuncture on expression of matrix metalloproteinase and tissue inhibitor in cartilage of rats with knee osteoarthritis. Zhongguo Zhen Jiu 2011;31(3):241–6.

18. Wang D-H, Bao F, Wu Z, et al. Influence of acupuncture on IL-1beta and TNF-alpha expression in the cartilage of rats with knee arthritis. Zongguo Gu Shang 2011;24(9):775–8.
19. Rose WJ, Sargeant JM, Hanna WJB, et al. A scoping review of the evidence for efficacy of acupuncture in companion animals. Anim Health Res Rev 2017;18(2): 177–85.
20. Paley CA, Johnson MI. Acupuncture for the relief of chronic pain: a synthesis of systematic reviews. Medicina 2019;56(1):6.
21. Vickers AJ, Vertosick EA, Lewith G, et al. Acupuncture for chronic pain: update of an individual patient data meta-analysis. J Pain 2018;19(5):455–74.
22. Yuan Q-L, Wang P, Liu L, et al. Acupuncture for musculoskeletal pain: a meta-analysis and meta-regression of sham-controlled randomized clinical trials. Sci Rep 2016;6:30675.
23. Manheimer E, Cheng K, Linde K, et al. Acupuncture for peripheral joint osteoarthritis. Cochrane Database Syst Rev 2010. https://doi.org/10.1002/14651858.cd001977.pub2.
24. Li J, Li Y-X, Luo L-J, et al. The effectiveness and safety of acupuncture for knee osteoarthritis. Medicine 2019;98(28):e16301. https://doi.org/10.1097/md.0000000000016301.
25. Cao L, Zhang X-L, Gao Y-S, et al. Needle acupuncture for osteoarthritis of the knee: a systematic review and updated meta-analysis. Saudi Med J 2012; 33(5):526–32.
26. Zhang Q, Yue J, Golianu B, et al. Updated systematic review and meta-analysis of acupuncture for chronic knee pain. Acupunct Med 2017;35(6):392–403.
27. Manheimer E, Cheng K, Wieland LS, et al. Acupuncture for hip osteoarthritis. Cochrane Database Syst Rev 2018;5:CD013010. https://doi.org/10.1002/14651858.cd013010.
28. Jia P, Tang L, Yu J, et al. Risk of bias and methodological issues in randomised controlled trials of acupuncture for knee osteoarthritis: a cross-sectional study. BMJ Open 2018;8(3):e019847.
29. Li X, Wang R, Xing X, et al. Acupuncture for myofascial pain syndrome: a network meta-analysis of 33 randomized controlled trials. Pain Physician 2017;20(6): E883–902.
30. Lane DM, Hill SA. Effectiveness of combined acupuncture and manual therapy relative to no treatment for canine musculoskeletal pain. Can Vet J 2016;57: 407–14.
31. Baker-Meuten A, Wendland T, Shamir SK, et al. Evaluation of acupuncture for the treatment of pain associated with naturally-occurring osteoarthritis in dogs: a prospective, randomized, placebo-controlled, blinded clinical trial. BMC Vet Res 2020;16(1). https://doi.org/10.1186/s12917-020-02567-1.
32. Teixeira LR, Luna SPL, Matsubara LM, et al. Owner assessment of chronic pain intensity and results of gait analysis of dogs with hip dysplasia treated with acupuncture. J Am Vet Med Assoc 2016;249(9):1031–9.
33. Jæger GT, Larsen S, Søli N, et al. Two years follow-up study of the pain-relieving effect of gold bead implantation in dogs with hip-joint arthritis. Acta Vet Scand 2007;49(1). https://doi.org/10.1186/1751-0147-49-9.
34. Sharifi D, Sasani F, Bakhtiari J, et al. The effect of acupuncture therapy on the repair of the calcaneal tendon (tendo calcaneus communis) in dogs. Turk J Vet Anim Sci 2009;33(3):181–4.

35. Kapatkin AS, Tomasic M, Beech J, et al. Effects of electrostimulated acupuncture on ground reaction forces and pain scores in dogs with chronic elbow joint arthritis. J Am Vet Med Assoc 2006;228(9):1350–4.
36. Shmalberg J, Burgess J, Davies W. A randomized controlled blinded clinical trial of electr-acupuncture administered one month after cranial cruciate ligament repair in dogs. Am J Tradit Chin Vet Med 2014;9(2):43–51.
37. Naddaf H, Baniadam A, Esmaeilzadeh S, et al. Histopathologic and radiographic evaluation of the electroacupuncture effects on ulna fracture healing in dogs. Open Vet J 2014;4(1):44–50.
38. Epstein M, Rodan I, Griffenhagen G, et al. AAHA/AAFP pain management guidelines for dogs and cats. J Am Anim Hosp Assoc 2015;51(2):67–84.
39. Mathews K, Kronen PW, Lascelles D, et al. Guidelines for recognition, assessment and treatment of pain. J Small Anim Pract 2014;55(6):E10–68.
40. Willis J. Forerunners of the Chiropractic Adjustment. In: Fundamentals of chiropractic. Amsterdam: Elsevier Health Sciences; 2003. p. 33–5.
41. Cleveland A. The Chiropractic Paradigm. In: Fundamentals of chiropractic. Amsterdam: Elsevier Health Sciences; 2003. p. 59–72.
42. Henderson CNR. The basis for spinal manipulation: chiropractic perspective of indications and theory. J Electromyogr Kinesiol 2012;22(5):632–42.
43. Coulter ID, Crawford C, Hurwitz EL, et al. Manipulation and mobilization for treating chronic low back pain: a systematic review and meta-analysis. Spine J 2018; 18(5):866–79.
44. Paige NM, Miake-Lye IM, Booth MS, et al. Association of spinal manipulative therapy with clinical benefit and harm for acute low back pain: systematic review and meta-analysis. JAMA 2017;317(14):1451–60.
45. Qaseem A, Wilt TJ, McLean RM, et al. Noninvasive treatments for acute, subacute, and chronic low back pain: a clinical practice guideline from the American College of Physicians. Ann Intern Med 2017;166(7):514–30.
46. Palmgren PJ, Sandström PJ, Lundqvist FJ, et al. Improvement after chiropractic care in cervicocephalic kinesthetic sensibility and subjective pain intensity in patients with nontraumatic chronic neck pain. J Manipulative Physiol Ther 2006; 29(2):100–6.
47. Marshall P, Murphy B. The effect of sacroiliac joint manipulation on feed-forward activation times of the deep abdominal musculature. J Manipulative Physiol Ther 2006;29(3):196–202.
48. Langstone J, Ellis J, Cunliffe C. A preliminary study of the effect of manual chiropractic treatment on the splenius muscle in horses when measured by surface electromyography. Equine Vet J 2015;47:18. https://doi.org/10.1111/EVJ.12486_41.
49. Acutt EV, le Jeune SS, Pypendop BH. Evaluation of the effects of chiropractic on static and dynamic muscle variables in sport horses. J Equine Vet Sci 2019;73: 84–90. https://doi.org/10.1016/J.JEVS.2018.10.016.
50. Haussler KK, Martin CE, Hill AE. Efficacy of spinal manipulation and mobilisation on trunk flexibility and stiffness in horses: a randomised clinical trial. Equine Vet J 2010;42(SUPPL. 38):695–702.
51. Alvarez CBG, L'Ami JJ, Moffatt D, et al. Effect of chiropractic manipulations on the kinematics of back and limbs in horses with clinically diagnosed back problems. Equine Vet J 2008;40(2):153–9.
52. Sullivan KA, Hill AE, Haussler KK. The effects of chiropractic, massage and phenylbutazone on spinal mechanical nociceptive thresholds in horses without clinical signs. Equine Vet J 2008;40(1):14–20.

53. Haussler KK, Manchon PT, Donnell JR, et al. Effects of low-level laser therapy and chiropractic care on back pain in quarter horses. J Equine Vet Sci 2020;86: 102891. https://doi.org/10.1016/J.JEVS.2019.102891.
54. Halle KS, Granhus A. Veterinary chiropractic treatment as a measure to prevent the occurrence of spondylosis in boxers. Vet Sci 2021;8(9):199.
55. Haussler KK, Hesbach AL, Romano L, et al. A systematic review of musculoskeletal mobilization and manipulation techniques used in veterinary medicine. Anim 2021;11(10):2787. https://doi.org/10.3390/ANI11102787.
56. Church EW, Sieg EP, Zalatimo O, et al. Systematic review and meta-analysis of chiropractic care and cervical artery dissection: no evidence for causation. Cureus 2016;8(2). https://doi.org/10.7759/CUREUS.498.
57. Agricultural Improvement Act. HR, 2. 115 Congress. Session 2. Section 297A (2018).
58. Andre CM, Hausman JF, Guerriero G. Cannabis sativa: The plant of the thousand and one molecules. Front Plant Sci 2016;7(FEB2016):19. https://doi.org/10.3389/FPLS.2016.00019/BIBTEX.
59. Gaynor JS, Muir WW. Alternative Drugs and Novel Therapies. In: Handbook of veterinary pain management. 3rd edition. St. Louis: Elsevier; 2015. p. 290–1.
60. Gamble L-J, Boesch JM, Frye CW, et al. Pharmacokinetics, safety, and clinical efficacy of cannabidiol treatment in osteoarthritic dogs. Front Vet Sci 2018;5: 165. https://doi.org/10.3389/FVETS.2018.00165/BIBTEX.
61. Verrico CD, Wesson S, Konduri V, et al. A randomized, double-blind, placebo-controlled study of daily cannabidiol for the treatment of canine osteoarthritis pain. Pain 2020;161(9):2191–202.
62. Kogan LR. The use of cannabidiol-rich hemp oil extract to treat canine osteoarthritis-related pain: a pilot study. Available at: https://www.researchgate.net/publication/339698157. Accessed November 16, 2021.
63. Mejia S, Duerr FM, Griffenhagen G, et al. Evaluation of the effect of cannabidiol on naturally occurring osteoarthritis-associated pain: a pilot study in dogs. J Am Anim Hosp Assoc 2021;57(2):81–90. https://doi.org/10.5326/JAAHA-MS-7119.
64. Vaughn D, Kulpa J, Paulionis L. Preliminary investigation of the safety of escalating cannabinoid doses in healthy dogs. Front Vet Sci 2020;7:51. https://doi.org/10.3389/FVETS.2020.00051/BIBTEX.
65. McGrath S, Bartner LR, Rao S, et al. Randomized blinded controlled clinical trial to assess the effect of oral cannabidiol administration in addition to conventional antiepileptic treatment on seizure frequency in dogs with intractable idiopathic epilepsy. J Am Vet Med Assoc 2019;254(11):1301–8.
66. Wakshlag JJ, Schwark WS, Deabold KA, et al. Pharmacokinetics of cannabidiol, cannabidiolic ccid, Δ9-tetrahydrocannabinol, tetrahydrocannabinolic acid and related metabolites in canine serum after dosing with three oral forms of hemp extract. Front Vet Sci 2020;7:505. https://doi.org/10.3389/FVETS.2020.00505/BIBTEX.
67. Wakshlag JJ, Cital S, Eaton SJ, et al. Cannabinoid, terpene, and heavy metal analysis of 29 over-the-counter commercial veterinary hemp supplements. Vet Med Res Rep 2020;11:45. https://doi.org/10.2147/VMRR.S248712.
68. Comblain F, Serisier S, Barthelemy N, et al. Review of dietary supplements for the management of osteoarthritis in dogs in studies from 2004 to 2014. J Vet Pharmacol Ther 2016;39(1):1–15.
69. Henrotin Y, Priem F, Mobasheri A. Curcumin: A new paradigm and therapeutic opportunity for the treatment of osteoarthritis: curcumin for osteoarthritis management. Springerplus 2013;2(1):1–9.

70. Colitti M, Gaspardo B, Della Pria A, et al. Transcriptome modification of white blood cells after dietary administration of curcumin and non-steroidal anti-inflammatory drug in osteoarthritic affected dogs. Vet Immunol Immunopathol 2012; 147(3–4):136–46.
71. Gugliandolo E, Peritore AF, Impellizzeri D, et al. Dietary supplementation with palmitoyl-glucosamine co-micronized with curcumin relieves osteoarthritis pain and benefits joint mobility. Anim 2020;10(10):1827.
72. Daily JW, Yang M, Park S. Efficacy of turmeric extracts and curcumin for alleviating the symptoms of joint arthritis: a systematic review and meta-analysis of randomized clinical trials. J Med Food 2016;19(8):717–29.
73. Comblain F, Barthélémy N, Lefèbvre M, et al. A randomized, double-blind, prospective, placebo-controlled study of the efficacy of a diet supplemented with curcuminoids extract, hydrolyzed collagen and green tea extract in owner's dogs with osteoarthritis. BMC Vet Res 2017;13(1):1–11.
74. Caterino C, Aragosa F, della Valle G, et al. Clinical efficacy of Curcuvet and Boswellic acid combined with conventional nutraceutical product: An aid to canine osteoarthritis. PLoS One 2021;16(5):e0252279.
75. Innes JF, Fuller CJ, Grover ER, et al. Randomised, double-blind, placebo-controlled parallel group study of P54FP for the treatment of dogs with osteoarthritis. Vet Rec 2003;152(15):457–60.
76. Ammon HPT. Boswellic acids in chronic inflammatory diseases. Planta Med 2006; 72(12):1100–16.
77. Roy NK, Deka A, Bordoloi D, et al. The potential role of boswellic acids in cancer prevention and treatment. Cancer Lett 2016;377(1):74–86.
78. Qurishi Y, Hamid A, Zargar MA, et al. Potential role of natural molecules in health and disease: Importance of boswellic acid. J Med Plants Res 2010;4(25): 2778–86.
79. Yu G, Xiang W, Zhang T, et al. Effectiveness of boswellia and boswellia extract for osteoarthritis patients: a systematic review and meta-analysis. BMC Complement Med Ther 2020;20(1):1–16.
80. Reichling J, Schmökel H, Fitzi J, et al. Dietary support with Boswellia resin in canine inflammatory joint and spinal disease. Schweiz Arch Tierheilkd 2004; 146(2):71–9.
81. Moreau M, Lussier B, Pelletier JP, et al. A medicinal herb-based natural health product improves the condition of a canine natural osteoarthritis model: A randomized placebo-controlled trial. Res Vet Sci 2014;97(3):574–81. https://doi.org/10.1016/J.RVSC.2014.09.011.
82. Miscioscia E, Shmalberg J, Scott KC. Measurement of 3-acetyl-11-keto-beta-boswellic acid and 11-keto-beta-boswellic acid in Boswellia serrata supplements administered to dogs. BMC Vet Res 2019;15(1). https://doi.org/10.1186/s12917-019-2021-7.
83. Gongwang L. Drugs for Invigorating Yang. In: Chinese herbal medicine Beijing. HuaXia; 2000. p. 80.
84. Sui Z, Zhang L, Huo Y, et al. Bioactive components of velvet antlers and their pharmacological properties. J Pharm Biomed Anal 2014;87:229–40. https://doi.org/10.1016/J.JPBA.2013.07.044.
85. Xie WQ, Zhao YJ, Li F, et al. Velvet antler polypeptide partially rescue facet joint osteoarthritis-like phenotype in adult β-catenin conditional activation mice. BMC Complement Altern Med 2019;19(1):1–8.

86. Gilbey A, Perezgonzalez JD. The New Zealand Medical Journal. Health benefits of deer and elk velvet antler supplements: a systematic review of randomised controlled studies. J New Zeal Med Assoc NZMJ 2012;125:8716.
87. Moreau M, Dupuis J, Bonneau NH, et al. Clinical evaluation of a powder of quality elk velvet antler for the treatment of osteoarthrosis in dogs. Can Vet J 2004; 45(2):133.
88. Lall R, Srivastava AK, Gupta RC. A randomized, blinded, placebo-controlledsStudy of BVP-01, a proprietary nutraceutical formulation for the treatment of canine osteoarthritis. Int J Vet Heal Sci Res 2021;9(1):266–73.

Clinical Guide to Obesity and Nonherbal Nutraceuticals in Canine Orthopedic Conditions

Barbara Esteve Ratsch, PhD, DVM (Austria), CCRP[a,*],
David Levine, PT, PhD, DPT, CCRP[b,c], Joseph J. Wakshlag, DVM, PhD[d]

KEYWORDS

• Obesity • Activity • Exercise • Osteoarthritis • Nutraceutical

KEY POINTS

- Obesity can be addressed successfully using hypocaloric diets and increased physical activity.
- Physical activity for the obese/overweight patient has to be tailored to the patient and client and structured exercise programs can be helpful in weight loss and retention of lean body mass.
- Nutraceutical interventions to mitigate the clinical signs associated with osteoarthritis is well established in the form of marine oils and can help diminish the use of nonsteroidal anti-inflammatories.
- The use of disease-modifying nutraceuticals aimed at preservation of cartilage are in their infancy in canine orthopedic medicine with many short-term studies suggesting equivocal results, which can be implemented as part of patient management, yet longer term studies are needed.

COMPARATIVE OBESITY AND PHYSICAL ACTIVITY IN HUMAN MEDICINE

In humans, being overweight can be defined as excessive or abnormal accumulation of fat or adipose tissue in the body that impairs health and affects all body systems.[1–3] Body mass index (BMI) is commonly used, and a BMI of 25–29.9 is considered overweight with a BMI of 30 or greater considered obese.[2] Ways to measure obesity

[a] Department of Physical Medicine, Evidensia Sørlandet Animal Hospital, Krittveien 2, Hamresanden 4656, Norway; [b] Department of Health, Education and Professional Studies, University of Tennessee, Chattanooga, TN 37403, USA; [c] Department of Physical Therapy, The University of Tennessee at Chattanooga, 615 McCallie Avenue Department #3253, Chattanooga, TN 37403, USA; [d] Department of Clinical Sciences, Cornell University College of Veteinary Medicine, 930 Campus Road, CPC - 3-536, Ithaca, NY 14853, USA
* Corresponding author. Evidensia Sørlandet Animal Hospital, Krittveien 2, Hamresanden 4656, Norway
E-mail address: barbara.esteve@veterinary-academy-of-higher-learning.com

Vet Clin Small Anim 52 (2022) 939–958
https://doi.org/10.1016/j.cvsm.2022.03.002
0195-5616/22/

commonly include BMI, waist circumference, body fat percentage (determined in several different ways), and dual-energy X-ray absorptiometry (DEXA) and are different from the typical body condition scores (BCS) implemented in canine medicine.[4,5] Being overweight or obese is associated with a multitude of comorbidities including diabetes mellitus, dyslipidemia, hyperlipidemia, cardiovascular disease, obstructive sleep apnea, chronic obstructive pulmonary diseases, cancer, low back pain, osteoarthritis (OA), complications from COVID-19: coronavirus disease of 2019, chronic disease mortality and morbidity, and premature death.[3,4,6,7] Weight loss as little as 5%–10% can improve one's health and quality of life.[8] The most common weight loss approaches include interventions such as diet, exercise, or a combination of the two.[9–16]

Physical activity is positively associated with physical functioning and life satisfaction.[17] Increased body weight and global body weakness are associated with a sedentary lifestyle, which can impair one's physical function and quality of life. Different types of supervised physical exercise (endurance, strength, etc.) and following general physical activity recommendations had equal efficacy in reducing body weight, improving one's body composition, and restoring one's physical function. The current recommendation suggests that people of all ages should perform 30–60 min of physical activity of moderate intensity on most, if not all, days of the week.[18] Body fat loss can be associated with the intensity of the activity. The higher the intensity, the greater the loss.[19] Moderate to intense aerobic exercise has the highest potential to reduce adipose tissue in overweight or obese individuals without the inclusion of a hypocaloric diet.[20] Visser's found a reduction of visceral adipose tissue of 30 cm in women and 40 cm in men after 12 weeks of aerobic physical activity.

PHYSICAL ACTIVITY PLUS HYPOCALORIC DIETS FOR OVERWEIGHT/OBESE HUMANS

A combination of restricted energy consumption and increased energy expenditure has been proven to be efficient in managing obesity.[21] Physical activity increases the amount of calories the body burns (energy expenditure), and a hypocaloric diet restricts energy consumption. Weight loss can be achieved through increasing physical activity and following a hypocaloric diet. General physical activity recommendations when combined with a hypocaloric diet are effective at reducing body weight and modifying one's body composition.[18] A hypocaloric diet alone is adequate to lose weight in the short term, but physical activity is vital to modify the new body composition. Diet alone will result in a reduction in fat mass, but when combined with exercise, there is an increase in both muscle mass and bone mineral density. Weight loss following a hypocaloric diet resulted in decreased bone mineral density in the hip and lumbar spine, but when combined with exercise, bone mineral density did not decrease.[22] Physical activity decreases body fat but maintains muscle mass unlike diet alone.[19] Making hypocaloric approaches and increases in physical activity the gold standard for obesity intervention.

OBESITY AND PHYSICAL ACTIVITY IN DOGS

Like in humans, an excessive amount of fat in the body has been associated with a variety of metabolic disorders and further comorbidities in companion animals. These include insulin resistance, altered adipokine patterns, changes in lipid metabolism, ectopic fat accumulation, respiratory and cardiovascular diseases, skin pathologies, pancreatitis, neoplasms, urogenital disorders, OA, increased anesthetic risk, and premature death.[23–32]

In humans, criteria have been established for what constitutes "overweight" and "obesity".[26] There is currently no specific percentage information in dogs to define the reduced, ideal or excessive amount of fat in the body, as we lack baseline data.[33] Due to species, breed, size, gender, age, lifelong physical activity, and chosen evaluation technique, the diagnosis of an overweight or obesity state is complex in companion animals.[34–36] Female dogs may present approximately 3%–5% more fat content at ideal weight than males.[37] In the absence of rigorous epidemiologic studies, no standardized values exist regarding the distinction between overweight and obesity in dogs.[26,37–41] Although speculative, dogs are often presumed as being overweight if their body weight exceeds the ideal body weight by 10%–19% and obese when exceeding more than 20%.

Noninvasive techniques to diagnose and monitor fat content in pets include bodyweight recording, BCS, and less frequent morphometric measurements.[37,40,42–48] The muscle condition score (MCS) is also relevant in the tailored diagnosis and monitoring of obesity[38,49,50] More sophisticated noninvasive methods including DEXA, computed tomography (CT), and magnetic resonance imaging (MRI) are used for research purposes but have little utility for the general practitioner.[30,37,39,44,48,51–53]

Diagnosing and monitoring treatment by documenting the body weight alone may be misleading, as in humans and dogs no linear rate of body weight loss is to be expected in the course of a hypocaloric treatment.[54–56] A slow progress in the bodyweight loss may lead to frustration of the pet owner.[45] It is therefore important to inform owners about the expected rate of weight loss, which is expected to slowly diminish after initial expected weight loss as the patient advances in the weight loss protocol to avoid a premature dropout of the program.

The positive effect of weight loss has been subjectively described in dogs after a partial weight loss of 6%–10%.[31,55,57] Improvement in life quality has also been reported simply by reducing body weight from obese to overweight, and significantly better cardiorespiratory performance has been demonstrated in the process.[58] There are suggestions that partial weight loss programs might be more appropriate for some dogs.[46,54,55,59] But, although weight loss can have health benefits, current therapeutic strategies are not ideal. Many obese dogs that enroll in a weight loss program do not lose weight or regain it.[46,54]

When examining the literature there is a tendency to focus much on the outcomes of dogs that completed the trial in the literature, while ignoring for the relatively high percentage of dogs that did not enroll or dropped out of the program.[55] This large cohort of unsuccessful candidates is not taken into account, making global recommendations across clinical cohorts difficult since owners who complete these trials may be more heavily invested than the typical client and patient presenting to general practice clinics.

Other factors including size, age, and breed of the dog appear to be important when defining the energy requirements of dogs. Aging dogs may even require different daily energy requirements depending on their lifetime daily physical activity amount (sedentary vs physical active lifestyle).[60] There is currently one long-term prospective study in dogs to evaluate the extent to which weight loss could be sustained after initial weight loss programs.[61]

PHYSICAL ACTIVITY FOR OVERWEIGHT/OBESE DOGS

Poor evidence exists to describe an ideal exercise program for overweight/obese dogs[62] and the recommendations for pet owners regarding daily physical activity leading to a safe and efficient fat mass loss currently lack any scientific background.[47] Obesity enhances joint inflammation, mechanically impairs gait patterns, overloads the musculoskeletal and cardiorespiratory system, reduces the flexibility of the rib cage during inspiration, and causes heat intolerance.[24,31,58,63–65] Like in humans, ectopic fat deposition inside and around muscle fibers (myosteatosis) may have an impact in the muscular functionality, contractility strength, and oxidative capacity in overweight/obese dogs.[66] In sum, obesity significantly limits functional physical performance. A distinction is therefore recommended between the terms "physical activity" and "physical exercise". "Physical activity" is understood to be any form of workout and may happen in the context of amateur practice like daily walks, various sports, or lifestyle activities. "Physical exercise" defines a professional workout program, composed and prescribed qualitatively and quantitatively to improve physical fitness of an individual. Depending on the clinical indication and progression stage, physical exercise may vary in its frequency and duration as well as type and intensity of performed exercise.[67]

The subject of screening and monitoring cardiorespiratory fitness in the context of physical activity capacity and/or physical exercise capacity has not been widely explored even in healthy sporting dogs. Also, little is known about the direct physiologic blood flow effect in the adipose tissue in dogs during physical exercise. Although blood flow may increase in all adipose tissue depots, it seems to happen to different degrees, and it is not proven whether this consistently occurs in all signalments and clinical conditions.[68] Similar to humans, muscle fibers of obese dogs may also present a reduced mitochondrial density and hence reduced oxidative capacity compared with lean dogs, impairing the cell's ability to oxidize lipids.[66] The physical activity offered to the companion dog probably may also depend on the physical effort the pet owner is willing to make for themselves, which partly depends on the climatic conditions.[69] The size and the skull shape of the animal may also determine the ability of a pet owner to provide physical activity in an efficient and safe way. As a general rule, owner participation in the therapy should be maximized. Nevertheless, the owner should not bear the responsibility alone to perform the suitable physical performance for the chronically diseased pet. Still waiting for more evidence, the AAHA's recommendations for required daily physical activity for obese dogs are transferred from human recommendations.[62,70]

The 6-minute walk test (6MWT) is a useful diagnostic and monitoring tool for physical performance in dogs with various conditions, such as brachycephalic obstructive airway syndrome (BOAS) and obesity. The primary measurement is the patient's comfortable walking distance, but data can also be collected on blood oxygen saturation and perception of respiratory distress during and after performance.[58,71,72] The 6MWT showed significant changes in heart and respiratory rate and oxygen saturation (SpO_2) during progressing fat loss in dogs and may be a worthwhile clinical test to assess progress and physiologic improvements during weight loss.[58]

PHYSICAL ACTIVITY PLUS HYPOCALORIC DIET FOR THE OVERWEIGHT/OBESE CANINE

The effectiveness of physical exertion on body weight loss management continues to be the subject of much debate and the opinions appear controversial and even contradictory in recent studies. **Table 1** chronologically lists studies that have incorporated exercise in dog weight loss management over the last 15 years. Some of the studies were prospective in nature and lasted between 1 and 6 months.[47,63,69,73–75] The prospective trials were commonly carried out on few animals and the canine population varied in age, breed, size, skull shape, gender, sexual status, and overweight/obese degree. The data describing the diagnosis and the monitoring of physical capacity performance were mostly not reported, except by one.[75] The description of

Table 1
Studies on exercise in weight loss management of dogs

Study	Duration	n	Age	SM	HC Diet Only	HC Diet and PA	Home PA	Structured PE	Diagnostic and Monitoring Tools	Outcomes	mBCS Initial	mBCS Outcome	% Drop out rate
Mlacnik et al. (2006)[63] PR	24 wk	29	8.4 y ± 3.2 y	M & FAL & SI		X(Ctrl & Exp)	X(Ctrl & Exp)	X(Exp)	CE, CBC, CB, BW, BCS	Increased PA may have facilitated BW loss	≥ 4/5	Ideal 3/5 In 53% dogs (Ctrl) vs 86% dogs (Exp)	0%
Chauvet et al. (2011)[43] RS	12 wk	8	3 y– 10 y	M & FAL		X	X	X	CE, HR, CBC, CB, BW, BCS, MM	Mean performance on the UWTM increased significantly	5/5	ND	37.5%
Wakshlag et al. (2012)[73] PR	88 wk	61	1.5 y – 11 y	M & FAL & SI		X	X		HCT, CB, BW, BCS,pedometer	Steps/dayA: 9721 ± 3,105I: 4619 ± 1243	≥ 7/9	5–6/9	33%
Morrison et al. (2014)[69] PR	26 wk	16	1 y- < 9 y	M & FAL		X	X		BW, BCS, accelerometer	BW loss is not associated with a spontaneous change in PA	5/5	4/5	12.5%
German et al. (2015)[45] RS	352 wk	143	1.3 y – 19 y	M & FAL & SI		X	X		DEXA, CE, CBC, CB, BW, UA	ND	ND	25.5% BW loss	39%

(*continued on next page*)

Table 1
(continued)

Study	Duration	n	Age	SM	HC Diet Only	HC Diet and PA	Home PA	Structured PE	Diagnostic and Monitoring Tools	Outcomes	mBCS Initial	mBCS Outcome	% Drop out rate
Vitger et al. (2016)[75] PR	12 wk	19	2 y – 13 y	M & F AL & SI	X (Ctrl)	X (Exp)	X (Exp)		DEXA, CE, HR, CBC, CB, UA, BW, BCS, accelerometer	Mean accelero-meter counts increased in the Exp group and decreased in the Ctrl group	7–9/9 (Exp)vs. 6–8/9 (Ctrl)	5–8/9 (Exp) vs 5–8/9 (Ctrl)	15.8%
Porsani et al. (2020)[50] RS	156 wk	73	All ages	M & F AL & SI		X	X		MR, BW, BCS, MCS	No significant association between BW loss success and PA	$\geq$ 8/9	BCS outcome varied according to individual BW loss speed/wk	0%
Chapman et al. (2019)[47] PR	8 wk	13	1 y – 8 y	M & F AL	X (Ctrl)		X (Exp) PA increase of 30%		MR, BW, BCS, MM, accelerometer	No significant differences in mean accelero-meter counts between Ctrl and Exp groups	6–9/9 (Exp) vs 6–9/9 (Ctrl)	6–9/9 (Exp) vs 5–8/9 (Ctrl)	0%

Niese et al. (2021)[74] PR	8 wk	24	ND	ND	X (Ctrl)	X (Exp)	CE BCS, BW, H, pedometer	The number of pedometer steps increased significantly in both groups	6.5/9	5.7/9	31%

Abbreviations: A, active dogs; AL, altered; BCS, body condition score; BW, body weight; CB, clinical biochemistry; CBC, complete blood count; CE, clinical examination; Ctrl, control group; DEXA, dual-energy X-ray absorptiometry; Exp, experimental group; F, females; H, height; HC, hypocaloric; HCT, hematocrit; HR, heart rate; I, inactive dogs; M, males; mBCS, mean body condition score; MCS, muscle condition score; MM, morphometric measurements; MR, medical records; MWT, 6-min walk test; n, number of dogs; ND, not described; PA, physical activity; PE, physical exercise; PEx, physical exertion; PR, prospective study; RS, retrospective study; SI, sexually intact; SM, signalment; UA, urinalysis; UWTM, underwater treadmill; versus, versus; wk, week; wks, weeks; y, years 6.

the chosen physical exercise as well as its monitoring were often not reported. Clarifying the type of prescribed physical activity was made only in the minority of weight loss regimes.

The reevaluations determining success or failure were mainly performed by the exclusive evaluation of body weight. In cases of slow weight loss, the daily offered calories were often further reduced from baseline recommendations. Physical exercise combined with a hypocaloric diet significantly preserved lean mass in dogs compared with a hypocaloric diet as monotherapy, but it made no significant difference in the body weight reduction between both dog groups.[75,76]

In another trial, active dogs lost about the same amount of body weight toward the end of the study as the less active dogs although they were allowed to consume more calories than the sedentary dogs. The active dogs reached their ideal body weight in less weeks than the sedentary dogs.[73] In some trials, approximately 30% of the dogs that started the weight loss program dropped out before reaching the goal, providing some evidence of the difficulty of hypocaloric plans and increased physical activity for owners suggesting that compliance is often an issue for the clinician and patient (see **Table 1**).

Concluding with the limited evidence and standardization of physical exercise or physical activity regimens remains elusive regarding recommendations. However, physically active dogs may be able to consume a higher daily calorie amount compared with sedentary dogs and still lose weight suggesting that clinically we should be recommending home activity or structured physical exercise protocols to improve outcomes related to obesity management.[73,75]

CANINE NONHERBAL OSTEOARTHRITIS NUTRACEUTICALS

Marine Oils

Geriatric animals and postorthopedic surgical patients are predisposed to degenerative and/or chronic inflammatory joint pathologies and marine oils with elevated concentrations of long-chain omega three fatty acids have received significant attention with respect to decreasing the clinical signs associated with primarily inflammatory OA. Omega-3 fatty acids are polyunsaturated fatty acids. The most commonly studied include the 18-carbon alpha linolenic acid (ALA), the 20-carbon eicosapentaenoic acid (EPA), and the 22-carbon doxosohexaenoic acid (DHA). These dietary long-chain omega-3 fatty acids are incorporated in cellular membranes, and EPA serves as a substrate for the COX and LOX enzymes. Omega-6 fatty acids are required in normal physiologic processes but during inflammation are thought to contribute more to the formation of “proinflammatory” prostaglandins and leukotrienes, whereas omega-3 produces the less inflammatory 3-series prostaglandins and 5-series leukotrienes.[77] EPA and DHA are found most commonly in fish oils although algal forms of EPA and DHA are also used in foods and supplements; however, marine animal forms of oils are richest in EPA and DHA. Dogs and humans have limited ability to convert ALA (found in flax seed and other oils) to EPA, and little to no conversion of ALA to DHA occurs in dogs. ALA-enriched diets must provide a high percentage (>7 times that needed of EPA/DHA) of fat as this precursor omega-3, because conversion to the longer chain EPA and DHA is inefficient, making dosing impractical in a typical supplement regimen.[78] Fish oil supplementation with EPA and DHA has been studied in naturally occurring OA in dogs with several papers suggesting the benefits either through objective analysis such as client-specific outcomes and pain scale data and objective kinetics analysis.[79–85] These studies suggest that regardless of whether the fish oil is incorporated into food or used as a stand-alone nutraceutical, the addition diminishes clinical signs associated with OA. Any diet with elevated amounts of polyunsaturated fatty acids also requires increased amounts of vitamin E due to the increased lipid peroxidation from such supplementation.[77] This may not be particularly relevant unless super supplementing EPA and DHA from fish oils at the highest levels of efficacy. Diets containing elevated EPA and DHA at 2.5–4.0 g/1000 kcal, which translates into doses of around 100–275 mg/kg body weight as a starting dose that is feasible (i.e., 100 mg/kg body weight), and one study suggests that a dose of 50 mg of EPA/DHA per kg body weight may also be beneficial.[79,81,84] It must also be recognized that in much of the literature the dose is based on metabolic body weight (kg $^{0.75}$), which is not commonly used by the general practitioner therefore the recommendations in this text are converted to the common kilogram of body weight. Common fish oil capsules that are 1000 mg total fat content will contain about 250–300 mg of combined EPA and DHA. Therefore, a 25-kg dog requires eight or more capsules per day to reach the recommended intake if the diet is low in these fatty acids; therefore dosing with teaspoon quantities of similar fish oil is recommended (two to three teaspoons).

One study of a commercial therapeutic joint diet with additional fish oil found that the greatest effect on scoring systems occurred with an estimated 7.5 g/1000 kcal of EPA and DHA.[81] This study used relative doses of 100, 250, or 375 mg/kg based on relative maintenance energy requirements and revealed that although all three groups performed better on the subjective assessment that the highest dose performed better than the lowest dose suggesting a dose–response relationship. Although more may seem better in this case, the amount of liquid fish oil in the higher dose precludes its use clinically due to the large amount of fish oil needed particularly in cases of GI sensitivities or obese prone dogs (which is often the case) where the added calories may be more detrimental than the benefits to be gained. If attempting to supplement in the obese dog, then dosing should be done based on presumed ideal body weight as to not supply the dog with additional calories. The clinical response of patients can be highly variable as well depending on the dietary EPA and DHA that the dog is getting from typical commercial diets, which is usually less than 0.5 g/1000 kcal; however, some fish-based commercial diets may reach 1 g or more/1000 kcals. These discrepancies not addressed in studies suggest that the clinical effects of supplementation can vary depending on the base diet that the dog is already consuming. Importantly, from a clinical perspective, as most dogs with OA are on nonsteroidal anti-inflammatories, it has been shown that supplementation with EPA and DHA may allow for lowering of NSAID doses in dogs: A multicenter study of a therapeutic joint diet reported to contain about 2.5 g of EPA and DHA per 1000 kcal, resulted in a decrease of carprofen dose from 4.4 mg/kg per day to 3.3 mg/kg per day in the treatment group. The control group in this study decreased from 4.2 mg/kg per day to 3.6 mg/kg per day over a 12-week period.[80] When fed for 90 days, the diet reportedly increased peak vertical force (PVF) by 5.6% in dogs versus 0.4% in dogs fed a control diet.[81]

A variety of other nonbotanical supplements are marketed for the management of OA, some of which may be included in therapeutic diets labeled for such conditions. These include glucosamine and chondroitin, avocado and soybean unsaponifiables (ASUs), undenatured collagen II (UCII), green-lipped mussel, and egg shell membrane (EM), which have clinical trials data relevant to veterinary clinical practice, with fewer positive outcomes than fish oil in general and should also be considered particularly in the NSAID intolerant patient. A recent meta-analysis of canine supplements for this purpose documented clear benefits for omega-3 fatty acids but only limited evidence for all supplements examined.[86]

Glucosamine and Chondroitin

The most common joint supplements are products designed as chondroprotectants. Proteoglycans are thought to be critical in maintaining the features of cartilage, such as flexibility and elasticity, and are stabilized with long chains of hyaluronic acid. Glucosamine is a precursor to hyaluronic acid and other glycosaminoglycans. Chondroitin sulfate is also a precursor to major glycosaminoglycans, which in turn are conjugated to core proteins to form proteoglycans known as aggrecans. These precursors for glycosaminoglycans synthesis are commonly used in humans and in animals although efficacy has been significantly questioned in human meta-analyses.[87,88]

A double-blinded positive-controlled trial of a product dosed at 475 mg glucosamine HCl, 350 mg chondroitin sulfate per roughly 20 kg of body weight found that subjective OA scores were improved at 70 days with this product similarly to 42 days of treatment days carprofen.[89] A shorter study compared similar dosing of a different glucosamine and chondroitin product to meloxicam and to carprofen, but only for 60 days, and found improvements only with the NSAIDs as measured by ground reaction forces and subjective scores.[90] A recent evaluation of dogs with OA (n = 20+ per group) evaluated Dasuquin use versus placebo for 90 showing no significant benefits when assessing canine brief pain inventory or accelerometer activity measures throughout the study. These clinical findings suggest little benefit on OA-related pain; however, there have been no studies examining long-term cartilage integrity in dogs. In long-term human trials, there is evidence of retarded cartilage loss in knees 2 years from the institution of treatment compared with placebo in those taking 1500 mg of glucosamine or chondroitin once daily rather than splitting the dosing to twice a day.[91] Currently based on these findings, recommendations for slowing cartilage degeneration hover in the 40–50 mg/kg of either glucosamine or chondroitin sulfate or a mix of these two once a day in an effort to slow the progression of cartilage loss in canine orthopedic rehabilitation patients globally. Many pet foods provide additional glucosamine and chondroitin in commercial pet food formulations; unfortunately, the amounts added to commercial pet food would have to be over 3000 mg/kg of dry weight in the food, which is difficult to find. Additionally, we do not understand the bioavailability of glucosamine or chondroitin from these commercial pet foods, thus making recommendations outside of supplementation is tenuous at best.

Avocado and Soybean Unsaponifiables

The use of ASUs as a supplement has very little evidence surrounding its clinical use in naturally occurring canine OA. There is evidence in a model of surgically induced cranial cruciate disease that there may be some clinical utility. A dose of 10 mg/kg body weight daily was used showing that cartilage damage was lessened in dogs with unstable stifles compared with a placebo-controlled group with eight dogs in each group. Further assessment of inflammatory biomarkers and metalloproteases showed less upregulation of these markers of inflammation and cartilage degeneration in the group receiving ASU.[92,93] Again, humans appear to have more long-term assessments using this supplement, and studies have suggested that cartilage thickness in humans is improved with long-term supplementation compared with placebo when providing 300 mg of ASU daily.[94]

Undenatured Collagen Type II

The use of UCII has been growing in popularity as a nutritional supplement in humans, but the benefits of UCII may be unique due to the native form of collagen.

Mechanistically the use of UCII is an issue of immune tolerance similar to the use of other allergens used in dermatology to build T helper cell tolerance leading to a diminished inflammatory response, which in this case would be tolerance to byproducts of excessive cartilage degradation in the joint leading to less inflammation in the joint tissues.[95] The premise in dogs appears to show clinical utility in a number of placebo blinded or noninferiority studies compared with NSAIDs in naturally occurring OA in dogs. In earlier studies using UCII alone or in combination with other potential nutraceuticals in small groups of dogs (n-5 per group) using veterinary scoring suggested that within 60–90 days that dogs receiving 10 mg per day of UCII showed mild significant clinical improvements.[96] A follow-up study by the same research group from Murray State University using 10 mg of UCII alone or in combination with glucosamine and chondroitin showed similar findings using veterinary assessment of joint pain indices as well as objective ground reaction forces. Interestingly, as a single-component UCII performed better for pain relief compared with the combination of UCII and large doses of glucosamine and chondroitin sulfate.[97] Most importantly, in both studies, the effects of UCII were not immediate and required approximately 90 days to see significant results making it important for owners to be aware that immediate results are not to be expected.[96,97] A more recent examination of UCII using a dose of 10 mg per day of a specific product (also enriched with inconsequential small amounts of omega three fatty acids) in dogs with single or multijoint OA compared with the NSAID robenocoxib showed a similar reduction in standardized owner assessed scoring for both groups.[98] Although the power of this study was not sufficient to definitively show noninferiority due to dropouts in both treatment groups the results were positive like other studies using UCII. In addition, a recent examination in sporting Labradors suggest benefits of UCII supplementation including longer distances traveled during training and improved speed of performing tasks, alterations in lymphocyte and neutrophil counts, decreased IL-6 as a marker of inflammation, and decreased markers of cartilage degradation in the serum of dogs receiving UCII.[99] It is important to note that there are a plethora of collagen products on the market today and only undenatured collagen type 2 or the trademarked UCII is thought to be effective. More surprisingly is that regardless of the size of the dogs studied the same dose of UCII was used across studies and a dose–response relationship has not been explored in dogs. Until further evidence, the common dose is 10 mg once a day.

Green-Lipped Mussel

The use of green-lipped mussels (GLMs), otherwise known as *perna canaliculus,* is nearly 4 decades old in the treatment of OA; however, evidence did not surface in the scientific literature until the early 2000s where four different studies examined the efficacy of GLM. An initial study examined a top dressing of GLM supplement, a specifically formulated treat and a pet food incorporating GLM as part of treatment protocols compared with placebo (approximately 15 subjects per group) at approximately 75 mg/kg or greater dose based on size ranges of the subjects. Veterinary assessments of pain, joint swelling of affected joint, and crepitus were assessed blindly and scores were totaled in a poorly described methodology showing that regardless of delivery vehicle, total arthritis scores were different from placebo suggesting efficacy in a 6-week study.[100] Similarly, a follow-up study by the same research group using a GLM enriched dog food in a placebo blinded study showed similar efficacy using a predicted relative dose of approximately 45 mg/kg based on normal maintenance energy requirements for dogs using similar veterinary scoring lameness and pain estimates.[101] Further placebo blinded studies using lower doses of GLM as a supplement at 11 mg/kg body weight compared with placebo showed no improvements over the placebo groups suggesting that this lower dose was not particularly effective and the higher doses are recommended.[102] A more comprehensive assessment of GLM compared with carprofen and placebo groups was performed in dogs with naturally occurring OA. In this study, a proprietary extract called Lyproflex was dosed based on relative size with dogs over 40 kg receiving 3000 mg per day and dogs under 40 kg receiving 2000 mg per day for 10 days followed by half the initial dose for the remainder of the 12-week study with subjective and objective assessment performed every 4 weeks. Veterinary assessments, client vertical analog scoring for locomotion and pain, as well as objective ground reaction forces of the most affected limb were assessed. Although vertical analog assessments were significantly different from placebo treatment, ground reaction forces were not significant from the placebo group for GLM. However, across all outcome measures, carprofen at 2 mg/kg twice daily showed significant improvements globally.[103] Finally, a 120-day open-label study examined GLM at approximately 12.5 $\pm$ 10 mg/kg versus placebo showed no significant improvement compared with placebo more than 56 days with possible differences in subjective veterinary and client scoring at day 56, but not day 28. Extension of all dogs from the placebo and GLM treatment groups for another 56 days showed further improvements in scores at 128 days for both groups of dogs.[104]

These data and somewhat ambiguous dosing regimens and an understanding of dietary factors that might be influencing efficacy to leave gaps in our understanding of the clinical utility of GLM, particularly as the mechanisms for efficacy are elusive. Much of the literature suggests that the fatty acid fraction from GLM includes omega three fatty acids and potential intermediate chain derivatives with anti-inflammatory effects similar to fish oil. This is underscored by a recent paper in canine clinical OA using the fatty acid fraction of GLM called PCSO-524 showing the potential efficacy of this fatty acid supplement in a noninferiority study compared with firocoxib. Approximately 25 dogs per group were enrolled into PCSO-524 plus firoxocib placebo, firocoxib, and PCSO-524 placebo or a combination of PCSO-524 and firocoxib. All dogs were more than 20 kg, and all dogs received four capsules per day (200 mg of GLM-derived omega three fatty acids, 400 mg olive oil, and 900 mg alpha tocopherol) of the PCSO-524 or a placebo PCSO-524 (sesame oil base). Although there were no significant differences between groups regarding veterinary scoring or force plate kinetics, all three groups showed improvements on objective and subjective assessments, and most interestingly, the combination proved beneficial for decreasing serum prostaglandin E2 levels that are a potent inflammatory mediator.[105] These collective data suggest that GLM may be similar in action to fish oil and may prove to be an effective nutraceutical to augment standard NSAID dosing and potentially provide means to decrease NSAID dosing.

Egg Shell Membrane

More recent trends in supplements being used in humans have led to the use of the inner collagenous membrane found in egg shells, which have been touted as a similar supplement to UCII and have made it into the canine supplement market. There are only two studies examining the efficacy in naturally occurring OA in dogs. The first study examined the use of EM at approximately 13.5 mg/kg in a placebo blinded supplement trial for 12 weeks. Although the statistical analysis used in this study was suspect, they suggest a decrease in canine brief pain inventory between groups at the 1 week mark, which was no longer found at the 6-week mark. Similarly, veterinary assessment pain and lameness scores were no different between the groups at week 1 or 6; however, the biomarker of cartilage degradation did show less CTX-II

Table 2
Evidence based nonherbal nutraceuticals for canine degenerative joint disease/OA subjective and objective outcome data with dosing range of studies, potential starting dose and frequency of administration

Nutraceutical	References	Subjective Outcome[b]	Objective Outcome[b]	Range of Dosing	Starting Dose	Frequency
Marine Oil	79–85	Positive	Positive	50–375 mg/kg	100 mg/kg[a]	SID
Glucosamine/Chondroitin Sulfate	89–91	Positive	Negative	20–50 mg/kg	40 mg/kg	SID
ASU	93–94	Positive	Positive	10 mg/kg	10 mg/kg	SID
Green-Lipped Mussel	101–106	Positive	Negative	11–75 mg/kg	50 mg/kg	SID
UCII	97–100	Positive	Positive	10 mg per dog	10 mg per dog	SID
Egg Shell Membrane	107–108	Positive	Negative	3.5–7.5 mg/kg	6 mg/kg	SID

[a] Dose is recommended EPA/DHA, which is usually 13%–25% of the total marine oil source depending on fish or algal extract.
[b] Subjective outcomes are client-specific outcome surveys (i.e., canine brief pain inventory, etc.), objective outcome is force kinetics using pressure mats/plates or histopathological analysis of joint tissues.

metabolite in the bloodstream of dogs being supplemented EM at week 6.[106] A more recent pilot study using less than 12 dogs in the placebo and treatment groups each, assessed a proprietary EM supplement with other botanicals, vitamins, and minerals that were dosed based on the manufacturer's instructions (Movoflex).[107] In this study, there appears to be no difference between treatment and placebo when assessing validated canine brief pain inventory owner responses at week 6 or week 12. However, a difference between groups at week 12 was noted when assessing client-specific data using the Liverpool Osteoarthritis in Dog assessment at the 12-week point compared with placebo. Further serum cytokine and biomarkers of joint health showed no differences between groups.[107,108] These two studies suggest that the dosing regimen being used in dogs may not be optimal or that the preparations of these supplements are not yet optimized for clinical response. Regardless, there appear to be more effective nutraceutical treatments that can be used to treat naturally occurring OA in dogs.

In conclusion, nonherbal use of nutraceuticals has its place in the management of the OA patient with sufficient evidence to consider using marine oils to help mitigate the inflammation and progression of OA (**Table 2**). Other supplements such as UCII, ASU, and GLM appear to have utility and may be considered depending on the response to fish oil enrichment and are likely to improve the clinical response and hasten progression, even if only slightly. Supplements such as glucosamine, chondroitin, and EM show a little short-term benefit (see **Table 2**). The long-term effects of these supplements on cartilage integrity in the dog have not been performed; therefore any long-term recommendations for joint integrity are tenuous considering all of the aforementioned studies in general were short-term studies of 4 months or less.

CLINICS CARE POINTS

- Obesity is a difficult disease to mitigate with exercise alone but may have utility for maintaining lean mass during weight loss.
- Hypocaloric diets remain to be the mainstay for managing weight loss in patients.
- Prevailing evidence points to the use of long chain omega three fatty acids from marine sources in mitagation of the inflammatory response of OA.
- Newer evidence suggest there may be utility in providing nutraceuticals like green lipped mussel, UC-II and egg shell membrane for managemnt of OA.
- The use of glucosamine and/or chondroitin does not appear to mitigate clinical signs of OA, but could be useful for chondroprotections.

DISCLOSURE

The authors have nothing to disclose.

REFERENCES

1. Wong MCS, Huang J, Wang J, et al. Global, regional and time-trend prevalence of central obesity: a systematic review and meta-analysis of 13.2 million subjects. Eur J Epidemiol 2020;35:673–83.
2. Nuttall FQ. Body mass index: obesity, bmi, and health: a critical review. Nutr Today 2015;50:117–28.

3. Djalalinia S, Qorbani M, Peykari N, et al. Health impacts of obesity. Pak J Med Sci 2015;31:239–42.
4. Endalifer ML, Diress G. Epidemiology, predisposing factors, biomarkers, and prevention mechanism of obesity: a systematic review. J Obes 2020;2020: 6134362.
5. Duren DL, Sherwood RJ, Czerwinski SA, et al. Body composition methods: comparisons and interpretation. J Diabetes Sci Technol 2008;2:1139–46.
6. Global BMIMC, Di Angelantonio E, Bhupathiraju Sh N, et al. Body-mass index and all-cause mortality: individual-participant-data meta-analysis of 239 prospective studies in four continents. Lancet 2016;388:776–86.
7. Malik VS, Ravindra K, Attri SV, et al. Higher body mass index is an important risk factor in COVID-19 patients: a systematic review and meta-analysis. Environ Sci Pollut Res Int 2020;27:42115–23.
8. Blackburn G. Effect of degree of weight loss on health benefits. Obes Res 1995; 3(Suppl 2):211s–6s.
9. Robson EK, Hodder RK, Kamper SJ, et al. Effectiveness of weight-loss interventions for reducing pain and disability in people with common musculoskeletal disorders: a systematic review with meta-analysis. J Orthop Sports Phys Ther 2020;50:319–33.
10. Stoner L, Rowlands D, Morrison A, et al. Efficacy of exercise intervention for weight loss in overweight and obese adolescents: meta-analysis and implications. Sports Med 2016;46:1737–51.
11. Stoner L, Beets MW, Brazendale K, et al. Exercise dose and weight loss in adolescents with overweight-obesity: a meta-regression. Sports Med 2019;49: 83–94.
12. Dombrowski SU, Knittle K, Avenell A, et al. Long term maintenance of weight loss with non-surgical interventions in obese adults: systematic review and meta-analyses of randomised controlled trials. Bmj 2014;348:g2646.
13. Johnston BC, Kanters S, Bandayrel K, et al. Comparison of weight loss among named diet programs in overweight and obese adults: a meta-analysis. JAMA 2014;312:923–33.
14. Franz MJ, VanWormer JJ, Crain AL, et al. Weight-loss outcomes: a systematic review and meta-analysis of weight-loss clinical trials with a minimum 1-year follow-up. J Am Diet Assoc 2007;107:1755–67.
15. Truby H, Haines TP. Comparative weight loss with popular diets. Bmj 2020;369: m1269.
16. Ma C, Avenell A, Bolland M, et al. Effects of weight loss interventions for adults who are obese on mortality, cardiovascular disease, and cancer: systematic review and meta-analysis. Bmj 2017;359:j4849.
17. Jepsen R, Aadland E, Andersen JR, et al. Associations between physical activity and quality of life outcomes in adults with severe obesity: a cross-sectional study prior to the beginning of a lifestyle intervention. Health Qual Life Outcomes 2013;11:187.
18. Benito PJ, Bermejo LM, Peinado AB, et al. Change in weight and body composition in obese subjects following a hypocaloric diet plus different training programs or physical activity recommendations. J Appl Physiol (1985) 2015;118: 1006–13.
19. Hernández-Reyes A, Cámara-Martos F, Molina-Luque R, et al. Changes in body composition with a hypocaloric diet combined with sedentary, moderate and high-intense physical activity: a randomized controlled trial. BMC Womens Health 2019;19:167.

20. Vissers D, Hens W, Taeymans J, et al. The effect of exercise on visceral adipose tissue in overweight adults: a systematic review and meta-analysis. PLoS One 2013;8:e56415.
21. Hall M, Castelein B, Wittoek R, et al. Diet-induced weight loss alone or combined with exercise in overweight or obese people with knee osteoarthritis: A systematic review and meta-analysis. Semin Arthritis Rheum 2019;48:765–77.
22. Soltani S, Hunter GR, Kazemi A, et al. The effects of weight loss approaches on bone mineral density in adults: a systematic review and meta-analysis of randomized controlled trials. Osteoporos Int 2016;27:2655–71.
23. Brunetto MA, Sá FC, Nogueira SP, et al. The intravenous glucose tolerance and postprandial glucose tests may present different responses in the evaluation of obese dogs. Br J Nutr 2011;106(Suppl 1):S194–7.
24. Chandler ML. Impact of obesity on cardiopulmonary disease. Vet Clin North Am Small Anim Pract 2016;46:817–30.
25. Kealy RD, Lawler DF, Ballam JM, et al. Effects of diet restriction on life span and age-related changes in dogs. J Am Vet Med Assoc 2002;220:1315–20.
26. German AJ. The growing problem of obesity in dogs and cats. J Nutr 2006;136: 1940s–6s.
27. Maranesi M, Di Loria A, Dall'Aglio C, et al. Leptin system in obese dog skin: a pilot study. Animals (Basel) 2020;10.
28. Tropf M, Nelson OL, Lee PM, et al. Cardiac and metabolic variables in obese dogs. J Vet Intern Med 2017;31:1000–7.
29. Cortese L, Terrazzano G, Pelagalli A. Leptin and immunological profile in obesity and its associated diseases in dogs. Int J Mol Sci 2019;20.
30. German AJ, Ryan VH, German AC, et al. Obesity, its associated disorders and the role of inflammatory adipokines in companion animals. Vet J 2010;185:4–9.
31. Marshall W, Bockstahler B, Hulse D, et al. A review of osteoarthritis and obesity: current understanding of the relationship and benefit of obesity treatment and prevention in the dog. Vet Comp Orthop Traumatol 2009;22:339–45.
32. Clark M, Hoenig M. Metabolic effects of obesity and its interaction with endocrine diseases. Vet Clin North Am Small Anim Pract 2016;46:797–815.
33. Markwell PJ vEW, Parkin GD, Sloth CJ, et al. Obesity in the dog. J Small Anim Pract 1990;31:533–7.
34. Chandler M, Cunningham S, Lund EM, et al. Obesity and associated comorbidities in people and companion animals: a one health perspective. J Comp Pathol 2017;156:296–309.
35. Sandøe P, Palmer C, Corr S, et al. Canine and feline obesity: a one health perspective. Vet Rec 2014;175:610–6.
36. Finke MD. Evaluation of the energy requirements of adult kennel dogs. J Nutr 1991;121:S22–8.
37. D L. Development and validation of a body condition score system for dogs. Canine Practice 1997;22:10-15.
38. Joshua JO. The obese dog and some clinical repercussions. J Small Anim Pract 1970;11:601–6.
39. Laflamme DP, Kuhlman G, Lawler DF. Evaluation of weight loss protocols for dogs. J Am Anim Hosp Assoc 1997;33:253–9.
40. Burkholder WJ. Use of body condition scores in clinical assessment of the provision of optimal nutrition. J Am Vet Med Assoc 2000;217:650–4.
41. Courcier EA, Thomson RM, Mellor DJ, et al. An epidemiological study of environmental factors associated with canine obesity. J Small Anim Pract 2010;51: 362–7.

42. Carciofi AC, Gonçalves KNV, Vasconcellos RS, et al. A weight loss protocol and owners participation in the treatment of canine obesity. Ciência Rural 2005;35: 1331–8.
43. Chauvet A, Laclair J, Elliott DA, et al. Incorporation of exercise, using an underwater treadmill, and active client education into a weight management program for obese dogs. Can Vet J 2011;52:491–6.
44. A G. Obesity in companion animals. Practice 2010;32:42–50.
45. German AJ, Titcomb JM, Holden SL, et al. Cohort study of the success of controlled weight loss programs for obese dogs. J Vet Intern Med 2015;29: 1547–55.
46. German AJ. Obesity prevention and weight maintenance after loss. Vet Clin North Am Small Anim Pract 2016;46:913–29.
47. Chapman M, Woods GRT, Ladha C, et al. An open-label randomised clinical trial to compare the efficacy of dietary caloric restriction and physical activity for weight loss in overweight pet dogs. Vet J 2019;243:65–73.
48. Tvarijonaviciute A, Muñoz-Prieto A, Martinez-Subiela S. Obesity in humans and dogs: similarities, links, and differences. In: Pets as sentinels, forecasters and promoters of human health. Springer; 2020.
49. Freeman LM. Cachexia and sarcopenia: emerging syndromes of importance in dogs and cats. J Vet Intern Med 2012;26:3–17.
50. Porsani MYH, Teixeira FA, Amaral AR, et al. Factors associated with failure of dog's weight loss programmes. Vet Med Sci 2020;6:299–305.
51. Mawby DI, Bartges JW, d'Avignon A, et al. Comparison of various methods for estimating body fat in dogs. J Am Anim Hosp Assoc 2004;40:109–14.
52. Adolphe JL, Silver TI, Childs H, et al. Short-term obesity results in detrimental metabolic and cardiovascular changes that may not be reversed with weight loss in an obese dog model. Br J Nutr 2014;112:647–56.
53. Kim SP, Ellmerer M, Van Citters GW, et al. Primacy of hepatic insulin resistance in the development of the metabolic syndrome induced by an isocaloric moderate-fat diet in the dog. Diabetes 2003;52:2453–60.
54. German AJ. Outcomes of weight management in obese pet dogs: what can we do better? Proc Nutr Soc 2016;75:398–404.
55. Flanagan J, Bissot T, Hours MA, et al. Success of a weight loss plan for overweight dogs: The results of an international weight loss study. PLoS One 2017;12:e0184199.
56. Newburgh LH, Johnston MW. Endogenous obesity—a misconception. Ann Intern Med 1930;3:815–25.
57. Saker KE, Remillard RL. Performance of a canine weight-loss program in clinical practice. Vet Ther 2005;6:291–302.
58. Manens J, Ricci R, Damoiseaux C, et al. Effect of body weight loss on cardiopulmonary function assessed by 6-minute walk test and arterial blood gas analysis in obese dogs. J Vet Intern Med 2014;28:371–8.
59. German AJ. Weight management in obese pets: the tailoring concept and how it can improve results. Acta Vet Scand 2016;58:57.
60. Harper EJ. Changing perspectives on aging and energy requirements: aging, body weight and body composition in humans, dogs and cats. J Nutr 1998; 128:2627s–31s.
61. German AJ, Holden SL, Morris PJ, et al. Long-term follow-up after weight management in obese dogs: the role of diet in preventing regain. Vet J 2012;192: 65–70.

62. Brooks D, Churchill J, Fein K, et al. AAHA weight management guidelines for dogs and cats. J Am Anim Hosp Assoc 2014;50:1–11.
63. Mlacnik E, Bockstahler BA, Muller M, et al. Effects of caloric restriction and a moderate or intense physiotherapy program for treatment of lameness in overweight dogs with osteoarthritis. J Am Vet Med Assoc 2006;229:1756–60.
64. Brady RB, Sidiropoulos AN, Bennett HJ, et al. Evaluation of gait-related variables in lean and obese dogs at a trot. Am J Vet Res 2013;74:757–62.
65. Bruchim Y, Horowitz M, Aroch I. Pathophysiology of heatstroke in dogs - revisited. Temperature (Austin) 2017;4:356–70.
66. Malenfant P, Joanisse DR, Thériault R, et al. Fat content in individual muscle fibers of lean and obese subjects. Int J Obes Relat Metab Disord 2001;25:1316–21.
67. Preedy V. Handbook of anthropometry: physical measures of human form in health and disease. Springer Science & Business Media; 2012.
68. Bülow J, Tøndevold E. Blood flow in different adipose tissue depots during prolonged exercise in dogs. Pflugers Arch 1982;392:235–8.
69. Morrison R, Reilly JJ, Penpraze V, et al. A 6-month observational study of changes in objectively measured physical activity during weight loss in dogs. J Small Anim Pract 2014;55:566–70.
70. Hunter GR, Brock DW, Byrne NM, et al. Exercise training prevents regain of visceral fat for 1 year following weight loss. Obesity (Silver Spring) 2010;18:690–5.
71. Enright PL. The six-minute walk test. Respir Care 2003;48:783–5.
72. Villedieu E, Rutherford L, Ter Haar G. Brachycephalic obstructive airway surgery outcome assessment using the 6-minute walk test: a pilot study. J Small Anim Pract 2019;60:132–5.
73. Wakshlag JJ, Struble AM, Warren BS, et al. Evaluation of dietary energy intake and physical activity in dogs undergoing a controlled weight-loss program. J Am Vet Med Assoc 2012;240:413–9.
74. Niese JR, Mepham T, Nielen M, et al. Evaluating the potential benefit of a combined weight loss program in dogs and their owners. Front Vet Sci 2021;8:653920.
75. Vitger AD, Stallknecht BM, Nielsen DH, et al. Integration of a physical training program in a weight loss plan for overweight pet dogs. J Am Vet Med Assoc 2016;248:174–82.
76. Herrera Uribe J, Vitger AD, Ritz C, et al. Physical training and weight loss in dogs lead to transcriptional changes in genes involved in the glucose-transport pathway in muscle and adipose tissues. Vet J 2016;208:22–7.
77. Bauer JE. Therapeutic use of fish oils in companion animals. J Am Vet Med Assoc 2011;239:1441–51.
78. Dunbar BL, Bigley KE, Bauer JE. Early and sustained enrichment of serum n-3 long chain polyunsaturated fatty acids in dogs fed a flaxseed supplemented diet. Lipids 2010;45:1–10.
79. Fritsch DA, Allen TA, Dodd CE, et al. A multicenter study of the effect of dietary supplementation with fish oil omega-3 fatty acids on carprofen dosage in dogs with osteoarthritis. J Am Vet Med Assoc 2010;236:535–9.
80. Fritsch D, Allen TA, Dodd CE, et al. Dose-titration effects of fish oil in osteoarthritic dogs. J Vet Intern Med 2010;24:1020–6.
81. Roush JK, Cross AR, Renberg WC, et al. Evaluation of the effects of dietary supplementation with fish oil omega-3 fatty acids on weight bearing in dogs with osteoarthritis. J Am Vet Med Assoc 2010;236:67–73.

82. Roush JK, Dodd CE, Fritsch DA, et al. Multicenter veterinary practice assessment of the effects of omega-3 fatty acids on osteoarthritis in dogs. J Am Vet Med Assoc 2010;236:59–66.
83. Hielm-Björkman A, Roine J, Elo K, et al. An un-commissioned randomized, placebo-controlled double-blind study to test the effect of deep sea fish oil as a pain reliever for dogs suffering from canine OA. BMC Vet Res 2012;8:157.
84. Mehler SJ, May LR, King C, et al. A prospective, randomized, double blind, placebo-controlled evaluation of the effects of eicosapentaenoic acid and docosahexaenoic acid on the clinical signs and erythrocyte membrane polyunsaturated fatty acid concentrations in dogs with osteoarthritis. Prostaglandins Leukot Essent Fatty Acids 2016;109:1–7.
85. Rialland P, Bichot S, Lussier B, et al. Effect of a diet enriched with green-lipped mussel on pain behavior and functioning in dogs with clinical osteoarthritis. Can J Vet Res 2013;77:66–74.
86. Gagnon A, Brown D, Moreau M, et al. Therapeutic response analysis in dogs with naturally occurring osteoarthritis. Vet Anaesth Analg 2017;44:1373–81.
87. Wandel S, Jüni P, Tendal B, et al. Effects of glucosamine, chondroitin, or placebo in patients with osteoarthritis of hip or knee: network meta-analysis. Bmj 2010; 341:c4675.
88. Vandeweerd JM, Coisnon C, Clegg P, et al. Systematic review of efficacy of nutraceuticals to alleviate clinical signs of osteoarthritis. J Vet Intern Med 2012;26: 448–56.
89. McCarthy G, O'Donovan J, Jones B, et al. Randomized double blind positive controlled trial to assess the efficacy of glucosamine/chondroitin sulfate for the treatment of dogs with osteoarthritis. Vet J 2007;174:54–61.
90. Moreau M, Dupuis J, Bonneau NH, et al. Clinical evaluation of a nutraceutical, carprofen and meloxicam for the treatment of dogs with osteoarthritis. Vet Rec 2003;152:323–9.
91. Scott RM, Evans R, Conzemius MG. Efficacy of an oral nutraceutical for the treatment of canine osteoarthritis. A double-blind, randomized, placebo-controlled prospective clinical trial. Vet Comp Orthop Traumatol 2017;30: 318–23.
92. Gallagher B, Tjoumakaris FP, Harwood MI, et al. Chondroprotection and the prevention of osteoarthritis progression of the knee: a systematic review of treatment agents. Am J Sports Med 2015;43:734–44.
93. Altinel L, Saritas ZK, Kose KC, et al. Treatment with unsaponifiable extracts of avocado and soybean increases TGF-beta1 and TGF-beta2 levels in canine joint fluid. Tohoku J Exp Med 2007;211:181–6.
94. Boileau C, Martel-Pelletier J, Caron J, et al. Protective effects of total fraction of avocado/soybean unsaponifiables on the structural changes in experimental dog osteoarthritis: inhibition of nitric oxide synthase and matrix metalloproteinase-13. Arthritis Res Ther 2009;11:R41.
95. Christensen R, Bartels EM, Astrup A, et al. Symptomatic efficacy of avocado-soybean unsaponifiables (ASU) in osteoarthritis (OA) patients: a meta-analysis of randomized controlled trials. Osteoarthritis Cartilage 2008;16:399–408.
96. Yoshinari O, Moriyama H, Shiojima Y. An overview of a novel, water-soluble undenatured type II collagen (NEXT-II). J Am Coll Nutr 2015;34:255–62.
97. Peal A, D'Altilio M, Simms C, et al. Therapeutic efficacy and safety of undenatured type-II collagen (UC-II) alone or in combination with (-)-hydroxycitric acid and chromemate in arthritic dogs. J Vet Pharmacol Ther 2007;30:275–8.

98. D'Altilio M, Peal A, Alvey M, et al. Therapeutic efficacy and safety of undenatured type ii collagen singly or in combination with glucosamine and chondroitin in arthritic dogs. Toxicol Mech Methods 2007;17:189–96.
99. Stabile M, Samarelli R, Trerotoli P, et al. Evaluation of the effects of undenatured type ii collagen (uc-ii) as compared to robenacoxib on the mobility impairment induced by osteoarthritis in dogs. Vet Sci 2019;6.
100. Varney JL, Fowler JW, Coon CN. Undenatured type II collagen mitigates inflammation and cartilage degeneration in healthy Labrador Retrievers during an exercise regimen. Transl Anim Sci 2021;5:txab084.
101. Bierer TL, Bui LM. Improvement of arthritic signs in dogs fed green-lipped mussel (Perna canaliculus). J Nutr 2002;132:1634s–6s.
102. Bui LM, Bierer RL. Influence of green lipped mussels (Perna canaliculus) in alleviating signs of arthritis in dogs. Vet Ther 2001;2:101–11.
103. Dobenecker B, Beetz Y, Kienzle E. A placebo-controlled double-blind study on the effect of nutraceuticals (chondroitin sulfate and mussel extract) in dogs with joint diseases as perceived by their owners. J Nutr 2002;132:1690s–1s.
104. Hielm-Björkman A, Tulamo RM, Salonen H, et al. Evaluating complementary therapies for canine osteoarthritis part I: green-lipped mussel (perna canaliculus). Evid Based Complement Alternat Med 2009;6:365–73.
105. Pollard B, Guilford WG, Ankenbauer-Perkins KL, et al. Clinical efficacy and tolerance of an extract of green-lipped mussel (Perna canaliculus) in dogs presumptively diagnosed with degenerative joint disease. N Z Vet J 2006;54:114–8.
106. Vijarnsorn M, Kwananocha I, Kashemsant N, et al. The effectiveness of marine based fatty acid compound (PCSO-524) and firocoxib in the treatment of canine osteoarthritis. BMC Vet Res 2019;15:349.
107. Ruff KJ, Kopp KJ, Von Behrens P, et al. Effectiveness of NEM(®) brand eggshell membrane in the treatment of suboptimal joint function in dogs: a multicenter, randomized, double-blind, placebo-controlled study. Vet Med (Auckl) 2016;7:113–21.
108. Muller C, Enomoto M, Buono A, et al. Placebo-controlled pilot study of the effects of an eggshell membrane-based supplement on mobility and serum biomarkers in dogs with osteoarthritis. Vet J 2019;253:105379.

Joint Injection Techniques and Indications

Chris W. Frye, DVM*, Allison Miller, DVM, CCRP

KEYWORDS

• Joint • Diagnostic • Therapeutic • Injection

KEY POINTS

- Intra-articular (IA) injections may be used for both diagnostic and therapeutic purposes in canine medicine.
- Patient selection and sterile technique throughout the procedure minimize adverse effects.
- Risks of IA injections may include transient soreness, cartilage damage, and, rarely, septic arthritis.

INDICATIONS AND CONSIDERATIONS

Indications for injecting joints may include diagnostic, therapeutic, or a combination. Diagnostic injectates aim to reduce or eliminate the contribution of pain to lameness and may be assessed both subjectively andobjectively by the clinician. Blocking procedures are common in equine medicine and may involve targeted blocking of specific nerves that innervate a distal area of concern or a synovial structure suspected to be the most likely source of the lameness. Blocking of horse synovial structures or nerves is conducted in a sequential manner from more distal to more proximal with the intent of ruling out specific potential pathologic contributions along the way through repeated gait analysis in the conscious animal.[1] For intra-articular (IA) blocking, unlike whereby tissue sensation may be directly tested in perineural procedures, the known onset of action of the local anesthetic is used as the time point when to re-assess the patient for any clinical improvement in lameness.[2,3]

Typical short-acting anesthetic agents are most often used in the acute setting and include lidocaine, bupivacaine, or mepivacaine. In some countries, the availability of these medications may be limited and other agents, such as ropivacaine may be used. Some of these agents may have more of a detrimental effect on articular cartilage than others.[4–6] A study looking at a small population of horses in vivo, showed there was less evidence of single-dose damage of such medications.[7] A recent

Cornell University College of Veterinary Medicine, 930 Campus Road, Ithaca, NY 14853, USA
* Corresponding author.
E-mail address: cwf37@cornell.edu

Vet Clin Small Anim 52 (2022) 959–966
https://doi.org/10.1016/j.cvsm.2022.02.004

in vitro canine study supports the likelihood of minimal damage to chondrocytes when dosing clinically relevant concentration of nonliposomal.[8] Overall, mepivacaine seems to have less of an adverse effect on articular cartilage in many studies and therefore it is often preferred; however, many of these studies were ex vivo and controversy exists. Despite the limitations of diagnostic anesthesia, such strategies remain helpful to 1. discern a primary area of concern contributing to lameness when multiple potential contributors exist; 2. be implemented in situations when other diagnostics are unavailable. Although IA anesthesia may be helpful in localizing lameness, it fails to provide a specific diagnosis of lameness and may have a false-negative result—it remains imperfect.

Similar diagnostic blocks have been conducted in canine medicine; however, for reasons described later, a degree of sedation is recommended by these authors. Only a paucity of data has been published regarding the use of local anesthetics in diagnostic canine joint injection therapy[9–11]; however, Van Vynckt and colleagues demonstrated that IA mepivacaine into the cubital joint during sedation helped identify lameness due to medial coronoid disease.[9] Mepivacaine was selected in that study due to its quick onset of action (5–10 minutes) and intermediate duration (120–150 minutes) with most dogs showing an improvement in lameness within 2 to 25 minutes. Sedation with/without manual restraint was required to perform the joint injections,[12] and it was concluded that a protocol involving acepromazine and methadone or dexmedetomidine with atipamezole reversal was effective and did not interfere with lameness detection. It should be noted that these studies only investigated the elbow joint for a specific disease process that was causing lameness and dogs were subjectively graded with a reduction of 2 points (1–10 point lameness scale) being considered significant.

Although IA anesthesia may be conducted on appendicular joints, there is a reported near 10% false-negative result (no response despite pathology).[9,10] This clinical team has experienced false negatives in the face of advanced imaging confirmation using the previously prescribed techniques and incorporating kinetic gait analysis. However, it should be noted that the severity or tissues of the joint involved with the disease (subchondral bone for example) may interfere with the full effect of a diagnostic joint block. Using a corticosteroid may provide longer lasting results of which sedation cannot interfere, as well as therapeutic pain relief; however, such intervention, like IA anesthetics, still neglects to provide a definitive diagnosis. Furthermore, corticosteroids may have a degree of systemic absorption that could theoretically influence musculoskeletal pain elsewhere in the body.[13]

Therapeutic injections are numerous and described elsewhere but may include corticosteroids, visco-supplements, orthobiologics, radioisotopes, and TRPV1 agonists among others.[14–19] Some of these therapeutics combat pain alone and others may also modify the disease process. They comprise the most common reason to inject a joint and are often applied after a definitive diagnosis. Furthermore, they are considered to be a local intervention and may help augment or even reduce the need for other treatments.

Safety

Intra-articular injections are considered relatively safe in the veterinary patient but some risk is still present and should be discussed with owners before injection. Such risks are limited but may include, transient soreness, dermatitis (if the injection area is clipped), iatrogenic cartilage damage, and infection.

Iatrogenic damage to articular cartilage is a possibility any time a needle is introduced into a joint. A recent equine study found that a certain approach to the proximal interphalangeal joint resulted in less iatrogenic cartilage damage than other approaches.[20] The preferred technique also conveniently required fewer attempts to obtain synovial fluid, thereby decreasing the number of times a needle was introduced to the region. Specific cartilage studies following IA injections in canines are limited: when evaluating needle and traditional arthroscopy for the diagnosis of medial coronoid disease, iatrogenic damage from needle introduction was found in 6 out of 27 elbow joints.[21] Needle size in arthroscopy was larger than that commonly recommended for IA injections, however. Such findings add support for the use of ultrasound needle guidance when possible.

Transient soreness following an IA injection is a commonly reported side effect in humans and is likely related to both the trauma induced by the needle to the skin and joint capsule, as well as the distension of the synovial cavity itself with an injectate.[22,23] Changes to both the pH of the synovial fluid as well as an expected altered cytokine profile following injection with local anesthetics, corticosteroids, or orthobiologics likely also contribute to a transient soreness (such as joint flare). Transient soreness should not be confused for the more serious condition of septic arthritis as joint flares are typically seen within the first 3 days after injection, signs of septic arthritis generally occur later on (about a week out).

Numerous large-scale retrospective studies regarding the occurrence of septic arthritis following IA injection exist for horses and people. Equine studies have reported an occurrence of 2 to 7 septic joints per 10,000 injections and large-scale human studies report an even lower risk of 1 per 70 to 100,000 injections.[24–27] Risks in humans, while minimal, remain higher in some patients such as those that are immune compromised, have experienced prior joint surgery, or possess certain comorbidities, such as diabetes. The general overall lower risk in humans is theorized to be related to both improved experience and comfort of clinicians with IA injections as well as an improvement in sterile technique over the years. The routine availability of single-dose corticosteroid in sterile syringes may also decrease the risk compared with the use of a multi-dose vial. Septic arthritis typically presented within 10 days following IA injections in equine studies and within a week for people.[26,28]

While large-scale studies following IA injection are absent, several studies have evaluated the occurrence of canine septic arthritis. Various routes including prior penetrating or surgical wounds, extension from nearby diseased tissue, or hematogenous spread from a distant infection have all been described in the dog.[29–31] In this clinical team's experience, the likelihood of septic arthritis with appropriate candidate selection and joint injection technique remains minimal in the dog. If suspicion of joint infection exists based on history and examination, a standard workup may be indicated and could include imaging followed by arthrocentesis for fluid analysis, cytology, and culture, as well as ruling out other potential sources of infection unrelated to injection therapy.

Preparation

Once the site of joint injection has been selected, common preparation includes patient sedation, clipping of hair, and antiseptic preparation.[16] Therapeutic joint injections for people are most commonly performed in conscious patients with or without a topical analgesic like eutectic lidocaine/prilocaine gel; however, conscious sedation may be used.[32] To achieve the desirable analgesic effect, it is recommended the gel be applied 1 to 1.5 hours in advance of the procedure. Furthermore, discomfort may still be noted regardless of the application in people and deeper tissues may require further infiltration with local anesthetic.[33,34] Because veterinary patients remain greatly unaware of our good intentions, we believe that sedation, if not contraindicated, is advisable for any arthrocentesis or joint injection procedure as it should reduce patient fear, discomfort, and motion that increases the chances of iatrogenic tissue damage.

Some debate over the benefit of hair clipping has been investigated in many species.[16,35,36] A recent study examined the effects of clipping when using a 3 minute 4% chlorhexidine gluconate scrub with alcohol rinse and found no difference in microbial load cultured between clipped and unclipped skin over joints after preparation.[36] Although this study provides reasonable support for unclipped arthrocentesis in short-haired dogs, the sterile field is not obviously demarcated and application of ultrasound guidance, if indicated, would be greatly impeded to impossible. Regardless of clipping, the procedural area should be visually screened for evidence of skin disease or infection before proceeding with injection.

Various studies in human and animal medicine have examined such aseptic preparations and it should be noted that all techniques aim to reduce but cannot eliminate all flora.[16] Regardless, minimizing the risk of therapeutic injection-related joint infections through such preparation is essential. Comparisons between various common aseptic agents have been studied in dogs including those that are most commonly used (a povidone-iodine surgical scrub, 4% chlorhexidine gluconate followed by saline rinse, and 4% chlorhexidine gluconate followed by 70% alcohol rinse) and seem relatively equivalent in reducing microbial loads over clipped skin.[37] Our clinical team tends to clip the injection site and use 3 to 4 applications of a 4% chlorhexidine gluconate scrub for 30 seconds followed by alcohol gauze rinse. The same application is used to prepare an ultrasound transducer when indicated and 70% alcohol is then used as a conductive medium.

Technique

Traditionally, sound anatomic landmark knowledge and percutaneous palpation have been relied on for both arthrocentesis and therapeutic injection of canine appendicular synovial joints.[38] Systematic reviews and meta-analyses in human medicine support the use of ultrasound in that there is greater accuracy in needle placement within the joint, patients experience less pain, and more synovial fluid may be consistently obtained.[39–42] Given that respective canine joints are relatively smaller than their adult human counterparts, such imaging guidance may be of further benefit. Training and experience with musculoskeletal ultrasound and needle guidance, however, may be limiting for most practitioners. Few ultrasound-guided joint injection procedures have been described in dogs; however, we frequently practice this technique for many joints and soft tissue structures for the benefits mentioned.[43–45]

Regardless of imaging guidance, needle selection may depend on the patient size, joint, and desired injectate. Larger gauge needles (19 gauge) have been shown to have a significantly greater risk of hair contamination into horse fetlock joints that were not clipped.[46] For most medium to larger dogs, a 22 gauge 1 to 1.5″ needle is used in the shoulder, elbows, and stifle, while a 22 to 25 gauge 1″ needle is used in the carpi, tarsi, as well as distal joints. More viscous injectates such as hyaluronic acid are easier to inject through 22 gauge needles; however, a 25 gauge is adequate but slower for the distal locations. For large to giant dogs, we prefer a spinal needle to access the deeper coxofemoral joint.[38]

Sterile procedure should also include the use of sterile gloves. This will further allow the clinician to identify or palpate helpful landmarks over the aseptically prepared site and avoid certain superficial vessels and possibly nerves (such as the ulnar nerve during approach to the elbow). Attaining synovial fluid feedback to ensure proper needle placement before injection is ideal, particularly without imaging guidance. Some circumstances indicate the collection of synovial fluid before injectate as a diagnostic sample and have been described elsewhere.[16,38] The benefit of removing joint fluid volume equivalent to that of the injectate is unexplored and may be situationally dependent. Avoiding transient acute stretching of the joint capsule can help to reduce periprocedural discomfort or altered joint fluid dynamics[47,48]; on the other hand, fluid may help distribute medication throughout the area. We often incorporate passive range of motion of the joint to assist with injectate distribution. Regardless, injectate volumes will be more restricted in smaller synovial joints and acute discomfort can be noted when injectate volumes pressurize the capsule. We often rest the patient 5–7 days after therapeutic injections before weaning back toward prior activity over another week. Follow-up 1 to 2 weeks after a therapeutic injection is recommended but may be situationally dependent.

SUMMARY

Intra-articular injections have been an important tool when working to diagnose and treat canine synovial joint lameness. The procedure is not without risks. The most common mild side effect seen is postinjection transient soreness; however, the rare but more serious possibility of septic arthritis still exists. Such risks can be minimized by adhering to appropriate techniques and patient selection. Ultrasound guidance with a trained clinician may provide further benefit. The removal of some synovial fluid before administering an IA injection should be considered to confirm needle placement, provide diagnostic sampling, and help accommodate injectate volume. Diagnostic joint injections are not specific to a disease and their limitations must be remembered when interpreting a response.

CLINICS CARE POINTS

- Diagnostic joint injections are not specific for a disease and their limitations must be remembered when interpreting a response.
- Ultrasound-guided needle introduction into joints allows for more precise injectate placement, limits iatrogenic needle damage, decreases periprocedural discomfort, and improves synovial fluid volume feedback.
- Arthrocentesis before injection should be considered to help confirm needle placement, minimize transient soreness from capsular filling, provide a fluid sample for diagnostic purposes.
- Appropriate technique and patient selection help reduce both mild and major risks associated with joint injection from the more common complaint of transient soreness to the rare case of septic arthritis.

DISCLOSURE

The authors have nothing to disclose.

REFERENCES

1. Dyson S. Problems associated with the interpretation of the results of regional and intra-articular anaesthesia in the horse. Vet Rec 1986;118(15):419–22.
2. Schumacher J, Boone L. Local anaesthetics for regional and intra-articular analgesia in the horse. Equine Vet Educ 2021;33(3):159–68.

3. Bassage LH, Ross MW. Diagnostic Analgesia. Diagnosis and management of lameness in the horse. 2003. p. 93–123.
4. Piper SL, Kramer JD, Kim HT, et al. Effects of local anesthetics on articular cartilage. Am J Sports Med 2011;39(10):2245–53.
5. Park J, Sutradhar BC, Hong G, et al. Comparison of the cytotoxic effects of bupivacaine, lidocaine, and mepivacaine in equine articular chondrocytes. Vet Anaesth Analg 2011;38(2):127–33.
6. Hennig GS, Hosgood G, Bubenik-Angapen LJ, et al. Evaluation of chondrocyte death in canine osteochondral explants exposed to a 0.5% solution of bupivacaine. Am J Vet Res 2010;71(8):875–83.
7. Piat P, Richard H, Beauchamp G, et al. In vivo effects of a single intra-articular injection of 2% lidocaine or 0.5% bupivacaine on articular cartilage of normal horses. Vet Surg 2012;41(8):1002–10.
8. Rengert R, Snider D, Gilbert PJ. Effect of bupivacaine concentration and formulation on canine chondrocyte viability in vitro. Vet Surg 2021;50(3):633–40.
9. Van Vynckt D, Verhoeven G, Saunders J, et al. Diagnostic intra-articular anaesthesia of the elbow in dogs with medial coronoid disease. Vet Comp Orthop Traumatol 2012;25(04):307–13.
10. Van Vynckt D, Samoy Y, Mosselmans L, et al. The use of intra-articular aneshesia as a diagnostic tool in canine lameness. Vlaams Diergeneeskd Tijdschr 2012; 81(5):290–7.
11. Van Vynckt D, Verhoeven G, Samoy Y, et al. Anaesthetic arthrography of the shoulder joint in dogs. Vet Comp Orthop Traumatol 2013;26(04):291–7.
12. Van Vynckt D, Samoy Y, Polis I, et al. Evaluation of two sedation protocols for use before diagnostic intra-articular anaesthesia in lame dogs. J Small Anim Pract 2011;52(12):638–44.
13. Gamble LJ, Boesch JM, Wakshlag JJ, et al. Assessing the systemic effects of two different doses of intra-articular triamcinolone acetonide in healthy dogs. Vet Comp Orthop Traumatol 2020;3(02):e96–102.
14. Pelletier JP, Martel-Pelletier J. Protective effects of corticosteroids on cartilage lesions and osteophyte formation in the Pond-Nuki dog model of osteoarthritis. Arthritis Rheum 1989;32(2):181–93.
15. Kumar A, Walz A, Garlick D, et al. A single intra-articular dose of Fx006, an extended-release formulation of triamcinolone acetonide, has a similar effect on cartilage in healthy dogs as the commonly used kenalog-40® suspension. Osteoarthritis Cartilage 2014;22:S463–4.
16. Johnston SA, Tobias KM. Veterinary surgery: small animal expert consult-E-book. Elsevier Health Sciences; 2017.
17. Lattimer JC, Selting KA, Lunceford JM, et al. Intraarticular injection of a Tin-117 m radiosynoviorthesis agent in normal canine elbows causes no adverse effects. Vet Radiol Ultrasound 2019;60(5):567–74.
18. Iadarola MJ, Sapio MR, Raithel SJ, et al. Long-term pain relief in canine osteoarthritis by a single intra-articular injection of resiniferatoxin, a potent TRPV1 agonist. Pain 2018;159(10):2105–14.
19. Franklin SP, Pozzi A, Frank E. Biological therapies in canine sports medicine. Canine Sports Medicine and Rehabilitation. 2018. p. 404–24.
20. Mereu M, Hawkes C, Cuddy LC, et al. Evaluation of four techniques for injection of the proximal interphalangeal joint in horses. Vet Surg 2019;48(8):1437–43.
21. Hersch-Boyle RA, Chou PY, Kapatkin AS, et al. Comparison of needle arthroscopy, traditional arthroscopy, and computed tomography for the evaluation of medial coronoid disease in the canine elbow. Vet Surg 2021;50(S1):O116–27.

22. Plastaras CT, Joshi AB, Garvan C, et al. Adverse events associated with fluoroscopically guided sacroiliac joint injections. PM R 2012;4(7):473–8.
23. Plastaras C, McCormick Z, Macron D, et al. Adverse events associated with fluoroscopically guided zygapophyseal joint injections. Pain Physician 2014;17(4): 297–304.
24. Gillespie CC, Adams SB, Moore GE. Methods and variables associated with the risk of septic arthritis following intra-articular injections in horses: a survey of veterinarians. Vet Surg 2016;45(8):1071–6.
25. Steel CM, Pannirselvam RR, Anderson GA. Risk of septic arthritis after intra-articular medication: a study of 16, 624 injections in Thoroughbred racehorses. Aust Vet J 2013;91(7):268–73.
26. Seror P, Pluvinage P, Lecoq d'Andre F, et al. Frequency of sepsis after local corticosteroid injection (an inquiry on 1,160,00 injections in rheumatological private practice in France). Rheumatology 1999;38(12):1272–4.
27. Charalambous CP, Tryfonidis M, Sadiq S, et al. Septic arthritis following intra-articular steroid injection of the knee – a survey of current practice regarding antiseptic technique used during intra-articular steroid injection of the knee. Clin Rheumatol 2003;22(6):386–90.
28. Lapointe JM, Laverty S, Lavoie JP. Septic arthritis in 15 Standardbred racehorses after intraarticular injection. Equine Vet J 1992;24(6):430–4.
29. Marchevsky AM, Read RA. Bacterial septic arthritis in 19 dogs. Aust Vet J 1999; 77(4):233–7.
30. Stern L, McCarthy R, King R, et al. Imaging diagnosis – Discospondylitis and septic arthritis in a dog. Vet Radiol Ultrasound 2007;48(4):335–7.
31. Clements DN, Owen MR, Mosley JR, et al. Retrospective study of bacterial infective arthritis in 31 dogs. J Small Anim Pract 2005;46(4):171–6.
32. Lennard TA, Vivian DG, Walkowski SD, et al. Pain procedures in clinical practice E-book. Elsevier Health Sciences; 2011.
33. Uziel Y, Berkovitch M, Gazarian M, et al. Evaluation of eutectic lidocaine/prilocaine cream (EMLA) for steroid joint injection in children with juvenile rheumatoid arthritis: a double blind, randomized, placebo controlled trial. J Rheumatol 2003; 30(3):594–6.
34. Weiss JE, Haines KA, Chalom EC, et al. A randomized study of local anesthesia for pain control during intra-articular corticosteroid injection in children with arthritis. Pediatr Rheumatol 2015;13(1):1–8.
35. Hague BA, Honnas CM, Simpson RB, et al. Evaluation of skin bacterial flora before and after aseptic preparation of clipped and nonclipped arthrocentesis sites in horses. Vet Surg 1997;26(2):121–5.
36. Lavallée JM, Shmon C, Beaufrère H, et al. Influence of clipping on bacterial contamination of canine arthrocentesis sites before and after skin preparation. Vet Surg 2020;49(7):1307–14.
37. Osuna DJ, DeYoung DJ, Walker RL. Comparison of three skin preparation techniques in the dog Part 1: experimental trial. Vet Surg 1990;19(1):14–9.
38. Torres BT, Duerr FM. Arthrocentesis technique. Canine Lameness; 2020. p. 95–102.
39. Wu T, Dong Y, Song Hx, et al. Ultrasound-guided versus landmark in knee arthrocentesis: a systematic review. Semin Arthritis Rheum 2016;45(5):627–32.
40. Hoeber S, Aly AR, Ashworth N, et al. Ultrasound-guided hip joint injections are more accurate than landmark-guided injections: a systematic review and meta-analysis. Br J Sports Med 2016;50(7):392–6.

41. Aly AR, Rajasekaran S, Ashworth N. Ultrasound-guided shoulder girdle injections are more accurate and more effective than landmark-guided injections: a systematic review and meta-analysis. Br J Sports Med 2015;49(16):1042–9.
42. Wiler JL, Costantino TG, Filippone L, et al. Comparison of ultrasound-guided and standard landmark techniques for knee arthrocentesis. J Emerg Med 2010;39(1):76–82.
43. Jones JC, Gonzalez LM, Larson MM, et al. Feasibility and accuracy of ultrasound-guided sacroiliac joint injection in dogs. Vet Radiol Ultrasound 2012;53(4):446–54.
44. Levy M, Gaschen L, Rademacher N, et al. Technique for ultrasound-guided intra-articular cervical articular process injection in the dog. Vet Radiol Ultrasound 2014;55(4):435–40.
45. Bergamino C, Etienne AL, Busoni V. Developing a technique for ultrasound-guided injection of the adult canine hip. Vet Radiol Ultrasound 2015;56(4):456–61.
46. Waxman SJ, Adams SB, Moore GE. Effect of needle brand, needle bevel grin, and silicone lubrication on contamination of joints with tissue and hair debris after arthrocentesis. Vet Surg 2015;44(3):373–8.
47. Weitoft T, Uddenfeldt P. Importance of synovial fluid aspiration when injecting intra-articular corticosteroids. Ann Rheum Dis 2000;59(3):233–5.
48. Tarasevicius S, Kesteris U, Gelmanas A, et al. Intracapsular pressure and elasticity of the hip joint capsule in osteoarthritis. J Arthroplasty 2007;22(4):596–600.

Intra-articular Injectates

What to Use and Why

Peter J. Lotsikas, DVM

KEYWORDS

- Intra-articular injection • Injectate • Osteoarthritis • Synovitis

KEY POINTS

- Currently available intra-articular injectates can be used for short- to medium-term (less than a year) relief from joint discomfort stemming from acute or chronic inflammation.
- Many injectate options exist, although the majority have low-level literature support.
- No one injectate option is considered to be the gold standard, and individual patient considerations should guide which agent is most appropriate to use.

INTRODUCTION

Osteoarthritis (OA) affects a vast array of species, including all mammals, and can be a painful and severely debilitating condition Any joint or numerous joints may be affected. The progression of the disease process is influenced by extrinsic factors (trauma, joint impact from various types of exercise, and use) as well as intrinsic factors, such as immune-mediated conditions, metabolic dysfunction secondary to obesity, and endocrine disorders. Currently, there is no "cure" for OA; therefore, treatment is aimed at reducing the manifestations of pain and inflammation and the often ensuing negative cycle of disuse and immobility that follows as a consequence. OA is ideally managed with a multimodal approach, with the pillars of care being (1) achieving and maintenance of a lean body mass, (2) exercise modification, and (3) oral medications, with nonsteroidal anti-inflammatory medication being the preferred first-line medication.

Beyond these at-home strategies, intra-articular treatment is a joint-specific option and is gaining more widespread acceptance in veterinary medicine. Dogs serve as an excellent model for studying OA in humans, as they are anatomically, biochemically, and molecularly similar. Dogs also have similarities in clinical presentation and progression of disease.[1,2] This has led to a large amount of literature on the treatment of OA in dogs as an experimental animal model, but a rather limited amount of data from a naturally occurring OA clinical trial perspective.

Skylos Sports Medicine, 434 Prospect Boulevard, Frederick, MD 21701, USA
E-mail address: plotsika@yahoo.com

Vet Clin Small Anim 52 (2022) 967–975
https://doi.org/10.1016/j.cvsm.2022.03.004
0195-5616/22/

Intra-articular injections are nonoperative modalities that can be used to treat the clinical manifestations of OA, naturally occurring or surgical-induced acute synovitis, or intra-articular ligamentous or tendon injury. They may be reserved for patients in which other conservative modalities are ineffective or as a primary treatment. Injectable medications labeled for use or that have literature support for use in companion animal joints include corticosteroids, viscosupplements, orthobiologics (including platelet-rich plasma and stem cell therapy), and most recently, a radioisotope of Tin-117m, which is labeled as a veterinary device.[3–5] Mechanism of action varies between compounds, and thus, indications for which agent and when to use a specific therapy should be dictated by both patient characteristics and the underlying disease process. Intra-articular injections offer the advantage over oral medication in that they can target a specific affected joint or joints or tissue, have limited systemic absorption, and are tolerated in a wide array of patients with either comorbidities or oral medication intolerances.

Indications for intra-articular injections are as follows:

- Treatment of OA
- Treatment of naturally occurring or surgically induced acute synovitis
- Treatment of intra-articular ligamentous or tendon injury
- Potential advantage over oral medication in that they can target a specific affected joint or joints or tissue and have limited systemic absorption, which may benefit patients, of whom oral medications are not tolerated or effective

CORTICOSTEROIDS

Corticosteroids are powerful anti-inflammatory medications, with analgesic and antipyretic properties. The 2 main corticosteroid injectates that have current Food and Drug Administration (FDA) approval in dogs are triamcinolone acetonide and methylprednisolone acetate.

Mechanism of Action

Corticosteroids are reported to have both anti-inflammatory and immunosuppressive effects.[6] They are thought to reduce vascular permeability and inhibit accumulation of inflammatory cells, phagocytosis, production of neutrophil superoxide, metalloproteases, and metalloprotease activator and prevent the synthesis and secretion of several inflammatory mediators, such as prostaglandins and leukotrienes.[6] The clinical effect of steroids is reduced inflammation of the synovium, thereby reducing effusion and increasing the viscosity of joint fluid by stimulating production of endogenous hyaluronic acid (HA) concentrations.[6,7]

Uses

Corticosteroids are most appropriate to use to reduce active inflammation, either acute or chronic. Controversy over use of intra-articular corticosteroids exists with the long-standing belief that they can be harmful to articular cartilage. More than 35 in vivo animal studies have been performed looking at the effects of corticosteroids on joints.[8] Four relevant studies have been published in dogs, and all concluded that there were beneficial effects of methylprednisolone acetate and triamcinolone acetonide intra-articularly with few side effects.[8,9] However, other studies, particularly in horses, suggest methylprednisolone causes significant toxicity to the synovium and articular cartilage.[10] Therefore, methylprednisolone is often reserved for end-stage joints when there is minimal remaining articular cartilage. The label dose for methylprednisolone is 20 mg for a "large synovial space," which would equate to a stifle or coxofemoral joint of a large breed dog. Smaller spaces will require a correspondingly lesser dose. Triamcinolone is thought to be a safer option for preservation of articular cartilage and is thus used more frequently in small animals as a "first-line" injectable.[10] The labeled dose of triamcinolone is 1 to 3 mg per joint, with studies reporting doses as high as 40 mg per joint.[10] Local side effects are uncommon, with a low-level joint flare possible for 1 to 3 days postinjection. Although transient adrenocortical suppression has been documented with administration of 0.25 mg/kg and 0.5 mg/kg of triamcinolone acetonide, systemic and biochemical side effects are usually minimal, as long as the medication is appropriately delivered to the joint.[11] In this author's experience, one may see an increase in systemic absorption in patients with severe synovial proliferation and angiogenesis and often manifests as polyuria and polydipsia for 48 to 72 hours. It is the author's opinion that repeat injections of steroid should ideally be at least 3 to 4 months apart and not occur more than twice a year. Corticosteroids can also be administered in conjunction with hyaluronan, with positive improvement in mobility and comfort based on the Canine Brief Pain Inventory (CBPI) and Liverpool Osteoarthritis for Dogs questionnaires reported up to 6 months after administration in both the elbow and the hip joint.[4,12]

VISCOSUPPLEMENTS

Agent

Hyaluronic acid (also known as hyaluronan or hyaluronate) is a naturally occurring glycosaminoglycan and a component of synovial fluid and cartilage matrix. HA provides the viscosity and elastic properties of synovial fluid, functioning as viscous lubrication during slow joint movement and elastic shock absorption during rapid loading.[6,13] HA and its molecular weight (MW) decline as OA progresses with aging.[14] Manufactured HA is a frequently used viscosupplement intra-articular injectate used in dogs. HA is produced from harvested rooster combs or via bacterial fermentation and is manufactured both as low MW HA and as high-molecular-weight hyaluronic acid (HMWHA), with the literature favoring HMWHA with regard to efficacy.[6]

Mechanism of Action

Manufactured HA has similar viscoelastic properties to that of naturally occurring HA of synovial fluid and acts as a "replacement HA" in diseased synovial fluid whereby the normal viscosity may be decreased.[15] Furthermore, HA is thought to have disease-modifying effects, such as inducing endogenous HA synthesis, reducing synovial inflammation, protecting cartilage by obstructing oxygen-derived free radicals and degradative enzymes, and antinociceptive properties.[6,15] The challenge with HA is that it is rapidly eliminated from the joint space through synovial capillaries (for low-molecular HA) or the lymphatic vessels (for high-molecular HA), thus does not remain within the joint for a sustained period of time, which likely effects the duration of action.[6]

Use

Several studies have reported beneficial effects of HA on the articular cartilage in surgically induced OA dog models.[16,17] Marshall and colleagues[18] reported that a series of 3 weekly injections of 0.5 mL (4 mg) of HA (MW 6,000,000 Da) alleviated the severity of discomfort and progression associated with OA in a surgically induced canine cruciate ligament tear model. In a meta-analysis performed by Wang and colleagues,[19] HA was found to be beneficial in the management of OA of the human knee, with younger patients (<65 years old) with mild to moderate OA responding better to treatment than older patients or patients with more severe changes on radiographs (complete loss of joint space).

Recently, Alves and colleagues[1] reported benefit from a single injection of a high-molecular-weight hyaluronan in a randomized controlled trial using naturally occurring canine hip dysplasia models. The study group included dogs with mild, moderate, and severe radiographic OA. Significant improvement was reported in all groups with regard to stance symmetry index as well as several Clinical Metrology Instrument scores, particularly pain scores, which improved from 90 to 180 days.[1] However, radiographic signs progressed in both groups.[1] The author of this article finds a series of 3 injections, spaced 3 weeks apart, is most beneficial when HA is used as a sole agent. The typical dosing is 10 mg per "large synovial space."

POLYACRYLAMIDE HYDROGELS

Agent

Polyacrylamide hydrogels (PAAG) are newer viscosupplements. They are a highly viscous, nonsoluble, nontoxic, and nonimmunogenic biocompatible polymer gel consisting of 96% to 97.5% sterile water and 2.5% to 4% cross-linked polyacrylamide.[20]

Mechanism of Action

PAAGs are designed to form a thin inner lining on the synovium and joint surfaces. Hydrogels are reported to make the joint capsule stronger and more elastic.[20] These benefits help load-bearing through the joint and reduce inflammation. Because of its high molecular mass and aqueous cross-linking, hydrogels are more slowly broken down and removed from the joint by phagocytizing synoviocytes, rather than capillaries or lymphatics like HA.[20]Although there are several hydrogels on the market for horses, its use in dogs is still considered off-label usage in the United States. Promising results with longer-term alleviation of clinical signs in horses with naturally occurring OA in a single joint was reported by Tnibar and colleagues.[20] There was a significant decrease in lameness grade from baseline to 1, 3, 6, 12, and 24 months and a significant positive association with joint effusion reduction. Estimates for odds ratio showed that the effect of treatment increased over time.[20] The author of this article has used 4.0% polyacrylamide off label on numerous patients with mixed response and has noted several dogs to experience acute joint flare (joint effusion, worsening of lameness). This type of reaction has not often been reported in horses or other species (rabbit) tested.[19] It is interesting to note that a product available in Europe and elsewhere for use in small animals is a 2.5% polyacrylamide.[21] The difference in concentration of the hydrogel may be responsible for the joint flare noted by the author.

ORTHOBIOLOGICS

Agent

The term orthobiologics can be further divided into 2 broad categories, blood-derived products and stem cells. Blood-derived products include platelet-rich plasma, autologous conditioned plasma, autologous conditioned serum/interleukin-receptor antagonist protein (IRAP), and autologous conditioned protein. Stem cells can be further subdivided into stromal vascular fraction (SVF) from fat, cultured (expanded) SVF cell therapy, bone marrow aspirate, and bone marrow aspirate concentrate. Orthobiologics are considered "drugs" and fall under the jurisdiction of the FDA. There are currently no FDA-approved cellular therapies for use in animals, and the use of orthobiologics is considered off label/experimental. Platelet-rich plasma is specifically discussed in greater detail in Brittany Jean Carr's article, "Platelet Rich Plasma as an Orthobiologic: Clinically Relevant Considerations," in this issue.

Mechanism of Action

Intra-articular use of orthobiologics is thought to provide relief of discomfort and potentially reduce OA development through immune-modulation of the host joint environment and/or stimulation of endogenous progenitors enabling migration to sites of injury and inflammation. For example, IRAP blocks interleukin-1 (IL-1) from binding to IL-1 receptors on tissues within the joint. Of the cytokines identified in osteoarthritic joints, IL-1 is thought to be a major proinflammatory cytokine induced by joint injury. Prevention of binding of IL-1 blocks its degradative action and stops or slows the damage caused by IL-1 within the joint.

Mesenchymal stem cells (MSC), in the current available delivery method, are thought to promote tissue regeneration primarily through stimulation of endogenous progenitors rather than engraftment.[22,23] MSCs have been shown to disappear from the target tissue quickly after administration.[23,24] However, this agent is involved in the paracrine mediation process of stimulation of dormant host pericytes.[25] Once the pericytes are activated, they secrete factors, including chemokines and cytokines, to establish a regenerative environment. Tissue-intrinsic progenitors are prompted to proliferate and differentiate, whereas chemoattractants recruit endogenous progenitors to the site of injury. Antiapoptotic and antifibrotic factors may also limit the extent of damage to improve tissue healing.[26] Concurrently, activated MSCs are capable of modulating the immune response locally by selectively inhibiting the proliferation of immune cells.[23,27]

Uses

Although numerous studies involving orthobiologic agents exist, in the author's opinion, high-quality studies are currently lacking to support the routine use of IRAP and MSC for OA in the dog. There is more data to support the clinical use of intra-articular platelet-rich plasma; thus, it will be discussed in greater detail in Brittany Jean Carr's article, "Platelet Rich Plasma as an Orthobiologic: Clinically Relevant Considerations," in this issue.

RADIONUCLIDES FOR RADIOSYNOVIORTHESIS

Radiosynoviorthesis (ROS) is a process in which a radionuclide is administered intra-articularly to reduce the degree of synovial hypertrophy, thereby mitigating pain and the development of inflammation and arthritis.[28] ROS has been used in human medicine for decades, particularly in Europe. It is an approved human treatment option for early-stage chronic synovitis in rheumatoid arthritis, psoriatic arthritis, and OA patients.[28–30]

Agent

Currently, tin-117m is the only veterinary-approved radionuclide for ROS. It is considered a device rather than a drug, thus has not undergone the scrutiny of the FDA-approval process. Tin-117m is an artificially produced radionuclide of tin with a half-life of 14 days.[31] Two principal forms of the energy that it emits are (1) conversion electrons that have a short penetration range in tissue (~300 μm), and (2) imageable gamma radiation, which enables monitoring of local distribution in tissue. Tin-117m is metastable, indicated by the "m" suffix, meaning that it is a radioisotope with an energetic nucleus and a relatively long half-life and therefore distinct from highly unstable radionuclides with shorter half-lives.[31,32]

Mechanism of Action

The tin-117m radionuclide is combined with a homogeneous colloid.[31] These colloidal objects form microparticles (1.5–20 μm) that are small enough to be phagocytized by synovial macrophages in the synovial lining, after which they emit therapeutically active radiation within the synovial tissue until the radionuclide decays to its stable state.[31] During this process, the number of inflammatory cells causing synovitis is reduced, and inflamed tissue is replaced with a fibrotic synovial membrane. It is reported that this corresponds with alleviation of pain and improvement in function.[29–31]

Uses

Clinical use data with regard to ROS are limited in dogs. In a pilot study involving naturally occurring grade 1 to 2 OA of the elbow in dogs, 3 dosing levels of a single injection of Tin-117m were evaluated.[33] CBPI scores improved at most of the time points in all dose groups.[33] However, peak vertical force improvement was only noted in the high-dose group (2.5 mCl).[33] The improvement was noted at both 3- and 9-month marks as compared with pretreatment values. No adverse reactions were documented in any of the 23 dogs.[33] A smaller pilot study has also been performed on dogs with radiographic or MRI grade 3 OA (defined as well-developed degenerative joint disease with new bone proliferation > 5 mm along the proximal border of the anconeal process).[32] Significant improvement was noted by owners and on veterinary examination at day 90 and day 180 time points.[31] In neither of these studies was gait analysis was used in the first study, but not in the second. Niether study had a control group.[32] Use of radionuclide for ROS does require special radioactive material facility licensing, and regulations can vary from state to state and country to country. Dogs that have received treatments with Tin-117m may be released from radiation safety isolation immediately after treatment from the standpoint of external exposure. People should avoid prolonged close proximity, such as sleeping with a treated dog, for a month following Tin-117m ROS.[31,33,34]

SUMMARY

With a vast array of possible sources of discomfort stemming from joints and the etiopathogenesis of said conditions, it can be difficult to formulate a "best choice" for a specific patient. Rather, consideration should be given to patient individualities and clinical presentation for decision making. Based largely on literature regarding intra-articular therapy use in humans, treatments are in general most effective at providing relief in younger to middle-aged patients suffering from mild to moderate OA and less effective once OA is severe.[1,19,35] Based on clinical experience and the literature, the author considers a good response to intra-articular therapy to be a reduction in pain and improvement in mobility for 6 to 12 months. An average response would be 4 to 6 months of relief, and a poor response would be less than 4 months. A poor response would influence the decision making regarding the substance injected, concentration, and/or frequency of injections moving forward. Poor response to one substance does not predict how an individual animal will respond to another.

Corticosteroids are an appropriate choice for acute inflammation of a joint or chronic persistent synovitis but are effective for a relatively short duration. HA injections either as a single injection or in a series of 2 to 3 injections depending on the condition being treated and the substance injected can be beneficial for acute inflammation or chronic OA, with the duration of effect being variable.[1,18,36] Newer therapies, including orthobiologics, targeting inflammation at a cellular level may provide longer-lasting relief by truly immune modulating the joint environment. Injections can be used as stand-alone therapy or in conjunction with other treatments to allow for reduction in oral medication use.

CLINICS CARE POINTS

- Triamcinolone is an FDA approved corticosteroid for intra-articular use in dogs that is thought to be safe and efficacious. It can be administered as a sole agent or in conjunction with hyaluronic acid. High-molecular weight hyaluronic acid is option for replacing diseased synovial fluid thereby improving the viscosity of the fluid in an affected joint. It is classically administered in a series of injections, although a recent study indicated a single injection can improve pain scores in patients for up to 6 months. Orthobiologics and radiosynoviorthesis provide other options for reducing inflammation by immune modulating the cells of the synovial lining.

DISCLOSURE

The author has nothing to disclose.

REFERENCES

1. Alves JC, Dos Santos AMMP, Jorge P, et al. Effect of a single intra-articular high molecular weight hyaluronan in a naturally occurring canine osteoarthritis model: a randomized controlled trial. J Orthop Surg Res 2021;16(1):290.
2. Gregory MH, Capito N, Kuroki K, et al. A review of translational animal models for knee osteoarthritis. Arthritis 2012;2012:764621.
3. Bozynski C, Stannard J, Smith P, et al. Acute management of anterior cruciate ligament injuries using novel canine models. J Knee Surg 2015;29(07):594–603. https://doi.org/10.1055/s-0035-1570115.
4. Franklin SP, Cook JL. Prospective trial of autologous conditioned plasma versus hyaluronan plus corticosteroid for elbow osteoarthritis in dogs. Can Vet J 2013; 54(9):881–4.
5. Lattimer JC, Selting KA, Lunceford JM, et al. Intraarticular injection of a Tin-117 m radiosynoviorthesis agent in normal canine elbows causes no adverse effects. Vet Radiol Ultrasound 2019;60(5):567–74.
6. Ayhan E, Kesmezacar H, Akgun I. Intraarticular injections (corticosteroid, hyaluronic acid, platelet rich plasma) for the knee osteoarthritis. World J Orthop 2014;5(3):351–61.
7. Ostergaard M, Halberg P. Intra-articular corticosteroids in arthritic disease: a guide to treatment. BioDrugs 1998;9(2):95–103.
8. Vandeweerd JM, Zhao Y, Nisolle JF, et al. Effect of corticosteroids on articular cartilage: have animal studies said everything? Fundam Clin Pharmacol 2015; 29(5):427–38.
9. Murphy DJ, Todhunter RJ, Fubini SL, et al. The effects of methylprednisolone on normal and monocyte-conditioned medium-treated articular cartilage from dogs and horses. Vet Surg 2000;29(6):546–57. https://doi.org/10.1053/jvet.2000.17854.

10. Sherman SL, James C, Stoker AM, et al. In vivo toxicity of local anesthetics and corticosteroids on chondrocyte and synoviocyte viability and metabolism. Cartilage 2015;6(2):106–12.
11. Gamble LJ, Boesch JM, Wakshlag JJ, et al. Assessing the systemic effects of two different doses of intra-articular triamcinolone acetonide in healthy dogs. VCOT Open 2020;03(02):e96–102.
12. Franklin SP, Franklin AL. Randomized controlled trial comparing autologous protein solution to hyaluronic acid plus triamcinolone for treating hip osteoarthritis in dogs. Front Vet Sci 2021;8. https://doi.org/10.3389/fvets.2021.713768.
13. Brockmeier SF, Shaffer BS. Viscosupplementation therapy for osteoarthritis. Sports Med Arthrosc 2006;14(3):155–62.
14. Gupta RC, Lall R, Srivastava A, et al. Hyaluronic acid: molecular mechanisms and therapeutic trajectory. Front Vet Sci 2019;6:192.
15. Kuroki K, Cook JL, Kreeger JM. Mechanisms of action and potential uses of hyaluronan in dogs with osteoarthritis. J Am Vet Med Assoc 2002;221(7):944–50.
16. Abatangelo G, Botti P, Del Bue M, et al. Intraarticular sodium hyaluronate injections in the Pond-Nuki experimental model of osteoarthritis in dogs. I. Biochemical results. Clin Orthop Relat Res 1989;241:278–85.
17. Schiavinato A, Lini E, Guidolin D, et al. Intraarticular sodium hyaluronate injections in the Pond-Nuki experimental model of osteoarthritis in dogs. II. Morphological findings. Clin Orthop Relat Res 1989;241:286–99.
18. Marshall KW, Manolopoulos V, Mancer K, et al. Amelioration of disease severity by intraarticular hylan therapy in bilateral canine osteoarthritis. J Orthop Res 2000;18(3):416–25.
19. Wang CT, Lin J, Chang CJ, et al. Therapeutic effects of hyaluronic acid on osteoarthritis of the knee. A meta-analysis of randomized controlled trials. J Bone Joint Surg Am 2004;86(3):538–45.
20. Tnibar A, Schougaard H, Camitz L, et al. An international multi-centre prospective study on the efficacy of an intraarticular polyacrylamide hydrogel in horses with osteoarthritis: a 24 months follow-up. Acta Vet Scand 2015;57:20.
21. Christensen L, Camitz L, Illigen KE, et al. Synovial incorporation of polyacrylamide hydrogel after injection into normal and osteoarthritic animal joints. Osteoarthritis Cartilage 2016;24(11):1999–2002.
22. Jeong SY, Kim DH, Ha J, et al. Thrombospondin-2 secreted by human umbilical cord blood-derived mesenchymal stem cells promotes chondrogenic differentiation. Stem Cells 2013;31(10):2136–48. https://doi.org/10.1002/stem.1471.
23. Mancuso P, Raman S, Glynn A, et al. Mesenchymal stem cell therapy for osteoarthritis: the critical role of the cell secretome. Front Bioeng Biotechnol 2019;7:9.
24. ter Huurne M, Schelbergen R, Blattes R, et al. Antiinflammatory and chondroprotective effects of intraarticular injection of adipose-derived stem cells in experimental osteoarthritis. Arthritis Rheum 2012;64(11):3604–13.
25. Crisan M, Yap S, Casteilla L, et al. A perivascular origin for mesenchymal stem cells in multiple human organs. Cell Stem Cell 2008;3(3):301–13.
26. Ryan A, Murphy M, Barry F. Mesenchymal stem/stromal cell therapy. The biology and therapeutic application of mesenchymal cells. 2016:426-440. https://doi.org/10.1002/9781118907474.ch29.
27. Aggarwal S, Pittenger MF. Human mesenchymal stem cells modulate allogeneic immune cell responses. Blood 2005;105(4):1815–22.
28. Brenner W. Radionuclide joint therapy. In: Nuclear medicine therapy. CRC Press; 2007. p. 33–56.

29. Kampen WU, Voth M, Pinkert J, et al. Therapeutic status of radiosynoviorthesis of the knee with yttrium [90Y] colloid in rheumatoid arthritis and related indications. Rheumatology 2006;46(1):16–24.
30. Karavida N, Notopoulos A. Radiation synovectomy: an effective alternative treatment for inflamed small joints. Hippokratia 2010;14(1):22–7.
31. Donecker JM, Stevenson NR. Radiosynoviorthesis: a new therapeutic and diagnostic tool for canine joint inflammation. Technical Bulletin Exubrion Therapeutics. 2019.
32. Donecker J, Fabiani M, Gaschen L, et al. Treatment response in dogs with naturally occurring grade 3 elbow osteoarthritis following intra-articular injection of 117mSn (tin) colloid. PLoS One 2021;16(7):e0254613.
33. Aulakh KS, Lopez MJ, Hudson C, et al. Prospective clinical evaluation of intra-articular injection of Tin-117m (117mSn) radiosynoviorthesis agent for management of naturally occurring elbow osteoarthritis in dogs: a pilot study. Vet Med (Auckl) 2021;12:117–28.
34. Wendt RE 3rd, Selting KA, Lattimer JC, et al. Radiation safety considerations in the treatment of canine skeletal conditions using 153Sm, 90Y, and 117mSn. Health Phys 2020;118(6):702–10.
35. Battaglia M, Guaraldi F, Vannini F, et al. Efficacy of ultrasound-guided intra-articular injections of platelet-rich plasma versus hyaluronic acid for hip osteoarthritis. Orthopedics 2013;36(12):e1501–8.
36. Concoff A, Sancheti P, Niazi F, et al. The efficacy of multiple versus single hyaluronic acid injections: a systematic review and meta-analysis. BMC Musculoskelet Disord 2017;18(1):542.

Platelet-Rich Plasma as an Orthobiologic

Clinically Relevant Considerations

Brittany Jean Carr, DVM, CCRT

KEYWORDS

- Platelet-rich plasma • Orthobiologic • Biologic agent
- Autologous blood-derived product • Regenerative medicine
- Pure platelet-rich plasma • Leukocyte-rich platelet-rich plasma
- Leukocyte-poor platelet-rich plasma

KEY POINTS

- Platelet-rich plasma (PRP) is an autologous blood-derived product processed to concentrate platelets and the associated growth factors that have been used to treat wounds, osteoarthritis, and soft tissue injury in the canine.
- There are multiple commercial products and formulations of autologous blood-derived products available.
- It is imperative that future research adhere to a standardized universal nomenclature to describe autologous blood-derived products so that indications are able to be identified and evidence-based protocols can be established.

INTRODUCTION

Platelets play an integral role in both hemostasis and wound healing as they contain alpha granules with a number of associated growth factors and cytokines.[1,2] By definition, platelet-rich plasma (PRP) is a biological product containing the plasma fraction of autologous blood with a concentration of platelets and the associated growth factors and cytokines that is higher than baseline.[1,2] The associated growth factors and cytokines that have been correlated to tissue healing include platelet-derived growth factor (PDGF), transforming growth factor-α (TGF-α), transforming growth factor-β (TGF-β), vascular endothelial growth factor (VEGF), basic fibroblastic growth factor (bFGF), epidermal growth factor (EGF), connective tissue growth factor (CTGF), insulin-like growth factor (IGF), hepatocyte growth factor (HGF), and keratinocyte growth factor (KGF) (**Table 1**).[3] These various growth factors and cytokines have been shown to work individually and/or synergistically to promote cell recruitment, cell migration, cell proliferation, angiogenesis, and osteogenesis.[1–5] Furthermore, PRP has also

The Veterinary Sports Medicine and Rehabilitation Center, 4104 Liberty Highway, Anderson, SC 29621, USA
E-mail address: dr.brittcarrbenson@gmail.com

Vet Clin Small Anim 52 (2022) 977–995
https://doi.org/10.1016/j.cvsm.2022.02.005
0195-5616/22/

Table 1
Partial list of PRP-based growth factors and cytokines

Growth Factors and Cytokines	Function
PDGF	Mitogenic for mesenchymal cells and osteoblasts. Stimulates chemotaxis and mitogenesis in fibroblast, glial cells, and smooth muscle cells. Regulates collagenase secretion and collagen synthesis. Stimulates macrophage and neutrophil chemotaxis.
TGF-α, TGF-β	Stimulates undifferentiated mesenchymal cell proliferation. Regulates endothelial, fibroblastic, and osteoblastic mitogenesis. Regulates collagen synthesis and collagenase secretion. Regulates mitogenic effects of other growth factors. Stimulates endothelial chemotaxis and angiogenesis. Inhibits macrophage and lymphocyte proliferation.
TNF	Regulates monocyte migration, fibroblast proliferation, macrophage activation, and angiogenesis.
VEGF	Stimulates angiogenesis and mitogenesis for endothelial cells
bFGF	Promotes growth and differentiation of chondrocytes and osteoblasts. Mitogenic for mesenchymal cells, chondrocytes, and osteoblasts.
EGF	Proliferation of keratinocytes and fibroblasts. Stimulates mitogenesis for endothelial cells.
CTGF	Stimulates angiogenesis, cartilage regeneration, fibrosis, and platelet adhesion.
IGF-1	Chemotactic for fibroblasts and promotes protein synthesis. Augments proliferation and differentiation of osteoblasts.
HGF	Stimulates epithelial repair and neovascularization during wound healing.
KGF	Regulates epithelial migration and proliferation.
Ang-1	Supports angiogenesis and proliferation of endothelial cells.

Modified from Everts et al.[3]

Abbreviations: PDGF: platelet-derived growth factor; TGF-α: transforming growth factor-α; TGF-β: transforming growth factor-β; TNF: tumor necrosis factor; VEGF: vascular endothelial growth factor; bFGF: basic fibroblastic growth factor; EGF: epidermal growth factor; CTGF: connective tissue growth factor; IGF: insulin-like growth factor; HGF: hepatocyte growth factor; KGF: keratinocyte growth factor; Ang-1: angiopoietin-1

been shown to recruit, stimulate, and provide a scaffold for stem cells.[6–10] Thus, PRP has been used to manage numerous conditions including wound healing, osteoarthritis, and soft tissue injury in humans and equines as well as canines.[11–46]

Platelet-Rich Plasma Applications in the Canine: Wound Healing

Almost immediately following injury to the skin, platelets play a critical role in clotting and providing scaffolds for cell migration as well as providing cytokines and growth factors to support and regulate tissue regeneration.[11] Various PRP products, most commonly platelet-rich fibrin (PRF) and autologous platelet gel (APG), have been applied to wound margins in humans, horses, and dogs to support and stimulate healing.[12–17] Multiple studies on wound healing in people and dogs have found that PRP promotes wound epithelialization, reduces scar formation, exhibits antimicrobial activity, and stimulates angiogenesis.[12–17] Thus, PRP is currently being used in the canine as a biological wound healing enhancer.

Platelet-Rich Plasma Applications in the Canine: Osteoarthritis

Osteoarthritis affects more than 20% of the canine population.[18] The alpha granules of platelets contain various growth factors and cell mediators that are known to modulate inflammation and promote tissue healing.[19–21] Thus, autologous blood-derived products have been used to manage osteoarthritis in humans, horses, and dogs to alleviate pain, reduce inflammation, and improve function.[19–33] Further, recent studies have shown that PRP seems to be beneficial in dogs with osteoarthritis.[22–29] Multiple studies have reported that dogs with osteoarthritis treated with a single injection of PRP may have improvement in validated client survey results and subjective pain and gait scores as well as objective kinetic gait findings for anywhere from 30 to 180 days.[23,24,26–28] One study performed in dogs with moderate and severe osteoarthritis that were treated with 2 intra-articular injections of PRP 14 days apart found that the PRP group had significantly better clinical metrology instruments than saline control group at multiple time points, some up to 180 days.[29] Numerous studies have also been performed in dogs with cranial cruciate ligament (CCL) injury and have also shown that PRP has beneficial effects in improving pain, lameness, effusion, and/or overall inflammation within the stifle.[25,26,30–33] Thus, PRP is thought to be beneficial in dogs with stifle osteoarthritis secondary to CCL injury.[25,26,30–33] In summary, either a single injection or series of PRP have been used in dogs to help manage symptoms associated with osteoarthritis.

Platelet-Rich Plasma Applications in the Canine: Soft Tissue Injury

Tendons and ligaments are known have poor self-repair capability.[3,34–37] Histologic specimens often reveal that tendinosis is not an acute inflammatory condition, but rather a failure of normal tendon repair mechanism associated with angiofibroblastic degeneration.[3,34–37] Concentrated growth factors and inflammatory mediators within PRP are believed to induce a transient inflammatory event that triggers tissue regeneration by stimulating cell recruitment and proliferation.[3,35–38] Furthermore, PRP has been shown to have a beneficial immunomodulatory effect on tenocytes to stimulate the secretion of angiogenic proteins in injured tenocytes.[3,36–38] Thus, the growth factors released by PRP work in concert to initiate a healing response within damaged tissues.[3,35–38] Numerous human and equine studies have shown PRP has a beneficial effect on tissue healing.[3,35–45] A recent canine study showed that dogs with supraspinatus tendinopathy treated with a single PRP ultrasound-guided injection had subjective improvement in lameness and function in 40% of dogs with improved tendon fiber pattern and in 60% of dogs with improved tendon echogenicity 6 weeks following treatment.[46] However, there is still limited evidence available regarding the use of PRP in the canine for tendinopathy.

PLATELET-RICH PLASMA CONSTITUENTS

Multiple formulations of PRP have been developed and studied in humans, equines, and canines (**Table 2**). There is still debate as to what the ideal formulation of PRP is; however, as the name implies, PRP products concentrate platelets while including or removing various other constituents. Further, recent studies have found that red blood cells (RBC), neutrophils, and mononuclear cells may also affect a PRP product is contributing to the inflammatory response following PRP administration.[36,47–62]

Platelets

PRP should contain enough concentrated platelets to contribute to cell proliferation, cell migration, and cell immunomodulatory activities. Numerous studies have indicated that the ideal PRP product should increase platelets anywhere from 2- to 6-fold compared with baseline CBC, depending on the clinical application.[48–50,63–66] In vitro, in vivo, and clinical studies have shown PRP formulations with both a

Table 2
PRP product terminologies and abbreviations used in veterinary medicine

ACP	Autologous Conditioned Plasma
ACS	Autologous conditioned serum
APG	Autologous platelet gel
LP-PRP	Leukocyte-poor platelet-rich plasma
LR-PRP	Leukocyte-rich platelet-rich plasma
PFC	Platelet-derived factor concentrate
P-PRP	Pure platelet-rich plasma
PRF	Platelet-rich fibrin
PRFM	Platelet-rich fibrin matrix
PRGF	Plasma rich in growth factors

moderate (2- to 3-fold increase) and high (4- to 6-fold increase) platelet concentrations are beneficial for soft tissue and bone healing.[66] However, there is still no consensus on the ideal platelet concentration for specific applications.[3,67]

While the increase in platelet fold is commonly referenced, absolute platelet concentration is important as recent studies have concluded that cells respond to PRP in a dose-dependent manner.[3,67] In fact, recent studies have shown that growth factor concentrations beyond a certain level may not necessarily be advantageous for cell stimulatory processes as there seems to be a ceiling effect.[3,47,68,69] Further, in the human literature it has been proposed that platelet concentration greater than 6x baseline (or >1800 x 10^3 platelets/μ) may be detrimental and lead to cellular apoptosis as well as the downregulation and desensitization of growth factor receptors.[57,65,69,70] Thus, there has been a recent shift in focus to defining absolute platelet concentration rather than platelet fold increase.[3,65,67] This is important as when processed appropriately smaller volumes of blood may yield an acceptable absolute platelet concentration in the PRP product. It is imperative that future studies define the absolute platelet concentration of the PRP product used so that evidence-based protocols can be established.

Red Blood Cells

Most recent studies agree that it is best to reduce RBC in PRP as they have been shown to have a deleterious inflammatory effect.[48,54,55,61] RBCs are known to damage cartilage and synovium directly via iron-catalyzed formation of reactive oxygen species.[48,54,55,61] Further, an increased RBC concentration in PRP has been shown to increase concentrations of unwanted inflammatory mediators IL-1 and TGF-α.[55] One recent study demonstrated that synoviocytes treated with RBC concentrate demonstrated significantly more synoviocyte death when compared with a leukocyte-rich PRP (LR-PRP, defined as having an overall WBC count greater than the WBC count in whole blood, average 26.6 K/μL), leukocyte poor PRP (LP-PRP, defined as having an overall WBC count less than the WBC count in whole blood, average 6.1 K/μL), and phosphate-buffered saline (PBS).[54] Thus, most agree it is best to reduce RBCs in PRP. Many of the commercially available PRP systems reduce the RBC concentration in the PRP product produced.

Leukocytes (Neutrophils)

There is still much debate regarding whether or not leukocytes should be included in PRP, particularly neutrophils. Multiple studies have shown that neutrophils increase concentrations of inflammatory mediators IL-1β, TNF-α, IL-6, IL-8, and MMP-9.[48,51–56,58] Previous reports have indicated that LR-PRP causes significantly more synoviocyte death when compared with LP-PRP and PBS.[54,61] Thus, many argue that neutrophil concentration should be decreased for intra-articular applications. However, some studies suggest that leukocytes should be included in PRP for soft tissue applications as in tendinosis there is a failure of normal tendon repair in which case concentrated growth factors and inflammatory mediators within PRP work together to re-initiate a healing response.[36,37,39–43] However, one recent study compared an LR-PRP product to an LP-PRP product and found that while both LR-PRP and LP-PRP seem to induce tendon stem/progenitor cell differentiation into active tenocytes, LR-PRP may be detrimental to the healing of injured tendons because it induces catabolic and inflammatory effects on tendon cells and may prolong the effects in healing tendons.[62] However, this study also concluded that when LP-PRP is used to treat acutely injured tendons, it may result in the formation of excessive scar tissue due to the strong potential of LP-PRP to induce inordinate cellular anabolic effects.[62] Thus, there is still debate as to whether leukocytes should or should not be included in PRP.

Mononuclear Cells

While the direct effect of mononuclear cells remains unclear, recent studies indicate they may be beneficial.[62,71,72] Monocytes are associated with an increase in cellular metabolism and collagen production in fibroblast as well as a decreased release of antiangiogenic cytokines interferon-γ and IL-12.[71,72] Previous studies have shown that platelets activate lymphocytes to help stimulate collagen production via an increase in IL-6 expression.[71,72] Thus, while their significance in PRP is unknown, the current thought is that mononuclear cells may be beneficial in PRP.

Platelet-Rich Plasma Activation

The concentration of growth factors in PRP has been shown to not only be affected by its composition but also its activation method.[73–76] Platelets in PRP are activated by physical or chemical stimuli that then cause the release of growth factors.[75] Commonly used exogenous activation methods include thermal activation, activation with thrombin solution, and activation with calcium.[67] The argument for exogenous PRP activation is that nonactivated PRP may release only a fraction of the growth factors contained within the platelets.[77]

A recent review of human PRP preparation methodology suggested that the activation of PRP by calcium gluconate 10% was associated with greater potential of inducing osteoblast and fibroblast proliferation, but it does not contribute to higher platelet or growth factor concentrations in some studies.[76] Thermal activation at 370°C was associated with higher platelet concentrations when compared with the activation by calcium gluconate 10%.[76] However, several studies have found that freezing/thawing PRP may negatively affect platelet morphology, function, and growth factor release.[78–81] One recent study specifically performed in canines showed that there are positive correlations between platelet and anabolic growth factor concentrations in canine PRP.[81] Furthermore, it was determined that intentional platelet activation has a greater effect on growth factor delivery than platelet concentration with thrombin providing a more robust activation than calcium chloride ($CaCl_{2}$).[81]

Photoactivation of PRP has also been used and shown to be safe.[82–85] Photoactivation is thought to increase anti-inflammatory cytokines and decrease proinflammatory cytokines (IL-2 and IL-6).[73] One recent in vitro study has shown that the photoactivation of PRP induced significantly more prolonged release and higher amount of PDGF, FGF, and TGF-β than PRP activated with $CaCl_2$.[85] However, there are no in vivo studies to date.

Extracorporeal shockwave therapy (ESWT) has also been used to activate PRP. A recent study in equine PRP demonstrated the application of ESWT to PRP significant increased growth factor concentrations.[86] Thus, the combination of ESWT and PRP is thought to potentially result in the synergism of these 2 modalities for tissue healing.[86]

Whole blood collection site has also been shown to affect platelet activation.[87] A recent canine study indicated that collecting whole blood from the jugular vein may cause more platelet activation and recommended that PRP should be processed in a timely manner following sample collection to avoid platelet activation and loss.[87] In human medicine, various other patient factors (such as body mass index, smoking status, regular exercise, nutrition, positioning during blood collection, and so forth) have been investigated as factors that may influence PRP composition; thus, patient factors could also be an area of future study in veterinary medicine.[3,87,88]

Finally, not all commercial PRP products are activated exogenously before administration as platelets are known to activate endogenously when placed in contact with collagen fibers or other coagulation factors within the extracellular matrix *in situ*.[67,89–91] There, unfortunately, remains debate as to whether or not PRP should be activated and if so, which activation agent is best.

Platelet-Rich Plasma Anticoagulation

Commonly used anticoagulants include ethylenediaminetetraacetic (EDTA), Anticoagulant citrate dextrose-A (ACD-A), and sodium citrate. There is great debate as to which anticoagulant is best for minimizing effects on platelet function and optimizing PRP formulation. One recent study found that EDTA suppresses platelet degranulation.[92] Thus, EDTA is not commonly recommended for PRP.[92,93] ACD-A is the most commonly used anticoagulant for PRP as it maintains the optimal pH for platelets at 7.2 while the citrate binds to calcium preventing the coagulation cascade.[92,93] A recent review has shown that ACD-A was associated with the preservation of platelet morphology with no effects on growth factor concentration.[76] Sodium citrate, while less commonly used, has been associated with greater induction of proliferation of mesenchymal cells.[76] One recent study in rabbits found that sodium citrate, when used in a pure platelet-rich gel, yielded a higher number of platelets and leukocytes; however, there was no difference in growth factor concentration when compared with ACD-A.[94] Most commercial PRP kits available for companion animals use ACD-A.

Frozen Storage of Platelet-Rich Plasma

To minimize cost, waste, and time, veterinarians often ask if PRP can be frozen and thawed for future use. Multiple studies have shown that once frozen the platelets are no longer viable.[81,95–99] However, while some studies suggest that freezing PRP changes levels of various growth factors as well as inflammatory mediators, canine freeze-thawed PRP has been shown to still contain high levels of TGF-β which may be of clinical value.[81,95–99] Nonetheless, there is limited information outlining the optimal procedure for freezing PRP and how long PRP can be stored for.[81] Finally, to date no studies have been performed to define the use of freeze-thawed PRP in the canine nor have studies been performed to compare the efficacy of freeze-thawed canine PRP and fresh canine PRP for various conditions.

PLATELET-RICH PLASMA IN CLINICAL PRACTICE

Platelet-Rich Plasma Processing

Over the years multiple methodologies have been developed to produce PRP with various characteristics. Typically a whole blood sample ranging anywhere from 5 to 60 mL is drawn from the patient into a syringe primed with the anticoagulant of choice. The whole blood sample is then processed via differential filtration or centrifugation to yield a platelet-rich end product.[93,100]

PRP filtration in the canine involves passing whole blood through a gravity filtration system, which is dependent on the pore size of the filter and gravity of isolate platelets. On the other hand, many commercially available PRP systems rely on differential centrifugation to separate various components of whole blood to produce the final PRP product. A blood sample ranging anywhere from 5 mL to 60 mL depending on the system used and patient size is collected and placed in a centrifuge for either 1 or 2 spins. Systems using a 'single spin' are thought to concentrate platelets but not to the degree that 'double spin' techniques are able to.[93,100,101] Systems using 2 spins or a 'double spin' technique often perform a 'soft' spin first to separate the RBCs. Once the RBCs have been removed, the supernatant plasma is then centrifuged a second time also known as the 'hard' spin, which is typically at a higher speed and/or longer duration to obtain the final platelet concentrate.

Commercial Platelet-Rich Plasma Products

Multiple studies have investigated the compositional differences of commercially available PRP systems in both the canine and feline.[102–106] Two recent studies compared different commercially available PRP systems.[102,103] Franklin and colleagues compared the following 5 systems: ProTec PRP, MediVet PRP, C-PET Platelet Enhancement Therapy, SmartPReP ACP+, and Arthrex Angel cPRP.[102] Carr and colleagues compared the following 5 systems: SmartPReP ACP+, Arthrex ACP, CRT PurePRP, ProTec PRP, and C-PET Platelet Enhancement Therapy.[103] Both studies found differences among platelet concentration and WBC concentration in the final PRP product.[107,108] In Franklin and colleagues, the Arthrex Angel cPRP and SmartPReP ACP + had the highest platelet concentration in the PRP product.[102] Both the Arthrex Angel cPRP and SmartPReP ACP + PRP products were leukocyte rich.[102] The MediVet PRP was the only product that increased platelets while reducing leukocytes.[102] This study only looked at total WBC count and did not specifically assess neutrophil content.[102] Similarly Carr and colleagues found that the SmartPReP ACP+ and CRT PurePRP had the highest platelet concentration in the PRP product; however, the CRT PurePRP PRP product was leukoreduced while the SmartPReP ACP+ was leukocyte rich.[103] This study assessed total WBC count as well as neutrophil content and found the SmartPReP ACP + PRP product to concentrate neutrophils.[103] Neither of these studies assessed growth factor content or made efficacy claims.[102,103]

Regarding growth factor concentration among the commercially available systems, a study was performed and compared transforming growth factor-β1 (TGF-β1), platelet-derived growth factor-BB (PDGF-BB), vascular endothelial growth factor, and tumor necrosis factor-alpha (TNF-α) as well as the leukocyte content between ProTec PRP, MediVet PRP, C-PET Platelet Enhancement Therapy, SmartPReP ACP+, and Arthrex Angel cPRP.[81] This study found that PRP made with C-PET Platelet Enhancement Therapy, SmartPReP ACP+, and Arthrex Angel cPRP had a notable leukocyte concentration.[81] However, approximately 40% of the leukocytes in the PRPs made with C-PET Platelet Enhancement Therapy and SmartPReP

ACP+ were neutrophils, while approximately 10% of the leukocytes in the PRP from Arthrex Angel cPRP were neutrophils and approximately 80% of the leukocytes in that PRP were lymphocytes.[81] Furthermore, this study found great variation in growth factor concentration among the PRP products.[81]

The use of PRP in feline patients has become increasingly more common. Performing PRP in feline patients is slightly more challenging as they are smaller in size and thus, larger blood samples are not feasible. Additionally, feline platelets tend to aggregate more than canine platelets, which can make PRP preparation and sample quantification difficult. Two recent studies assessed various commercial PRP systems for feline use.[104,105] In Ferrari and colleagues, the Arthrex ACP and CRT PurePRP systems were evaluated.[104] This study concluded that neither system was able to concentrate platelets as well in the feline and attributed this to significant platelet aggregation.[104] In Chun and colleagues the CRT PurePRP system was assessed.[105] This study assessed platelet concentration via a hematology analyzer as well as blood smears evaluated by a clinical pathologist.[105] This study found that the CRT PurePRP system was able to concentrate platelets by 2.5-fold and reduce both neutrophil and RBC concentration.[105] Neither of these studies assessed growth factor concentration or made efficacy claims.[104,105]

While the implications of differing PRP constituents are still unknown, the heterogeneity among differing commercial PRP systems is obvious (**Table 3**). Unfortunately, there is still no overall consensus on optimal component concentrations.[65,87,93,102–106] Further study is still needed to elucidate not only indications for PRP therapy but also optimal component concentrations for various indications. This may partly be due to a lack of the standardization of the PRP product. As previously discussed, there are great variations in PRP preparation and dosage among the various commercially available products, and this is not always well defined. Moving forward it is imperative that PRP terminology be standardized to accurately reflect the product being used and/or tested.

Various autologous blood-derived product classification schemes and standardized universal nomenclature systems have been proposed in the human literature for PRP, many of which account for platelet count, leukocyte content, RBC content, activation.[93,107–113] Most recently, the ISTH (International Society on Thrombosis and Hemostasis) has proposed a classification scheme that accounts for activation method, platelet count (<900 x 10^3 μL; 900–1700 x 10^3 μL; >1700 x 10^3 μL), preparation method, leukocyte content (as positive/negative, meaning the PRP sample has a greater or lower concentration of leukocytes compared with baseline CBC), RBC content (as positive/negative, meaning the PRP sample has a greater or lower concentration of RBC compared with baseline CBC).[114] Unfortunately there is no consensus yet. Ideally, a universal nomenclature system would be applied to all studies. It is imperative that future studies adhere to a standardized universal nomenclature to describe autologous blood-derived products so that the indications for various orthobiologics are able to be identified and evidence-based protocols can be established.

Platelet-Rich Plasma Administration

Once the PRP product is ready, it is injected using aseptic technique directly into the site of tissue injury, either via intra-articular injection or with ultrasound guidance for soft tissue lesions. It is crucial to deliver PRP directly to the site of tissue injury for it to be most effective; thus, appropriate intra-articular injection technique and ultrasound-guided soft tissue injection techniques are imperative for success.[25,34,45,46,114]

Table 3
Commercially available companion animal PRP systems overview

	Method (C, F, DS, SS, FC)[a]	Platelet Count (Cells/μL)	PRP PLT: WB PLT	Leukocyte Content	RBC Content	Activation	Anti-coagulant	Volume of Whole Blood Required	Species Validated
SmartPReP® ACP+	C, DS	1,340,667 ± 285,520[100,101]	3.2–5.0[100,101]	+	-	No	ACD-A	50 mL	Canine
Arthrex® ACP	C, SS	397,800 ± 121,600[104]	0.9–2.5[104]	-	-	No	ACD-A	16 mL	Canine, Equine
CRT PurePRP®	C, DS	1,559,600 ± 428,872[101]	5.5–6.5[101]	-	-	No	ACD-A	25–50 mL	Canine, Feline
ProTec PRP	C, SS	169,933 ± 3,695[100]	1.0[100]	-	-	No	Sodium citrate	9 mL	Canine, Equine
C-PET Platelet Enhancement Therapy	F	452,800 ± 185,747[100]	1.7[100]	+	-	No	ACD-A	55 mL	Canine, Equine
Arthrex Angel® cPRP	C, DS, FC	605,000–1,946,000[100]	3.9–7.4[100]	+/–	-	No	+/-ACD-A	35+mL	Canine, Equine
PureVet PRP	C, DS	743,000 ± 301,719[100]	3.3[100]	-	-	No	ACD-A	20 mL	Canine, Feline

[a] Method: C- centrifuge, F- filtration, DS- double spin, SS- single spin, FC- flow cytometry.

Platelet-Rich Plasma Contraindications and Adverse Events

While PRP is considered safe and well-tolerated, there are conditions in which PRP is contraindicated and should not be performed (**Box 1**).[114,115] In general, PRP is thought to be very well-tolerated with the vast majority of meta-analysis finding no statistically significant increase in adverse events following PRP injection compared with other injected products.[114,116] Regardless, though complications are uncommon (less than <1%), they should be monitored for.[116] There can be mild discomfort associated with the injection, which is typically managed with appropriate medical therapy. Less commonly, a sterile inflammatory response (ie, 'joint flare') has been reported in the human literature.[116] Typically this is seen in the first 24 hours following the injection, and patients can experience moderate to severe discomfort that usually improves within 72 hours. If noted, appropriate pain management should be initiated. Finally, septic arthritis could be a potential complication.[114,116] It is important to adhere to aseptic technique when injecting PRP to minimize the risk for this complication. If noted, the joint should be copiously lavaged, and a 4- to 8-week course of culture-directed antibiotic therapy is indicated.

Post–Platelet-Rich Plasma Therapy Recommendations

Following PRP therapy, exercise restriction is typically recommended for a minimum of 14 days; however, this recommendation may change based on the underlying condition that the patient is receiving treatment for. At this time patients should refrain from high-impact activity such as running, jumping, and playing roughly with other dogs.

Patients, are often prescribed, medications for discomfort as needed. It is not uncommon for there to be mild discomfort associated with the injection for the first 24 to 72 hours. Historically, antiplatelet therapies such as nonsteroidal anti-inflammatory drugs (NSAID) have been thought to be contraindicated due to the concern that they may negatively affect platelet function and diminish the effects of PRP. In the literature, antiplatelet therapies such as NSAID use before and during PRP therapy are controversial and most often not recommended.[117,118] However, a canine study showed that NSAID use does not inhibit platelet activation or growth factor release from PRP.[119] Additionally, a recent review concluded there are limited clinical data to support the general recommendation to discontinue antiplatelet therapies

Box 1
Contraindications for PRP therapy

Anemia

Anticoagulant Medications

Antiplatelet Therapy

Coagulopathy

Dermatitis

Immune-Mediated Disease

Neoplasia

Sepsis

Septic Arthritis

Thrombocytopenia

before or during PRP use.[118] Thus, while there is still much debate, NSAIDs are sometimes included in a patient's treatment plan if indicated.

Rehabilitation therapy is often encouraged following PRP therapy. One previous study found that dogs with osteoarthritis who were treated with plasma rich in growth factors (PRGF) and physical rehabilitation consisting of an exercise program maintained increased kinetic gait outcome measures throughout the 180-day study period, whereas dogs treated with PRGF had a decline in kinetic gait outcome measures after 90 days.[23] Low-level laser therapy is also commonly recommended following PRP as photoactivation is thought to support optimal growth factor and cytokine concentrations.[82–85]

Follow-up

A patient's progress should be monitored following PRP therapy. Both subjective and objective outcome measures should be used at each assessment to measure a patient's response. Typically the first reassessment is performed 14 days following PRP therapy or sooner if indicated. If no improvement is noted, another PRP injection may be performed. Human and canine studies suggest that 1 to 3 PRP injections should be performed in the same therapeutic cycle as multiple injections could increase and/or prolong treatment efficacy.[29,114,120–122] There are no recommendations for treatment frequency, but typically multiple PRP injections are performed 7 to 30 days apart.[29,31,114] If a patient has shown no improvement following 3 PRP injections, it is unlikely they will benefit from additional injections in that therapeutic cycle. Patients have been documented to show improvement following PRP therapy for up to 180 to 270 days.[23–33]

SUMMARY

PRP has been used to treat wounds, osteoarthritis, and soft tissue injury in the canine and has shown to be relatively safe and well-tolerated. PRP is widely available with multiple commercial systems validated for canine use that generate different PRP products. Further study is still needed to fully elucidate both indications for PRP therapy as well as optimal component concentrations for various indications. However, it is imperative that future studies adhere to a standardized universal nomenclature to describe PRP so that the indications are able to be clearly identified and evidence-based protocols can be established.

CLINICS CARE POINTS

- PRP formulations with both a moderate (2–3x) and high (4–6x) platelet concentrations are beneficial for soft tissue and bone healing.[66] Platelet concentration greater than 6x baseline (or >1800 x 10^3 platelets/μ) may be detrimental.[57,65,69,70] However, there is still no consensus on the ideal platelet concentration for specific applications.[3,67]
- Most recent studies agree that it is best to reduce red blood cells (RBC) in PRP as they have been shown to have a deleterious inflammatory effect.[48,54,55,61]
- There is still much debate regarding whether or not leukocytes should be included in PRP, particularly neutrophils as they increase concentrations of inflammatory mediators.[48,51–56,58] Many argue that neutrophil concentration should be decreased for intra-articular applications as an increased neutrophil concentration in PRP has been shown to cause synoviocyte death.[54,61] However, some studies suggest that leukocytes should be included in PRP for soft tissue applications as in tendinosis there is a failure of normal tendon repair in which case concentrated growth factors and inflammatory mediators within PRP work together to reinitiate a healing response.[36,37,39–43]

- Multiple studies have investigated the compositional differences of commercially available PRP systems, but there is still no overall consensus on optimal component concentrations.[65,87,93,102–106]
- It is crucial to deliver PRP directly to the site of tissue injury for it to be most effective; therefore, appropriate intra-articular injection technique and ultrasound-guided soft tissue injection techniques are crucial for success.[25,34,45,46,114]

DISCLOSURE

The author is a consultant for Companion Animal Health.

REFERENCES

1. Alves R, Grimalt R. A Review of Platelet-Rich Plasma: History, Biology, Mechanism of Action, and Classification. Skin Appendage Disord 2018;4(1):18–24.
2. Arnoczky SP, Sheibani-Rad S. The basic science of platelet-rich plasma (PRP): what clinicians need to know [published correction appears in Sports Med Arthrosc 2014;22(2):150. Shebani-Rad, Shahin [corrected to Sheibani-Rad, Shahin]]. Sports Med Arthrosc Rev. 2013;21(4):180-185.
3. Everts P, Onishi K, Jayaram P, et al. Platelet-Rich Plasma: New Performance Understandings and Therapeutic Considerations in 2020. Int J Mol Sci 2020;21(20):7794.
4. Hudgens JL, Sugg KB, Grekin JA, et al. Platelet-Rich Plasma Activates Proinflammatory Signaling Pathways and Induces Oxidative Stress in Tendon Fibroblasts. Am J Sports Med 2016;44(8):1931–40.
5. Andia I, Rubio-Azpeitia E, Maffulli N. Platelet-rich plasma modulates the secretion of inflammatory/angiogenic proteins by inflamed tenocytes. Clin Orthop Relat Res 2015;473(5):1624–34.
6. Lai F, Kakudo N, Morimoto N, et al. Platelet-rich plasma enhances the proliferation of human adipose stem cells through multiple signaling pathways. Stem Cell Res Ther 2018;9(1):107.
7. Tobita M, Tajima S, Mizuno H. Adipose tissue-derived mesenchymal stem cells and platelet-rich plasma: stem cell transplantation methods that enhance stemness. Stem Cell Res Ther 2015;6:215.
8. Ricco S, Renzi S, Del Bue M, et al. Allogeneic adipose tissue-derived mesenchymal stem cells in combination with platelet rich plasma are safe and effective in the therapy of superficial digital flexor tendonitis in the horse. Int J Immunopathol Pharmacol 2013;26(1 Suppl):61–8.
9. Martinello T, Bronzini I, Perazzi A, et al. Effects of in vivo applications of peripheral blood-derived mesenchymal stromal cells (PB-MSCs) and platlet-rich plasma (PRP) on experimentally injured deep digital flexor tendons of sheep. J Orthop Res 2013;31(2):306–14.
10. Zhang J, Wang JH. Platelet-rich plasma releasate promotes differentiation of tendon stem cells into active tenocytes. Am J Sports Med 2010;38(12):2477–86.
11. Pastar I, Stojadinovic O, Yin NC, et al. Epithelialization in Wound Healing: A Comprehensive Review. Adv Wound Care (New Rochelle) 2014;3(7):445–64.
12. Farghali HA, AbdElKader NA, Khattab MS, et al. Evaluation of subcutaneous infiltration of autologous platelet-rich plasma on skin-wound healing in dogs. Biosci Rep 2017;37(2):BSR20160503.
13. Farghali HA, AbdElKader NA, AbuBakr HO, et al. Antimicrobial action of autologous platelet-rich plasma on MRSA-infected skin wounds in dogs. Sci Rep 2019;9(1):12722.

14. Xu P, Wu Y, Zhou L, et al. Platelet-rich plasma accelerates skin wound healing by promoting re-epithelialization. Burns Trauma 2020;8:tkaa028.
15. Jee CH, Eom NY, Jang HM, et al. Effect of autologous platelet-rich plasma application on cutaneous wound healing in dogs. J Vet Sci 2016;17(1):79–87.
16. Iacopetti I, Patruno M, Melotti L, et al. Autologous Platelet-Rich Plasma Enhances the Healing of Large Cutaneous Wounds in Dogs. Front Vet Sci 2020; 7:575449.
17. Chicharro-Alcántara D, Rubio-Zaragoza M, Damiá-Giménez E, et al. Platelet Rich Plasma: New Insights for Cutaneous Wound Healing Management. J Funct Biomater 2018;9(1):10.
18. Marshall W, Bockstahler B, Hulse D, et al. A review of osteoarthritis and obesity: current understanding of the relationship and benefit of obesity treatment and prevention in the dog. Vet Comp Orthop Traumatol 2009;22(5):339–45.
19. Nie LY, Zhao K, Ruan J, et al. Effectiveness of Platelet-Rich Plasma in the Treatment of Knee Osteoarthritis: A Meta-analysis of Randomized Controlled Clinical Trials. Orthop J Sports Med 2021;9(3). 2325967120973284.
20. McCarrel TM, Mall NA, Lee AS, et al. Considerations for the use of platelet-rich plasma in orthopedics. Sports Med 2014;44(8):1025–36.
21. Cole BJ, Karas V, Hussey K, et al. Hyaluronic Acid Versus Platelet-Rich Plasma: A Prospective, Double-Blind Randomized Controlled Trial Comparing Clinical Outcomes and Effects on Intra-articular Biology for the Treatment of Knee Osteoarthritis. Am J Sports Med 2017;45(2):339–46. Erratum in: Am J Sports Med. 2017 Apr;45(5):NP10. PMID: 28146403.
22. Kazemi D, Fakhrjou A. Leukocyte and Platelet Rich Plasma (L-PRP) Versus Leukocyte and Platelet Rich Fibrin (L-PRF) For Articular Cartilage Repair of the Knee: A Comparative Evaluation in an Animal Model. Iran Red Crescent Med J 2015;17(10):e19594.
23. Cuervo B, Rubio M, Chicharro D, et al. Objective Comparison between Platelet Rich Plasma Alone and in Combination with Physical Therapy in Dogs with Osteoarthritis Caused by Hip Dysplasia. Animals (Basel) 2020;10(2):175.
24. Catarino J, Carvalho P, Santos S, et al. Treatment of canine osteoarthritis with allogeneic platelet-rich plasma: review of five cases. Open Vet J 2020;10(2): 226–31.
25. Venator KP, Frye CW, Gamble LJ, et al. Assessment of a Single Intra-Articular Stifle Injection of Pure Platelet Rich Plasma on Symmetry Indices in Dogs with Unilateral or Bilateral Stifle Osteoarthritis from Long-Term Medically Managed Cranial Cruciate Ligament Disease. Vet Med (Auckl) 2020;11:31–8.
26. Vilar JM, Manera ME, Santana A, et al. Effect of leukocyte-reduced platelet-rich plasma on osteoarthritis caused by cranial cruciate ligament rupture: A canine gait analysis model. PLoS One 2018;13(3):e0194752.
27. Okamoto-Okubo CE, Cassu RN, Joaquim JGF, et al. Chronic pain and gait analysis in dogs with degenerative hip joint disease treated with repeated intra-articular injections of platelet-rich plasma or allogeneic adipose-derived stem cells. J Vet Med Sci 2021;83(5):881–8.
28. Alves JC, Santos A, Jorge P, et al. A report on the use of a single intra-articular administration of autologous platelet therapy in a naturally occurring canine osteoarthritis model - a preliminary study. BMC Musculoskelet Disord 2020; 21(1):127.
29. Alves JC, Santos A, Jorge P. Platelet-rich plasma therapy in dogs with bilateral hip osteoarthritis. BMC Vet Res 2021;17(1):207.

30. Bozynski CC, Stannard JP, Smith P, et al. Acute Management of Anterior Cruciate Ligament Injuries Using Novel Canine Models. J Knee Surg 2016;29(7): 594–603.
31. Cook JL, Smith PA, Bozynski CC, et al. Multiple injections of leukoreduced platelet rich plasma reduce pain and functional impairment in a canine model of ACL and meniscal deficiency. J Orthop Res 2016;34(4):607–15.
32. Xie X, Wu H, Zhao S, et al. The effect of platelet-rich plasma on patterns of gene expression in a dog model of anterior cruciate ligament reconstruction. J Surg Res 2013;180(1):80–8.
33. Xie X, Zhao S, Wu H, et al. Platelet-rich plasma enhances autograft revascularization and reinnervation in a dog model of anterior cruciate ligament reconstruction. J Surg Res 2013;183(1):214–22.
34. Carr JB 2nd, Rodeo SA. The role of biologic agents in the management of common shoulder pathologies: current state and future directions. J Shoulder Elbow Surg 2019;28(11):2041–52.
35. Brossi PM, Moreira JJ, Machado TS, et al. Platelet-rich plasma in orthopedic therapy: a comparative systematic review of clinical and experimental data in equine and human musculoskeletal lesions. BMC Vet Res 2015;11:98.
36. Mishra A, Pavelko T. Treatment of chronic elbow tendinosis with buffered platelet-rich plasma. Am J Sports Med 2006;34(11):1774–8.
37. Fitzpatrick J, Bulsara M, Zheng MH. The Effectiveness of Platelet-Rich Plasma in the Treatment of Tendinopathy: A Meta-analysis of Randomized Controlled Clinical Trials. Am J Sports Med 2017;45(1):226–33. PMID: 27268111.
38. Zhou Y, Wang JH. PRP Treatment Efficacy for Tendinopathy: A Review of Basic Science Studies. Biomed Res Int 2016;2016:9103792.
39. de Jonge S, de Vos RJ, Weir A, et al. One-year follow-up of platelet-rich plasma treatment in chronic Achilles tendinopathy: a double-blind randomized placebo-controlled trial. Am J Sports Med 2011;39(8):1623–9.
40. Gosens T, Peerbooms JC, van Laar W, et al. Ongoing positive effect of platelet-rich plasma versus corticosteroid injection in lateral epicondylitis: a double-blind randomized controlled trial with 2-year follow-up. Am J Sports Med 2011;39(6): 1200–8.
41. Krogh TP, Fredberg U, Stengaard-Pedersen K, et al. Treatment of lateral epicondylitis with platelet-rich plasma, glucocorticoid, or saline: a randomized, double-blind, placebo-controlled trial. Am J Sports Med 2013;41(3):625–35.
42. Peerbooms JC, Sluimer J, Bruijn DJ, et al. Positive effect of an autologous platelet concentrate in lateral epicondylitis in a double-blind randomized controlled trial: platelet-rich plasma versus corticosteroid injection with a 1-year follow-up. Am J Sports Med 2010;38(2):255–62.
43. Thanasas C, Papadimitriou G, Charalambidis C, et al. Platelet-rich plasma versus autologous whole blood for the treatment of chronic lateral elbow epicondylitis: a randomized controlled clinical trial. Am J Sports Med 2011;39(10): 2130–4.
44. Montano C, Auletta L, Greco A, et al. The Use of Platelet-Rich Plasma for Treatment of Tenodesmic Lesions in Horses: A Systematic Review and Meta-Analysis of Clinical and Experimental Data. Animals (Basel) 2021;11(3):793.
45. Geburek F, Gaus M, van Schie HT, et al. Effect of intralesional platelet-rich plasma (PRP) treatment on clinical and ultrasonographic parameters in equine naturally occurring superficial digital flexor tendinopathies - a randomized prospective controlled clinical trial. BMC Vet Res 2016;12(1):191.

46. Ho LK, Baltzer WI, Nemanic S, et al. Single ultrasound-guided platelet-rich plasma injection for treatment of supraspinatus tendinopathy in dogs. Can Vet J 2015;56(8):845–9.
47. Wang SZ, Fan WM, Jia J, et al. Is exclusion of leukocytes from platelet-rich plasma (PRP) a better choice for early intervertebral disc regeneration? Stem Cell Res Ther 2018;9(1):199.
48. Dohan Ehrenfest DM, Doglioli P, de Peppo GM, et al. Choukroun's platelet-rich fibrin (PRF) stimulates in vitro proliferation and differentiation of human oral bone mesenchymal stem cell in a dose-dependent way. Arch Oral Biol 2010;55: 185–94.
49. Filardo G, Kon E, Roffi A, et al. Platelet rich plasma: why intra-articular? A systematic review of preclinical studies and clinical evidence on PRP for joint degeneration. Knee Surg Sports Traumatol Arthrosc 2013;23(9):2459–74.
50. McLellan J, Plevin S. Does it matter which platelet-rich plasma we use? Equine Vet Educ 2011;23(2):101–4.
51. Dragoo JL, Braun HJ, Durham JL, et al. Comparison of the acute inflammatory response of two commercial platelet- rich plasma systems in healthy rabbit tendons. Am J Sports Med 2012;40(6):1274–81.
52. McCarrel T, Fortier L. Temporal growth factor release from platelet-rich plasma, trehalose lyophilized platelets, and bone marrow aspirate and heir effect on tendon and ligament gene expression. J Orthop Res 2009;27(8):1033–42.
53. McCarrel TM, Minas T, Fortier LA. Optimization of leukocyte concentration in platelet-rich plasma for the treatment of tendinopathy. J Bone Joint Surg Am 2012;94(1–8):e143.
54. Braun HJ, Kim HJ, Chu CR, et al. The effect of platelet-rich plasma formulations and blood products on human synoviocytes. Am J Sports Med 2014;42(5): 1204–10.
55. Sundman EA, Cole BJ, Fortier LA. Growth factor and catabolic cytokine concentrations are influenced by the cellular composition of platelet-rich plasma. Am J Sports Med 2013;39(10):2135–40.
56. Sundman EA, Cole BJ, Karas V, et al. The anti-inflammatory and matrix restorative mechanisms of platelet- rich plasma in osteoarthritis. Am J Sports Med 2013;42(1):35–41.
57. Sundman EA, Boswell SG, Schnabel LV, et al. Increasing platelet concentrations in leukocyte-reduced platelet-rich plasma decrease collagen gene synthesis in tendons. Am J Sports Med 2013;42(1):35–41.
58. Boswell SG, Schnabel LV, Mohammed HO, et al. Increasing platelet concentrations in leukocyte-reduced platelet-rich plasma decrease collagen gene synthesis in tendons. Am J Sports Med 2013;42(1):42–9.
59. Castillo TN, Pouliot MA, Kim HJ, et al. Comparison of growth factor and platelet concentrations from commercial platelet-rich plasma separation systems. Am J Sports Med 2011;39(2):266–71.
60. Stief M, Gottschalk J, Ionita JC, et al. Concentration of platelets and growth factors in canine autologous conditioned plasma. Vet Comp Orthop Traumatol 2011;24:285–90.
61. Cavallo C, Filardo G, Mariani E, et al. Comparison of platelet-rich plasma formulations for cartilage healing. J Bone Joint Surg Am 2014;96:423–9.
62. Zhou Y, Zhang J, Wu H, et al. The differential effects of leukocyte-containing and pure platelet-rich plasma (PRP) on tendon stem/progenitor cells - implications of PRP application for the clinical treatment of tendon injuries. Stem Cell Res Ther 2015;6(1):173.

63. Hsu WK, Mishra A, Rodeo SR, et al. Platelet- rich plasma in orthopaedic applications: evidence-based recommendations for treatment. J Am Acad Orthop Surg 2013;21:739–48.
64. Pelletier MH, Malhotra A, Brighton T, et al. Platelet function and constituents of platelet rich plasma. Int J Sports Med 2013;34:74–80.
65. Oudelaar BW, Peerbooms JC, Huis In 't Veld R, et al. Concentrations of Blood Components in Commercial Platelet-Rich Plasma Separation Systems: A Review of the Literature. Am J Sports Med 2019;47(2):479–87.
66. Lansdown DA, Fortier LA. Platelet-rich plasma: formulations, preparations, constituents, and their effects. Oper Tech Sports Med 2017;25(1):7–12.
67. Mariani E, Pulsatelli L. Platelet Concentrates in Musculoskeletal Medicine. Int J Mol Sci 2020;21(4):1328.
68. Nguyen PA, Pham TAV. Effects of platelet-rich plasma on human gingival fibroblast proliferation and migration in vitro. J Appl Oral Sci 2018;26:e20180077.
69. Vahabi S, Yadegari Z, Mohammad-Rahimi H. Comparison of the effect of activated or non-activated PRP in various concentrations on osteoblast and fibroblast cell line proliferation [published correction appears in Cell Tissue Bank. Cell Tissue Bank 2017;18(3):347–53.
70. Weibrich G, Hansen T, Kleis W, et al. Effect of platelet concentration in platelet-rich plasma on peri-implant bone regeneration. Bone 2004;34(4):665–71.
71. Naldini A, Morena E, Fimiani M, et al. The effects of autologous platelet gel on inflammatory cytokine response in human peripheral blood mononuclear cells. Platelets 2008;19(4):268–74.
72. Yoshida R, Murray MM. Peripheral blood mononuclear cells enhance the anabolic effects of platelet-rich plasma on anterior cruciate ligament fibroblasts. J Orthop Res 2013;31(1):29–34.
73. Lana JFSD, Purita J, Paulus C, et al. Contributions for classification of platelet rich plasma - proposal of a new classification: MARSPILL. Regen Med 2017; 12(5):565–74.
74. Magalon J, Chateau AL, Bertrand B, et al. DEPA classification: a proposal for standardising PRP use and a retrospective application of available devices. BMJ Open Sport Exerc Med 2016;2(1):e000060.
75. Fukuda K, Kuroda T, Tamura N, et al. Optimal activation methods for maximizing the concentrations of platelet-derived growth factor-BB and transforming growth factor-β1 in equine platelet-rich plasma. J Vet Med Sci 2020;82(10):1472–9.
76. Pachito DV, Bagattini ÂM, de Almeida AM, et al. Technical Procedures for Preparation and Administration of Platelet-Rich Plasma and Related Products: A Scoping Review. Front Cell Dev Biol 2020;8:598816.
77. Textor JA, Norris JW, Tablin F. Effects of preparation method, shear force, and exposure to collagen on release of growth factors from equine platelet-rich plasma. Am J Vet Res 2011;72(2):271–8.
78. Roffi A, Filardo G, Assirelli E, et al. Does platelet-rich plasma freeze-thawing influence growth factor release and their effects on chondrocytes and synoviocytes? Biomed Res Int 2014;2014:692913.
79. Baldini M, Costea N, Dameshek W. The viability of stored human platelets. Blood 1960;16:1669–92.
80. Reid TJ, LaRussa VF, Esteban G, et al. Cooling and freezing damage platelet membrane integrity. Cryobiology 1999;38(3):209–24.
81. Franklin SP, Birdwhistell KE, Strelchik A, et al. Influence of Cellular Composition and Exogenous Activation on Growth Factor and Cytokine Concentrations in

Canine Platelet-Rich Plasmas. Front Vet Sci 2017;4:40. https://doi.org/10.3389/fvets.2017.00040.
82. Zhevago NA, Samoilova KA. Pro- and anti-inflammatory cytokine content in human peripheral blood after its transcutaneous (in vivo) and direct (in vitro) irradiation with polychromatic visible and infrared light. Photomed Laser Surg 2006; 24(2):129–39.
83. Freitag JB, Barnard A. To evaluate the effect of combining photo-activation therapy with platelet-rich plasma injections for the novel treatment of osteoarthritis. BMJ Case Rep 2013;2013:bcr2012007463. https://doi.org/10.1136/bcr-2012-007463.
84. Paterson KL, Nicholls M, Bennell KL, et al. Intra-articular injection of photo-activated platelet-rich plasma in patients with knee osteoarthritis: a double-blind, randomized controlled pilot study. BMC Musculoskelet Disord 2016;17:67. https://doi.org/10.1186/s12891-016-0920-3.
85. Irmak G, Demirtaş TT, Gümüşderelioğlu M. Sustained release of growth factors from photoactivated platelet rich plasma (PRP). Eur J Pharm Biopharm 2020; 148:67–76. https://doi.org/10.1016/j.ejpb.2019.11.011.
86. Seabaugh KA, Thoresen M, Giguère S. Extracorporeal Shockwave Therapy Increases Growth Factor Release from Equine Platelet-Rich Plasma *In Vitro*. Front Vet Sci 2017;4:205. https://doi.org/10.3389/fvets.2017.00205.
87. Frye CW, Enders A, Brooks MB, et al. Assessment of canine autologous platelet-rich plasma produced with a commercial centrifugation and platelet recovery kit. Vet Comp Orthop Traumatol 2016;29(1):14–9.
88. Alessio-Mazzola M, Lovisolo S, Sonzogni B, et al. Clinical outcome and risk factor predictive for failure of autologous PRP injections for low-to-moderate knee osteoarthritis. J Orthop Surg (Hong Kong) 2021;29(2). 23094990211021922.
89. Sano K, Takai Y, Yamanishi J, et al. A role of calcium-activated phospholipid-dependent protein kinase in human platelet activation. Comparison of thrombin and collagen actions. J Biol Chem 1983;258(3):2010–3.
90. Harrison S, Vavken P, Kevy S, et al. Platelet activation by collagen provides sustained release of anabolic cytokines. Am J Sports Med 2011;39(4):729–34.
91. Fufa D, Shealy B, Jacobson M, et al. Activation of platelet-rich plasma using soluble type I collagen. J Oral Maxillofac Surg 2008;66(4):684–90.
92. Arora S, Agnihotri N. Platelet-derived biomaterials for therapeutic use: review of technical aspects. Indian J Hematol Blood Transfus 2017;33:159–67.
93. Collins T, Alexander D, Barkatali B. Platelet-rich plasma: a narrative review. EFORT Open Rev 2021;6(4):225–35.
94. González JC, López C, Carmona JU. Implications of anticoagulants and gender on cell counts and growth factor concentration in platelet-rich plasma and platelet-rich gel supernatants from rabbits. Vet Comp Orthop Traumatol 2016; 29(2):115–24.
95. McClain AK, McCarrel TM. The effect of four different freezing conditions and time in frozen storage on the concentration of commonly measured growth factors and enzymes in equine platelet-rich plasma over six months. BMC Vet Res 2019;15:292. https://doi.org/10.1186/s12917-019-2040-4.
96. Kaux JF, Libertiaux V, Dupont L, et al. Platelet-rich plasma (PRP) and tendon healing: comparison between fresh and frozen-thawed PRP. Platelets 2020; 31(2):221–5.
97. Ljungkvist M, Lövdahl S, Zetterberg E, et al. Low agreement between fresh and frozen-thawed platelet-rich plasma in the calibrated automated thrombogram assay. Haemophilia 2017;23(3):e214–8.

98. Milants C, Bruyère O, Kaux JF. Responders to Platelet-Rich Plasma in Osteoarthritis: A Technical Analysis. Biomed Res Int 2017;2017:7538604.
99. Sonker A, Dubey A. Determining the Effect of Preparation and Storage: An Effort to Streamline Platelet Components as a Source of Growth Factors for Clinical Application. Transfus Med Hemother 2015;42(3):174–80.
100. Dhurat R, Sukesh M. Principles and methods of preparation of platelet-rich plasma: a review and author's perspective. J Cutan Aesthet Surg 2014;7: 189–97.
101. Gupta V, Parihar AS, Pathak M, et al. Comparison of Platelet-Rich Plasma Prepared Using Two Methods: Manual Double Spin Method versus a Commercially Available Automated Device. Indian Dermatol Online J 2020;11(4):575–9.
102. Franklin SP, Garner BC, Cook JL. Characteristics of canine platelet-rich plasma prepared with five commercially available systems. Am J Vet Res 2015;76(9): 822–7.
103. Carr BJ, Canapp SO Jr, Mason DR, et al. Canine Platelet-Rich Plasma Systems: A Prospective Analysis. Front Vet Sci 2016;2:73.
104. Ferrari JT, Schwartz P. Prospective Evaluation of Feline Sourced Platelet-Rich Plasma Using Centrifuge-Based Systems. Front Vet Sci 2020;7:322. https://doi.org/10.3389/fvets.2020.00322.
105. Chun N, Canapp S, Carr BJ, et al. Validation and Characterization of Platelet-Rich Plasma in the Feline: A Prospective Analysis. Front Vet Sci 2020;7:512. https://doi.org/10.3389/fvets.2020.00512.
106. Franklin SP. Canine autologous conditioned plasma using the Arthrex ACP® System: a brief review of the evidence. Fort Myers, FL: Arthrex® Vet Systems; 2018.
107. Dohan Ehrenfest DM, Rasmusson L, Albrektsson T. Classification of platelet concentrates: from pure platelet-rich plasma (P-PRP) to leucocyte- and platelet-rich fibrin (L-PRF). Trends Biotechnol 2009;27:158–67.
108. Delong JM, Russell RP, Mazzocca AD. Platelet-rich plasma: the PAW classification system. Arthroscopy 2012;28:998–1009.
109. Rossi LA, Murray IR, Chu CR, et al. Classification systems for platelet-rich plasma. Bone Joint J 2019;101-B(8):891–6. https://doi.org/10.1302/0301-620X.101B8.BJJ-2019-0037.R1.
110. Sharun Khan, M Pawde Abhijit. Universal Classification System for Platelet-Rich Plasma (PRP): A Method to Define the Variables in PRP Production. Burns 2021; 47.2:488–9.
111. Mautner K, Malanga GA, Smith J, et al. A call for a standard classification system for future biologic research: the rationale for new PRP nomenclature. PM R 2015;7. S53–S59.
112. Magalon J, Chateau AL, Bertrand B, et al. DEPA classification: a proposal for standardising PRP use and a retrospective application of available devices. BMJ Open Sport Exerc Med 2016;2:e000060.
113. Harrison P. Subcommittee on Platelet Physiology. The use of platelets in regenerative medicine and proposal for a new classification system: guidance from the SSC of the ISTH. J Thromb Haemost 2018;16(9):1895–900.
114. Eymard F, Ornetti P, Maillet J, et al. Correction to: Intra-articular injections of platelet-rich plasma in symptomatic knee osteoarthritis: a consensus statement from French-speaking experts. Knee Surg Sports Traumatol Arthrosc 2021; 29(10):3211–2.

115. Di Matteo B, Filardo G, Lo Presti M, et al. Chronic anti-platelet therapy: a contraindication for platelet-rich plasma intra-articular injections? Eur Rev Med Pharmacol Sci 2014;18(1 Suppl):55–9.
116. Eliasberg CD, Nemirov DA, Mandelbaum BR, et al. Complications Following Biologic Therapeutic Injections: A Multicenter Case Series. Arthroscopy 2021; 37(8):2600–5.
117. Frey C, Yeh PC, Jayaram P. Effects of Antiplatelet and Nonsteroidal Anti-inflammatory Medications on Platelet-Rich Plasma: A Systematic Review. Orthop J Sports Med 2020;8(4). 2325967120912841.
118. Magruder M, Rodeo SA. Is Antiplatelet Therapy Contraindicated After Platelet-Rich Plasma Treatment? A Narrative Review. Orthop J Sports Med 2021;9(6). 23259671211010510.
119. Ludwig HC, Birdwhistell KE, Brainard BM, et al. Use of a Cyclooxygenase-2 Inhibitor Does Not Inhibit Platelet Activation or Growth Factor Release From Platelet-Rich Plasma. Am J Sports Med 2017;45(14):3351–7.
120. Görmeli G, Görmeli CA, Ataoglu B, et al. Multiple PRP injections are more effective than single injections and hyaluronic acid in knees with early osteoarthritis: a randomized, double-blind, placebo-controlled trial. Knee Surg Sports Traumatol Arthrosc 2017;25(3):958–65.
121. Huang PH, Wang CJ, Chou WY, et al. Short-term clinical results of intra-articular PRP injections for early osteoarthritis of the knee. Int J Surg 2017;42:117–22.
122. Kavadar G, Demircioglu DT, Celik MY, et al. Effectiveness of platelet-rich plasma in the treatment of moderate knee osteoarthritis: a randomized prospective study. J Phys Ther Sci 2015;27(12):3863–7.

Physical Rehabilitation for Small Animals

Lauri-Jo Gamble, DVM, DACVSMR, CCRP, CVA

KEYWORDS

• Canine rehabilitation • Therapeutic exercises • Hydrotherapy • Manual therapy • Physical modalities

KEY POINTS

- Therapeutic exercise programs can address gait retraining, proprioception, balance, muscle strengthening, and endurance. Common therapeutic exercise equipment includes physioball, cavaletti rails, fitbone, balance disc, other balance block, rocker board, wobble board, resistance band, land treadmill, underwater treadmill, and swimming pool.
- Specialized manual skills are used extensively in evaluating and treating the rehabilitation patient. Manual treatment involves various soft tissue techniques, specific stretching techniques, passive range of motion, joint mobilization (including glides and traction), and massage.
- Physical modalities are tools that can be used to enhance a patient's rehabilitation treatment plan through use of thermal, sound, electrical, and light therapy to impact the physiology of the target tissue.

INTRODUCTION

Rehabilitation is a rapidly growing field in veterinary medicine; there is a strong interest on the part of the veterinary profession to learn more about sports medicine and rehabilitation to optimize patient outcomes following injury, surgery, and illness.

Rehabilitation can be offered in pre- and postoperative settings, as a conservative, nonoperative option, and to assist with management of palliative conditions. Investigators of multiple studies have reported beneficial effects of physical rehabilitation on the outcome of various disorders in veterinary patients. Studies have notably shown improved comfort and limb function following cranial cruciate ligament repair,[1–7] improved comfort in dogs with hip dysplasia,[8] improved weight loss rate,[9,10] increased survival time in dogs with degenerative myelopathy,[11] and improved outcome with spinal cord lesions in dogs[12–17] and in cats.[18] Rehabilitation therapy can facilitate recovery from surgery, improve functional status, alleviate pain, and result in a better quality of life.

The author has nothing to disclose; there are no commercial or financial conflicts of interest.
Sports Medicine and Rehabilitation Service, Ottawa Animal Emergency and Specialty Hospital, 1155 Lola Street, Suite 201, Ottawa K1K 4C1, Canada
E-mail address: lgamble@oaesh.com

Vet Clin Small Anim 52 (2022) 997–1019
https://doi.org/10.1016/j.cvsm.2022.03.005
vetsmall.theclinics.com

Abbreviations	
AROM	Active range of motion
NMES	Neuromuscular electrical stimulation
PEMF	Pulsed electromagnetic field
PROM	Passive range of motion
ROM	Range of motion
TENS	Transcutaneous electrical nerve stimulation
UWTM	Underwater treadmill

Physical rehabilitation, and more specifically formal physical rehabilitation in the clinic or hospital setting, can be subdivided into therapeutic exercises, manual therapy, and physical agent modalities. Some techniques are more useful at different stages in order to achieve optimum tissue healing and recovery of function (the reader is advised to view other sources[19–22]).

DISCUSSION

Therapeutic Exercises

Therapeutic exercises can be beneficial to postoperative patients, pets with osteoarthritis or soft tissue injury, and elite athletes with the goal of peak performance. Therapeutic exercises are used to improve active joint range of motion (AROM), weight bearing, posture, and gait, as well as build strength and muscle mass and increase conditioning (endurance, speed, proprioception). Therapeutic exercise programs should begin with low-level activities and progress to higher-level activities while incorporating various exercises to prevent boredom in the owner and patient while allowing appropriate progression of load to the tissues. They should be tailored to the activities the patient is expected to perform and focus on functional goals while also offering a broader comprehensive whole-body fitness. Exercise programs should be personalized individually to reflect the patient signalment and temperament, the owner compliance, the chronicity, type of injury, and level of required functional recovery.

Therapeutic exercises can either generate an isometric, concentric or eccentric muscular contraction. During an isometric contraction, the muscle generates tension without changing length; the muscle force is equal to the resistance. During a concentric contraction, the muscle force is greater than the resistance; therefore the length of the muscle shortens. While during an eccentric contraction, the muscle force is less than the resistance, and muscle lengthening occurs. Another way to classify exercises is based on their purpose, such as exercises aimed at promoting joint motion, core stability, proprioceptive, strength, endurance, and speed exercises. Strength exercises are performed with maximal or near-maximal muscle contraction, with relatively few repetitions, which results in muscle hypertrophy. Endurance exercises are performed with relatively little load applied to the muscle, but with repetitive contractions over a prolonged time, resulting in increased aerobic capacity.

Injury will cause a cascade of changes in the neuromuscular system, such as muscle recruitment patterns, neural firing patterns, neural firing rates, and more. This results in altered biomechanics and ineffective load distribution, resulting in a breakdown of the kinetic chain. Before creating any exercise program, the therapist should evaluate stance posture, transitions (sit to down, down to stand, sit to stand), and gait pattern in addition to usual orthopedic, neurologic, and muscular examinations. Strengthening alone is not an appropriate rehabilitation strategy; the cause of the weakness needs to be addressed, and the active use of the area needs to be restored. When designing an exercise protocol for a patient, the most important factor is to identify the patient's problems and limitations (specific impairments). Other patient considerations such as motivation, footing, assistive devices, and leash/harness control should also be assessed. After the patient is taught each exercise, these should be re-evaluated periodically, and the program should be modified accordingly.

Therapeutic exercises designed to improve joint motion (joint variable depending on the specific exercise) include incline walking, stair climbing, dancing, wheelbarrowing, sit-to-stand, cavalettis rails, underwater treadmill walking, and swimming.[19] Exercises improving strength include incline and decline walking, stair climbing, backward walking, side stepping, land treadmill and underwater treadmill activity with resistance, pulling or carrying weights, and jumping.[19] Conditioning exercises include jogging, running, playing ball, and sports-specific activities.[20] More information regarding home exercises for various conditions can be found elsewhere in this issue.

When performing therapeutic exercises and rehabilitation treatments in the clinic, special considerations regarding the design of the space is essential. Flooring with traction is paramount to avoid slipping, particularly for weak and neurologic patients. The hospital flooring can be modified by using yoga mats, runners, or foam puzzles. It is also important to have adequate space to perform treatments with as little interruption as possible, especially if other pets can be distractions to the patient. For the pets' safety, harness or leash should be used to guide them. Motivation should be provided with high-value treats. Timing of delivery of the treat is critical; it should be done immediately upon the patient demonstrating the correct behavior. For some exercises, where constant attention is desired, a frozen peanut butter mug or frozen cheese cup can be used. During therapeutic exercises, therapists should watch carefully for signs of fatigue, notably excessive panting, spade-shaped tongue, elevated heart rate, drooping tail or ears, trembling muscles, gait changes or refusal to continue. The patient should also be assessed the next day by their owner. If stiffness or soreness is reported, the intensity and/or the duration of the program should be decreased in the following session.

The following is a descriptive of some common therapeutic exercises and material used in the clinic.

Cavaletti rails

Cavalettis rails can be commercially purchased or created with broomstick, pool noodles, or PVC pipe and laundry basket, cone, or wood structure. Three to eight rails are ideal depending on available space, particularly if stride lengthening is a primary goal. The distance between rails is ideally just wide enough to allow for a single step between the rails at a normal gait speed; the faster the gait, the wider the poles should be placed. Height should be set slightly above the dog's carpus or below the tarsus, although with significantly paretic animals, the poles may need to be lower. Patients are asked to step over the poles without touching them for enhancing balance, coordination and proprioception, improving weight-bearing, and elongating stride length. Cavaletti rail walking has also been shown to increase range of motion (ROM), especially flexion, in elbow, carpus, stifle, and tarsus.[23] It can be performed first at a walk and for further challenge can be done at trot, over unstable surfaces or balance equipment (**Fig. 1**), over incline, into a circle or with various widths, heights, and patterns. Stepping over cavaletti rails has also been shown to increase engagement of the vastus lateralis and gluteus medius muscles, making it a valuable exercise for pelvic limb strengthening.[24] Cavaletti rails can also be raised to create a limbo dance to promote crawling. Crawling motion is beneficial to promote flexion while strengthening the supporting musculature that hold the joints into this more flexed position.

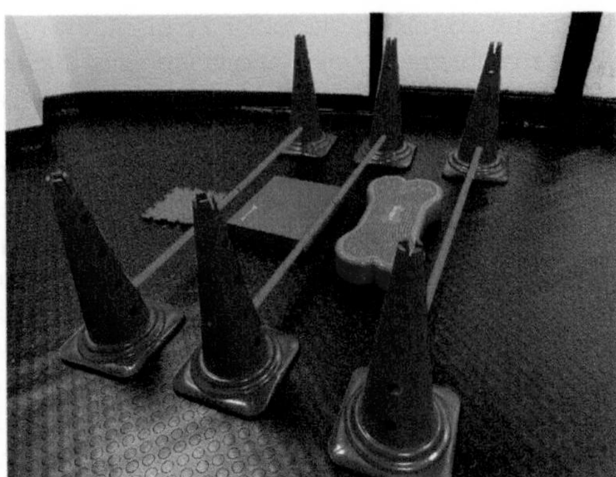

Fig. 1. Cavaletti rails. Standard cavaletti rails are here used in combination with unstable surfaces (fitbones, foam block, textured flooring) to increase difficulty.

Physioball and physioroll, foam block, wobble board, rocker board, fitbone, balance disc

Unstable surfaces (**Fig. 2**) can be used to focus on balance as well as core and stabilizer muscle strengthening. This can be achieved by performing various exercises such as sit-to-stands, down-to-stands, cookie stretches, planking, 2- or 3-legged

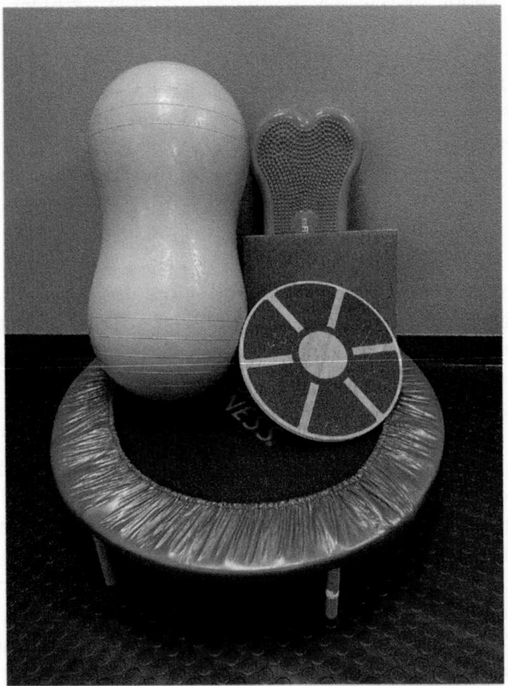

Fig. 2. Various unstable surfaces. This picture shows a physioball (in blue), a fitbone (in pink), a foam block (in purple), a wobble board (in wood) and a trampoline. These tools can be used to focus on balance and core and stabilizer muscle strengthening. Please also notice nonslippery flooring being using in the clinic setting.

standing, or elevated forelimbs on physiorolls, foam blocks, balance discs, or fitbones. Rocker boards and wobble boards differ in the directional movement they provide; rocker boards offer unidirectional movement, while wobble boards create a multidirectional movement. To make balance exercises more difficult, the patient may have 2 limbs on one unstable surface and the other 2 limbs elevated or on another unstable surface (**Fig. 3**). It has been demonstrated that these therapeutic exercises can increase muscle activity, to varying degrees, in the musculature of the pelvic limbs, especially vastus lateralis, biceps femoris, and gluteus medius.[25]

Physioball and trampoline can be used for rhythmic stabilization and perturbation exercises. Rhythmic stabilization is a technique used to strengthen postural muscles in dogs, particularly the triceps and quadriceps muscle groups, while also providing neuromuscular feedback to joints, ligaments, and muscle-tendon unit. This isometric exercise generates rapid firing of postural muscle, and it is ideal for non- to weakly ambulatory or significantly ataxic patients, but also for athletic patients. The animal should be standing squarely (supported by the physioball if weak) or directly on a trampoline or inflated mattress while the therapist provides gentle pressure over the pelvis or cranial thoracic region and gently bounces the animal up and down. Alternatively, weight shifting side to side can also be performed. The motion should be relatively rapid, with only enough recovery time to regain the normal standing position. It generates isometric contractions of agonist and antagonist muscles against resistance without movement intention.[19,20]

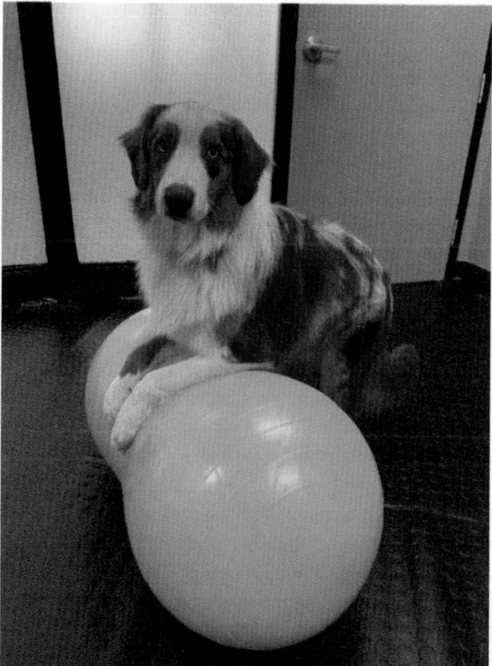

Fig. 3. A patient resting while performing rocking on a physioroll. A physioroll can be used with the thoracic or the pelvic limbs or even all 4 limbs to improve proprioception, balance, flexibility and core strength. In this case, the dog has its forelimbs on the physioroll with his hind limbs on the ground. The therapist would rock the dog back and forth to challenge his balance.

Incline, stairs, and ramps

Walking up an incline (either a ramp, hill or while walking on a land treadmill) results in increased flexion, extension, and ROM of the hip, shoulder extension and ROM, elbow flexion and extension, and carpal flexion while decreasing stifle extension.[23,26] Incline walking may also be useful to improve limb use or limb weight bearing due to the shift in the patient's center of gravity and engages pelvic limbs' musculature.[25,27] In contrast, decline walking causes less flexion and overall, less ROM of the hip joint.[23,28]

Similar to incline walking, climbing stairs can also be useful to improve ROM and strengthen the pelvic limbs' extensors (quadriceps and gluteals). More specifically, ascending stairs increases hip extension, stifle flexion, tarsal extension and flexion, shoulder flexion, and elbow and carpal flexion, extension, and ROM.[26,29] It has been shown that descending stairs affects ROM differently than decline walking on an equivalent ramp. Stair descent results in increased hip ROM, stifle flexion, and tarsal flexion and extension as well as greater elbow and shoulder ROM compared with ramp descent.[28,30]

Resistance bands

Resistance to a specific limb or muscle group can be added during therapeutic exercise by using an elastic resistance band. Theraband can be secure to the involved extremity, and the therapist can provide resistance on the opposite end. For example, lateral tension can be applied to the band while walking on a land treadmill to enhance contraction of the adductor muscles. Resistance bands may also be used in aquatic therapy.

Land treadmill

Land treadmills are excellent tools for various exercises ranging from improving limb use after surgery, to improving gait patterning in neurologic patients to increasing strength and endurance in high-level athletes.[19,20]

Canine-specific treadmills are ideal, as they have longer belts that enable medium and large dogs to trot comfortably and have railings on the sides to discourage jumping off while beginning at a lower speed (0.2 m/s or less). Incline and/or decline capacity and the ability to move the belt in reverse are useful features. One downside to canine treadmills is that the belt is narrower than human treadmill belts, so the therapist cannot walk on the belt with the patient. Instead, the handler is generally in front or beside the dog to ensure safety and provide positive rewards. Treadmills should not be facing a wall or have frequent distractions arising from behind them. Ideally, harnesses should be used as they are more comfortable and prevent excessive pulling on the neck.

Dogs can generally be easily trained to walk on a treadmill, especially with positive rewards in the form of food, praise, or toys. For introductory sessions to the treadmill, several repetitions of short intervals (5–15 seconds) are generally more successful than 1 prolonged episode. Release of pressure in the form of stopping the treadmill belt as soon as the dog voluntarily walks forward is also important. Patients should always be directly supervised and closely monitored for signs of fatigue, such as pulling on the harness, stumbling, or drifting side to side.

A warm-up period of walking and then fast walking is recommended before trotting on a treadmill. When changing speed of the treadmill, it is important to do it fairly rapidly to reach the speed of a comfortable trot from a walk to avoid an awkward transition for the dog. Most medium to large dogs can walk comfortably at a speed of 0.9 to 1.2 m/s, while they can trot at 1.7 to 2 m/s.[19] To target endurance, walking or jogging duration and speed can be increased; strengthening of the target limbs can

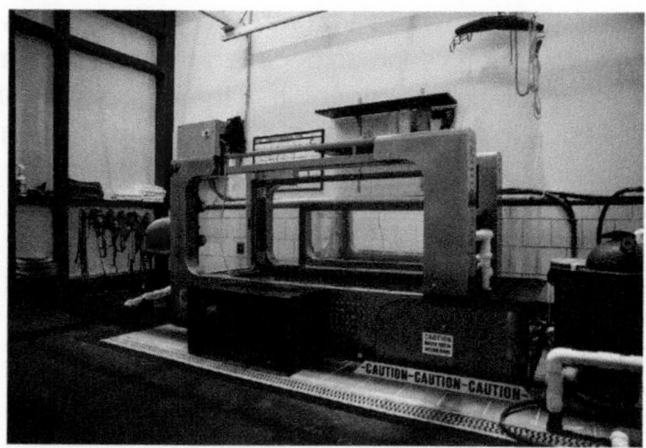

Fig. 4. Underwater treadmill room. Equipment frequently needed while using the underwater treadmill include harnesses, treats, bench, mirror, ceiling mounted hoist lift, equipment to clean and maintain water tank. Photo Darcy Rose/Cornell University College of Veterinary Medicine.

be achieved by inclining or declining the treadmill. Additional modifications can be applied by using resistance bands. Lateral work can also be accomplished placing the forelimbs on the treadmill and the hind limbs on a solid platform or vice versa. For added challenges, the solid platform can be replaced by an unstable surface, such as a paw pod or physioroll. These are high-level exercises that can be beneficial for isolated limb strengthening and core activation, but they should only be attempted once the dog is comfortable with regular treadmill exercise.

Aquatic therapies

Hydrotherapy has specific properties such as buoyancy, hydrostatic pressure, resistance (viscosity), and surface tension that result in decreased stress on the joints, improved strength, enhanced cardiorespiratory and muscular endurance, and greater range of motion. The metabolic requirements are also greater for exercises performed in water than on land. Incorporation of underwater treadmill (UWTM) exercise regimen in conventional canine weight management programs has been shown to be beneficial.[10] Hydrostatic pressure helps to reduce edema, while buoyance provides support, making water exercises less painful than exercise on land. Water is generally kept between 28 to 30°C.[31] Warmer temperatures can be beneficial for muscles relaxation, while cooler temperatures allow for more vigorous exercises. Warm water temperature also increases circulation, caloric expenditure, nerve conduction velocity, and coordination, and allows for increased soft tissue elasticity. However, a study in toy breed dogs recommended a temperature of 33°C or lower to prevent tachycardia, hyperventilation, and hyperthermia while swimming.[32]

Useful aquatic therapy equipment includes: UWTM, swimming pool or whirlpool (while bathtubs or plastic pools can be a cost-effective option for smaller dogs), pet life preserver, toys, harness, protective clothing for the therapist (wetsuit, gaiters), bench for the therapist, mirror to evaluate patients' gait, ceiling-mounted hoist lift to provide additional support in weak or nonambulatory patients, equipment to clean and maintain water tanks, and chlorine or bromine to sanitize the water (**Fig. 4**).

Aquatic therapy may be started at the earliest after suture removal, once the incision is sealed. Occasionally, early aquatic therapy is recommended, and sutures or staples are covered with a transparent film dressing (such as Tegaderm). For surgery such as total hip replacement, 4 weeks or more may be recommended before starting water therapy while for postsurgery neurologic rehabilitation, the timeframe will depend on the stabilization achieved. Conservative management of intervertebral disc disease should not have aquatic therapy prior to 1 month after initial insult, while medical management of neurologic conditions such as degenerative myelopathy or fibrocartilaginous emboli will often begin as soon as the patient is medically stable. Musculoskeletal conditions that do not respond well to water therapy include notably acute biceps tendinopathy and other severe muscle strains, fracture repair with external fixator, and open wounds. Precaution should be taken in patients with cardiac conditions, seizure, or incontinence.

Swimming and walking in UWTM differ in applications because of a variation in kinematics and kinetics. See **Table 1** for a comparison between swimming and underwater treadmill walking.

Underwater treadmill

Biomechanics research has shown that weight bearing can be reduced to 38% of body weight in the pelvic limbs with the water at the height of the greater trochanter. In a study performed on dogs, the amount of body weight borne when immersed in water (as a percentage of body weight on dry ground) was approximately 91% when the water was at the level of the lateral malleolus of the tibia, 85% at the level of the lateral condyle of the femur, and 38% at the level of the greater trochanter of the femur.[33] When the water is at the level of the greater trochanter, it also causes less extension of the pelvic limb joints. Joint flexion during underwater treadmill walking is greatest when the water level is at or slightly above the target joint.[34] Effect of water depth on limb kinematics should be considered when designing an exercise program, as it has a significant effect on stride frequency and stride length[35] and has an impact on gluteus medius and longissimus dorsi workload.[36] For example, one could extrapolate that patients with chronic biceps tendinopathy or medial shoulder instability may be worsened if the water level is set at or slightly above the shoulder, because increased flexion could excessively stress injured tissues. In these shoulder cases, the water level should be significantly higher than the point of the shoulder. In contrast, increased flexion is highly sought after following elbow arthroscopy, as maintaining normal elbow flexion is a primary goal. Therefore, the UWTM water level should be ideally set at or just above the elbow in those cases. Benefits from hydrotherapy have even been noted after as little as a single UWTM session in Labrador retrievers diagnosed with elbow dysplasia.[37]

UWTM walking can be beneficial for gait retraining in neurologic patients, as locomotor training promotes functional plasticity in locomotor central pattern generators

Table 1
Aquatic therapies–comparison between underwater treadmill walking and swimming

Walking in Underwater Treadmill	Swimming in Therapeutic Pool
Controlled activity allowing earlier intervention vs with swimming	Useful for weak and nonambulatory patient with severe paraparesis/paralysis
Partial weight-bearing (variable depending on water height)	Totally nonweight-bearing
Improve active range of motion compared with land (all 4 limbs)	Allow for maximum active ROM of joint (especially flexion)
Engage postural musculature and allow gait retraining	Antigravity muscles are inactive resulting in only concentric muscle contraction
Adjustable speed and water level allowing tailoring program for early postoperative conditions, moderate neurologic conditions, conditioning, and fitness	Improve endurance and cardiovascular fitness for cross-training

present in the spinal network while also affecting the characterization and quality of gait. Both land and underwater treadmill exercises have been associated with positive functional neurorehabilitation, especially with body weight-supported treadmill training in dogs with T11-L3 IVDH Hansen type I following decompressive surgery.[16,17] UWTM has also been associated with development of spinal walking (involuntary reflex gait) in paraplegic dogs and cats affected by irreversible thoracolumbar spinal cord lesion.[12,18] In the absence of superior control by the brain caused by complete spinal cord injury, the acquisition of spinal walking is made possible by dynamic interaction between the pelvic limb central pattern generator and proprioceptive feedback from the alpha-motor neurons stimulated by the rhythmicity of the gait patterning in the UWTM.

Even dogs that are fearful of water can be trained to walk in the UWTM. It can help to first have the dog walk into the underwater treadmill chamber without closing the door and without filling the water. Many newer units even have double doors, so the patient can walk through the treadmill for the first introduction. Ramps to enter and exit the treadmill are strongly recommended as even a small step up can be difficult for many patients with mobility impairments. Alternatively, some UWTM units can be recessed in relation to floor level for easier entry. Once the dog is comfortable into the contained space, starting to fill the water while a therapist is also in the UWTM with the dog can be beneficial. Most dogs learn to walk on the belt area without need for bumpers after just a few sessions, but initially floating bumpers or pool noodles can be used to prevent standing on the sides/front. Initial training steps in the UWTM are similar to the land treadmill training. Common speeds used for initiation to UWTM walking are between 0.3 and 0.5 m/s.[19] Intervals are often used during the first session for habituation (ie, 2 minutes of walking, repeated 3 times with 2-minute rest intervals). Over time, duration is increased, with a goal of up to 20 to 30 minutes of continuous walking in most cases. Additional challenge can be added by varying the speed, adding interval training, resistance jets, incline, or resistance bands (**Fig. 5**). Labored breathing or loss of the rhythmic gait pattern indicates stress or fatigue. Patients should be observed from the side, front, and back, or top. Therefore, mirrors are useful to assess the quality of joint movement and patient tolerance to activity.

Swimming

A swimming kinematics study has evaluated swimming motion in 6 breeds, ranging from Yorkshire Terrier to Newfoundland dog, and found the motion to be stereotypic

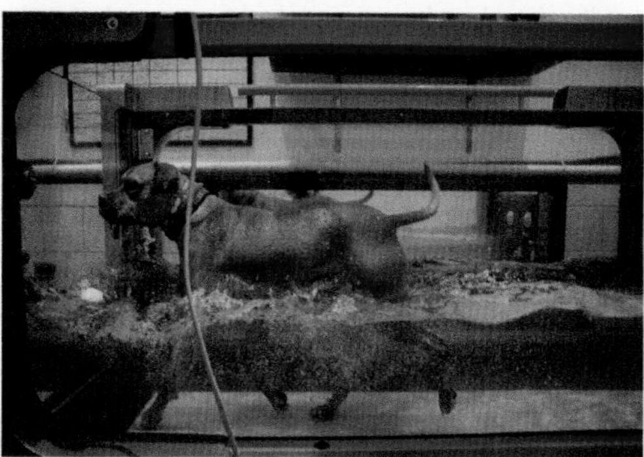

Fig. 5. Advanced patient trotting in the underwater treadmill. Notice that this patient is simply guided by praise and a ball. When first starting underwater treadmill therapy, guidance with a harness or even support from inside of the underwater treadmill is recommended. Photo Darcy Rose/Cornell University College of Veterinary Medicine.

among breeds.[38] Swimming increases pelvic limb overall ROM and individual joint flexion (especially stifle and tarsal flexion) compared with walking but may not be as useful in encouraging joint extension.[39] Swimming provides an increased cardiovascular exercise compared with UWTM walking. Therefore, weak or debilitated patients require assistance during swimming. During assisted swimming, the therapist can also provide additional perturbation by rolling the patient to stimulate a righting reflex, or create resistance to or assist with limb movement. Life-vests (personal flotation devices) can be used during swimming, especially while being introduced to swimming, not only as a safety measure, but also to provide a handle to guide the patient. However, it has been shown that usage of a flotation vest can alter ROM with less carpal and tarsal ROM, while an increase in current can generate greater ROM.[40] These factors should be considered during swimming-based rehabilitation. Challenge can be added by swimming against a current, by adding resistance, or interval swimming.

The recommended guidelines for length of time spent for aquatic exercise should be 15 to 30 minutes, depending on the breed (size) of dog.[41] Moreover, therapists should be well trained to observe sings of fatigue to prevent overexercise. Pushing the chin down, flattening the ears, and searching the pool perimeter are indicators of stress and fatigue. Other signs of fatigue include change in the swim stroke or change in the breathing pattern. Always remember to allow the dog to rest as needed.

Possible adverse effects of swimming in a chlorinated pool were evaluated in 412 dogs.[42] The reported complications included dry hair (20.63%), dry skin (18.93%), and abrasion wounds at the armpits (15.78%); these effects increased with increased frequency of swimming. Other adverse effects were red eyes (13.59%), otitis (6.31%), and a small number of respiratory problems (0.49%). No information regarding possible adverse effects of other common compounds used to disinfect swimming pool, such as bromine, ozone, and ultraviolet radiation, is available in dogs.

Vibration plate

Whole-body vibration is a platform that sends high-speed vibrations through all the body while the dog stands, sits, or lies on it. Several types of vibrating motions exist (vertical, oscillating, elliptical, 3-dimensional), as well as a large range of frequencies and intensities. As the machine vibrates, it transmits energy, forcing stabilizing muscles to contract and relax continuously. Advocates of vibration plate report improvement of flexibility, enhancement of blood flow, reduction of muscle soreness after exercises, muscle toning, and building strength. In people, vibration acceleration through whole-body vibration has been reported to promote fracture healing, prevent sarcopenia and possibly osteoporosis, improve strength in neurologic patients, and improve recovery following reconstructive anterior cruciate ligament (ACL) surgery.[43,44] However, comprehensive research is lacking, and no data are available at this time in canine patients.

Kinesiology taping

Kinesiology tape has been suggested to support the injured area by lightly adhering to the skin; it gently lifts the skin from the tissue below, which facilitates blood and lymphatic flow. It allows connective tissue surrounding the affected muscle or tendon to move along with the body. Although kinesiology taping has been shown to possibly be effective in aiding short-term pain, there is no firm evidence-based conclusion of the effectiveness for most movement disorders and in the prevention of sports injuries in people.[45,46] Despite various possible applications including tendon and ligament injuries, muscle imbalances, postural adjustments, lymphatic and circulatory condition, and acute and chronic pain, further scientific research is needed to fully understand the real effectiveness of application of kinesiology taping in animals, as little scientific evidence is available at this time.[47]

Manual Therapy

Specialized manual skills are used extensively in evaluating and treating the rehabilitation patient. Manual techniques can be used in an assessment to identify limitations in passive ROM, restrictions in arthrokinematic motion, muscle tightness, or other soft tissue abnormalities. Manual treatment involves a variety of soft tissue mobilization (including massage and myofascial release), specific stretching techniques, passive ROM (PROM), and joint mobilization (including glides and traction). Soft tissue treatments techniques are designed to address a specific tissue type and pathology, as, for example, techniques used to increase circulation and decrease edema are different than techniques used to address fascial adhesions or eliminate trigger points. Generally, using manual techniques first to resolve soft tissue and joint issues will expedite the active rehabilitation process.

Soft tissue mobilization

Soft tissue mobilization is the systematic application of manual pressure and movement of the soft tissues including skin, fascia, muscles, ligaments, and tendons. Massage performed in the morning generally helps to reduce stiffness, while evening massage relief muscular tension. Some studies have anecdotally suggested that soft tissue mobilization has a positive effect on circulation, driving fluid from the interstitial space to the vessel, which also decreases swelling.[19] Mobilization of connective tissue is also used to increase the extensibility of the tissue, to increase ROM, to prevent or reduce adhesion formation, and to increase scar mobility.[48] It has also been shown to promote healing, reduce pain, eliminate trigger points or tender areas, enhance postexercise recovery, increase function, and improve quality of life.[49,50] Commonly used massage techniques in animals include effleurage, petrissage, tapotement, cross-friction (deep friction massage), ischemic compression, trigger point pressure release, and myofascial release. The choice of technique for a particular patient will depend on the goal of treatment, the type of tissues, localization, and the pathologic state of the tissue (**Table 2**). Longitudinal strokes of moderate pressure (effleurage) will be effective for swelling, while ischemic compression will be ideal for muscle spasm treatment. There are a few contraindications to soft tissue mobilization, including over areas of mast cell tumors, thrombophlebitis, or dermatitis.

Passive range of motion, joint mobilization, and stretching

ROM is influenced by the joint type, the joint capsule, ligaments, and periarticular tendons and muscles. ROM is associated with flexibility (flexion and extension) and affected by activity, body condition, and joint health. When ROM is compromised, the body naturally compensates by increasing movement to another segment. Therefore, hypomobility to 1 joint may lead to hypermobility in the adjacent joint.

PROM is the motion of joints that results of the manipulation of the limbs by a caregiver. Early joint motion in the postoperative period has several benefits, including promoting cartilage nutrients, decreasing adhesion between tissue planes, decreasing edema, providing pain relief, and enhancing recovery.[19] Passive stretching has been shown to increase ROM, as assessed by goniometry of arthritic joints in Labrador retrievers.[51] During PROM, the therapist is moving the bony segments around a joint axis without active participation of the pet. PROM is used both as an assessment tool and a treatment technique. Normally, PROM is slightly greater than AROM, because each joint has a small amount of involuntary, end-range joint play motion

Table 2
Effects of different soft tissue mobilization techniques

Technique	Description	Effect
Effleurage	Long slow strokes Light-to-moderate pressure Parallel to the muscle fibers	Increase circulation Decrease swelling Decrease muscle spasm Increase soft tissue extensibility and ROM
Petrissage	Short, brisk strokes Moderate-to-deep pressure Parallel, perpendicular, or across the direction of the muscle fibers	Increase circulation Decrease muscle spasm Increase soft tissue extensibility and ROM
Tapotement	Rhythmic percussion Administered with tips of fingers with a stimulating stroke	Facilitate a weak muscle Increase circulation Decrease muscle spasm
Cross-friction massage	Maintained pressure Moderate digital pressure Perpendicular to desired tissue	Reduce adhesions Increase scar mobility Increase soft tissue extensibility and ROM
Ischemic compression	Sustained pressure Moderate-to-deep pressure Intentionally blocking blood flow	Eliminate trigger or tender points Decrease muscle spasm
Trigger point release	Gentle digital pressure As the trigger point tissue is released, digital pressure moves deeper into the trigger point until it resolves	Eliminate trigger or tender points Increase soft tissue extensibility and ROM
Myofascial release	Slow elongation Gentle pressure Applied in 3 planes of motion	Increase soft tissue extensibility and ROM Increase scar mobility

that the therapist can create with overpressure. To improve ROM, the end range of the movement is held for 10 to 20 seconds and repeated 3 to 5 times, while for postoperative cases, PROM involves gentle, repetitive motion of the joint in its midrange (away from full extension and full flexion) is performed for 10 to 20 repetitions, 3 to 6 times daily.[19] Previously, PROM was limited to bicycling motion of the limb, especially for home instruction; however, PROM is now explained with instructions regarding the direction of movement, the degree of force or stress to apply, and the number of repetitions and the frequency of treatment. When performing PROM, the pet should be as comfortable as possible, usually on a comfortable surface in lateral recumbency. However, PROM can also be performed in a standing position or while resting over a physioroll. Individual joints are gently flexed and extended (or abducted/adducted, rotate) through their comfortable ROM. The proximal limb of the joint of interested is stabilized, while the distal aspect is gently moved.

The goals of joint mobilization are to increase arthrokinematics ROM, improve joint alignment, decrease pain, and reduce muscle spasm by stimulating articular sensory receptors. Joint mobilization has been shown to have mechanical effects on the joint capsule that correspond with improve ROM. Different grades and techniques of mobilization can be used to treat hypomobility versus pain.

Stretching is a form of exercise in which a muscle or muscle group is maximally elongated. Stretching can be performed passively, in combination with soft tissue mobilization, or actively with specific exercise to increase muscle extensibility. Static stretching can either be the sustained elongation of muscle fibers for 10 to 60 seconds (this can be combined with PROM) or can be sustained over longer periods of time by the use of a splint or brace. A 30-second passive, static stretch is recommended, as human research has shown that carryover is more effective than a 15-second stretch.[20]

Physical Agent Modalities

Physical agent modalities are tools that can be used to enhance a patient's rehabilitation treatment plan through use of thermal, sound, electrical, and light therapy to impact the physiology of the target tissue. These tools should be used to augment and complement the treatment plan. These modalities can be effective toward reducing swelling, relieving pain, providing support, promoting tissue healing, and improving flexibility and articular ROM by affecting the elasticity of connective tissue. Understanding of the impact of each modality on different tissues is important but outside the scope of this article.

Superficial cold: cryotherapy

Cryotherapy is the therapeutic application of cold, including cold pack, ice massage, cold water baths, mechanical and electrical cold compression units, and vapocoolant sprays. Cryotherapy can be beneficial in acute inflammation, especially if pain reduction is the desired outcome. It causes vasoconstriction and decreases blood flow; it decreases both sensory and motor nerve conduction velocities. It reduces tissue metabolism and may diminish secondary hypoxic cellular injury, and it reduces swelling form acute trauma and reduces hemorrhage. Cold compression therapy is a safe modality following surgery (especially orthopedic surgeries) and tends to improve comfort and function.[3,4,21,52,53]

Cold application can provide tissue cooling 2 to 4 cm deep if applied for at least 10 minutes, but ideally 20 minutes for maximal cooling.[54] The superficial tissues such as skin and subcutaneous demonstrated the most rapid and profound cooling effect. The deeper tissues such as bone and muscle exhibited a smaller and more gradual decline in temperature.[55] However, cooling tissues for extended time or to less than 10°C can result in hunting response (arteriolar vasodilation.[19] To be safe and to avoid prolonged application, periodic inspection of the skin is recommended during treatment. Cryotherapy is rarely applied directly onto the animal skin; instead, a thin towel (moist or dry) or a protective sleeve is used.

Cryotherapy should not be used in a patient with compromised circulation, thermoregulatory disorders, or cold sensitivity, and precautions should be taken on areas of decreased sensation and open wounds. Caution should also be taken when using cryotherapy in the postoperative period, as it can delay warming.[53] Lastly, a growing body of human literature now indicates that following injury, pain-free movement through a full ROM as early as possible and gradually progressing to higher intensities and more complex movements should be prioritized as opposed to focusing solely on rest, ice, compression, elevation (acronym RICE) as historically recommended.[56]

Superficial heat: thermotherapy

Thermotherapy is the application of heat, especially through warm pack (superficial heat) and therapeutic ultrasound (superficial or deep depending on frequency). Thermotherapy is beneficial for chronic edema and during subacute or chronic inflammation. It can also be useful before exercise. Heat therapy relieves pain by reducing muscle tension, increasing blood flow and vasodilatation, increasing extensibility of fibrous tissues, and improving joint mobility while accelerating healing with increased metabolic rate.

There is relatively little information regarding heat therapy in dogs compared with cryotherapy. Superficial heat can increase tissue temperature down to 2 cm below the skin's surface if applied for 10 to 20 minutes.[57] The greatest effects occur within the first 1.5 cm, and tissue temperature with 20 minutes of application was not different at superficial or middle depth tissues compared with 10 minutes of application; therefore 10 minutes of application are generally recommended.[58] Effects of heat only occur if the tissue temperature rises by 1 to 4°C.

Thermotherapy should not be used during acute inflammation phase, over the infection site, during malignancy or active bleeding, or if the patient is experiencing a fever. Caution should be taken with patients sedated or under general anesthesia, areas of decreased circulation or sensation, in patients with pacemakers, and over growth plates.

Therapeutic ultrasound

Therapeutic ultrasound provides energy in the form of sound, which is absorbed by high protein content tissues, such as skeletal muscle. It can be a superficial or a deep heating agent depending on which frequency is being used. It can provide deeper heat (elevate tissue temperatures at depths of 2–5 cm) when low frequency is used (1 MHz), while more superficial heat (1–3 cm) is achieved with higher frequency (3.3 MHz).[59] Knowledge of the anatomy and the depth of the particular tissue being treated is important when choosing a therapeutic ultrasound protocol. When treating with therapeutic ultrasound, frequency, intensity, mode, and treatment time need to be established. Limited literature is available in dogs regarding the impact of each variable, but more information is available in human medical literature; however, this is beyond the scope of this article. The hair coat in dogs presents a problem not encountered with people, as the hair coat acts as a barrier to ultrasound. Therefore, shaving of the treatment area is required for both short- and long-hair coats[60] and a coupling agent (such as water-soluble gels or coupling gel pad cushion) must be used.

Therapeutic ultrasound is primarily used for the therapeutic effects of tissue temperature increase that leads to increased blood flow, decreasing pain and muscle spasm, improving tissue nutrition, improving the elasticity of fibrous structures and collagen, and improving joint mobility (ROM). If increased flexibility is the goal, stretching exercises should be performed during and immediately after therapeutic ultrasound, as impact on ROM is only transitory.[61]

Therapeutic ultrasound should not be used or should be used with caution directly over the heart or in animals with pacemakers, over areas of thrombophlebitis, neoplasm, metal implants, the spinal cord after laminectomy, and the epiphyseal area of growing bones.

Electrical stimulation

Electrical modalities include transcutaneous electrical nerve stimulation (TENS) and neuromuscular electrical stimulation (NMES), which focus respectively on pain control and muscle strengthening/activation. For both modalities, it is contraindicated to use high-intensity stimulation over the heart or in patients with a pacemaker, around the head and neck of patient with seizures, in areas with impaired sensation, over areas of thrombosis/thrombophlebitis, and over infected or neoplastic areas. To ensure good contact of the electrodes with the skin surface, the coat should be shaved over the treatment area. If rubber electrodes are used, a gel medium is needed to ensure adequate contact. Treatments should be initially short in duration and low in intensity to allow the animal to become accustomed to the sensation of electrical stimulation. Specific treatment parameters will not be covered into this article; the reader is referred to alternate sources for further information.[19,20]

Transcutaneous electrical nerve stimulation

TENS relieves pain by stimulating the release of endogenous opioids (beta-endorphin, met-enkephalin), activating segmental pain control mechanisms and relaxing musculature. The electrodes are generally placed directly over or along the edges of the painful area being treated. Alternatively, for more acute conditions or when local application of electrodes is not possible, electrodes can be placed along the side of the spine, near the nerve origins of the target treatment area.

A study evaluating the benefit of physical rehabilitation in conjunction with calorie restriction in the treatment of lameness in overweight dogs with osteoarthritis concluded that TENS treatment was a main factor associated with improvement in clinical signs (notably evaluation of ground reaction forces and lameness score).[9] Another study also concluded that TENS treatments improve ground reaction forces in osteoarthritic dogs.[62]

Neuromuscular electrical stimulation

NMES utilizes electrical stimulation to stimulate a muscle via an intact nerve. It causes a muscle contraction by depolarizing the motor nerve with an electrical current delivered via electrodes placed onto the skin. It is mostly used to address muscular weakness associated with either orthopedic or neurologic conditions, especially to slow disuse atrophy. It has been shown that at a frequency of 50 pulses per second at a duration of 175 microseconds, a muscle may contract up to 50% of the normal isometric contraction.[63] NMES recruit type II (fast twitch) fibers first, then type I (slow twitch), which is the reverse of the muscle recruitment pattern in a volitional contraction.[64] Thresholds for electrical stimulation of muscles in dogs (chronaxie) have been characterized in healthy beagles.[65] The usual procedure for delivering NMES is to place the electrodes over the muscle to be stimulated. The electrodes selected should be large to maximize comfort, but not so large that the current can affect adjacent muscles. The electrodes should also not contact each other, nor shoulder their coupling medium, as this allows the electric current to flow directly from 1 electrode to another instead of into the patient's tissue.

Evidence supporting NMES in dogs is scarce; however, some studies mention its usage in combination with other modalities, especially in neurologic patients,[66–69] as well as following surgical treatment of cranial cruciate ligament.[70]

Pulsed electromagnetic field

Pulsed electromagnetic field (PEMF) has been suggested to have anti-inflammatory properties by increasing the binding of calcium to calmodulin, a voltage-dependent process responsible for several biological cascades, leading to nitric oxide production.[71] PEMF should not be used in patients or manipulated by an owner with a pacemaker.[72]

PEMF is registered with the US Food and Drug Administration (FDA) in people for treatment of delayed and nonunion fractures, adjunctive treatment of postoperative pain, and musculoskeletal pain, notably secondary to osteoarthritis of the knee and plantar fasciitis; it has been shown to reduce the dosage of oral pain medication used. In dogs, PEMF has been shown to enhance callus formation and maturation in the late phase of bone healing,[73] to augment engineered cartilage growth and repair,[74] to improve comfort of dogs with osteoarthritis as per their owner assessment,[75] and even possibly yield an analgesic effect for up to 12 months in osteoarthritic dogs.[76] Two recent studies have also suggested benefits of PEMF therapy in the postoperative period of spinal decompressive surgeries. PEMF can reduce incisional pain in dogs postoperatively and may reduce extent of spinal cord injury and enhance proprioception recovery[14] and improved wound healing and reduction in owner-administered pain medications compared with control.[77]

Photobiomodulation

Photobiomodulation, or LASER therapy, is one of the more common physical agent modalities employed outside of specialty physical rehabilitation practice. One older estimate approximated about 20% of general practitioners use photobiomodulation;[78] however, a recent survey of Missouri veterinary practices revealed 43% of practices had a laser unit, so there is reason to believe this modality continues to gain popularity.[79] To clarify terminology, photobiomodulation best describes the physiologic effects of light on tissue; low-level light therapy, cold laser, and others introduce confusion and downplay the possible adverse effects associated with tissue heating.[80] LASER is an acronym representing the light amplification by the stimulated emission of radiation. This light differs from ordinary light based on its monochromatic, coherent, and collimated properties that facilitate tissue penetration. Additional relevant terminology includes: laser class, which is graded by capacity to induce retinal damage; power, as the rate at which energy is produced (W); and wavelength, as the color and electromagnetic classification of light energy. Laser dose is typically reported with respect to surface area of treated tissue (J/cm^2). All these parameters have the capacity to alter the light's absorption and potential therapeutic efficacy and impact the ultimate dose to tissues.

Photobiomodulation is theorized to induce an increase in cellular energy (ATP), nitric oxide, and reactive oxygen species, which in turn can function to promote tissue repair and angiogenesis, mediate vasodilation, modulate the immune and inflammatory response, and activate endogenous antioxidant enzymes. However, establishing an appropriate dose is challenging based on the possible differing response of tissue types and heterogeneity of treatment protocols and modality parameters. Furthermore, it is generally accepted that photobiomodulation follows a biphasic dose response where underdosing results in a lack of clinical effects and overdosing has the capacity to induce tissue damage.[81] The presence of a hair coat, particularly of darker color, can additionally impact the transmission of light to tissue below the epidermis, with darker hair coats and the presence of a hair coat significantly attenuating light penetration, likely necessitating a larger dose to reach the target tissue below.[82,83]

Precautions should be taken when manipulating a laser: use of protective eye wear specifically designed for the wavelength being used and caution when treating dark-colored skin and/or hair (as well as over tattoos). Metal examination tables or other metallic surfaces should be covered, as they will reflect light. It has been theorized that laser should not be used over open fontanels, pregnant uterus, open growth plates, or on patients receiving photosensitive medications.[78]

Despite increasing popularity, in vivo veterinary studies evaluating the effects of photobiomodulation are sparse, particularly with respect to its orthopedic applications. Three studies have examined the effects of photobiomodulation on dogs recovering from a tibial plateau leveling osteotomy (TPLO). One blinded, prospective, randomized clinical trial evaluated the effects of administration of class IV laser (800–900 nm dual wavelength, 3.5 J/cm^2, 6 W) or sham treatment to the stifle preoperatively noting that the peak vertical force on force plate objective gait analysis was greater in the treatment group at 8 weeks. No changes were noted in the other outcome measures including radiographic bone healing or assessment of lameness, behavior, movement, and response to manipulation.[84] Renwick and colleagues performed a similar randomized, double-blind, placebo-controlled clinical trial where laser therapy was applied pre- and postoperatively to the stifle and lumbosacral region using a class IV laser with different parameters, and ultimately a different total dose (660, 800, 905, and 970 nm wavelengths, maximum 15 W continuous wave, 20 W peak pulsed wave). Dogs in the photobiomodulation group had improved subjective outcomes for gait in the adjusted Canine Orthopedic Index, with no differences noted in the other clinical metrology instruments, radiographic bone healing, wound healing, or duration of nonsteroidal anti-inflammatory drug (NSAID) administration.[85] Lastly, Kennedy and colleagues investigated the effects of a class II laser applied pre- and post-operatively to the stifle and L6-7 lumbar region relative to placebo on Canine Brief Pain Inventory, objective ground reaction forces and accelerometry, radiographic bone healing, lameness, Glasgow Composite Pain Scale, and inflammatory markers in synovial fluid. The control group demonstrated greater mean ground reaction forces at 2 and 4 weeks after TPLO as well as lower owner-assigned pain scores during weeks 1 through 5. No other differences were noted among other outcome measures.[86] These 3 studies, while largely similar in design and evaluation of subjective and objective outcome measures, employed significantly different photobiomodulation protocols, which may have contributed to heterogeneity in their results.

Only 1 study has prospectively evaluated the effects of photobiomodulation in veterinary patients with osteoarthritis. The randomized, blinded, placebo-controlled trial demonstrated that twice-weekly photobiomodulation therapy at 10 to 20 J/cm2 per joint (5–10W, 980 nm, continuous wave) for 6 weeks improved lameness and pain scores and allowed dose reduction of NSAIDs in the treatment group. Although the data are promising, this study did have a low number of dogs (n = 20), and no objective outcome measures were assessed.[87] The paucity of literature on this topic in veterinary medicine is particularly relevant given that the survey of Missouri veterinary practices additionally revealed the most common application of laser treatment was osteoarthritis. Furthermore, the study demonstrated significant inconsistency in treatment protocols and level of training[79] Particularly given the routine use of this modality, further research is warranted to determine its efficacy and better define treatment protocols.

Other physical agents include extracorporeal shockwave therapy and acupuncture/electro-acupuncture treatments. More information about these tools is available elsewhere in this issue.

SUMMARY

Physical rehabilitation incorporates several aspects, notably therapeutic exercises, manual therapy, and physical modalities. Understanding of the effects, indications, contraindications, and precautions is essential for proper use, while understanding of the diagnosis, assessment of the stage of tissue healing and repair, and accurate clinical assessment of the functional limitations are essential when establishing a physical rehabilitation plan. Although there is a growing body of literature evaluating clinical efficacy of physical rehabilitation in dogs, many clinicians combine several technique and modalities in a single patient.[88] Wide variability exists in timing of initiation of treatment and in the type of therapy used, its frequency, and its intensity, although there is no head-to-head comparison to predict the best outcome. When reviewing the literature, there are also distinct outcomes depending on the surgical procedures used and type of patient cohort. There is also virtually no information regarding whether combining modalities results in an additive, synergistic, or negative benefit. A recent veterinary systematic review on the use of rehabilitation interventions following surgical repair of cranial cruciate ligament tear in dogs supports cold compression therapy and therapeutic exercises. However, there is a lack of class I level evidence, and many studies had a high risk of bias.[89] Therefore, at this time, it is recommended to identify impairments of each individual patient and set up specific goals reflecting the patient signalment and temperament, the owner compliance, the chronicity and type of injury, and the level of required functional recovery as opposed to relying on specific protocols.

CLINICS CARE POINTS

- During the acute inflammatory phase following orthopedic surgery (generally 72 hours), physical rehabilitation should focus on reduction of inflammation and pain, maintaining joint ROM and nutrition, and stimulating vascularization and tissue healing. At this stage, physical rehabilitation may include cryotherapy, PROM exercises, manual therapy/massage, and low-impact isometric therapeutic exercises.
- Following the initial recovery period, the goals of rehabilitation then should also include: restoring weight bearing, gait patterning, balance, proprioception and strength, and recovery of function. During this period, the focus of therapy may shift toward therapeutic exercises, aquatic therapies, and increasing general activity in the animal.
- Physical modalities can also be used to augment and complement the treatment plan based on stage of tissue healing and repair. Thermal, sound, electrical, and light therapy have been reported to reduce pain and inflammation, enhance healing, and reduce recovery time in the early and late stages following surgery.

ACKNOWLEDGMENTS

Dr. Gamble would like to thank Dr. Lindsay Elam (editor) for her contribution of the section on photobiomodulation (laser).

REFERENCES

1. Marsolais GS, Dvorak G, Conzemius MG. Effects of postoperative rehabilitation on limb function after cranial cruciate ligament repair in dogs. J Am Vet Med Assoc 2002;220(9):1325–30.
2. Monk ML, Preston CA, McGowan CM. Effects of early intensive postoperative physiotherapy on limb function after tibial plateau leveling osteotomy in dogs with deficiency of the cranial cruciate ligament. Am J Vet Res 2006;67(3):529–36.
3. Rexing J, Dunning D, Siegel AM, et al. Effects of cold compression, bandaging, and microcurrent electrical therapy after cranial cruciate ligament repair in dogs. Vet Surg 2010;39(1):54–8.
4. Drygas KA, McClure SR, Goring RL, et al. Effect of cold compression therapy on postoperative pain, swelling, range of motion, and lameness after tibial plateau leveling osteotomy in dogs. J Am Vet Med Assoc 2011;238(10):1284–91.
5. Wucherer KL, Conzemius MG, Evans R, et al. Short-term and long-term outcomes for overweight dogs with cranial cruciate ligament rupture treated surgically or nonsurgically. J Am Vet Med Assoc 2013;242(10):1364–72.
6. Romano LS, Cook JL. Safety and functional outcomes associated with short-term rehabilitation therapy in the post-operative management of tibial plateau leveling osteotomy. Can Vet J 2015;56(9):942–6.

7. Baltzer WI, Smith-Ostrin S, Warnock JJ, et al. Evaluation of the clinical effects of diet and physical rehabilitation in dogs following tibial plateau leveling osteotomy. J Am Vet Med Assoc 2018;252(6):686–700.
8. Greene LM, Marcellin-Little DJ, Lascelles BD. Associations among exercise duration, lameness severity, and hip joint range of motion in Labrador Retrievers with hip dysplasia. J Am Vet Med Assoc 2013;242(11):1528–33.
9. Mlacnik E, Bockstahler BA, Müller M, et al. Effects of caloric restriction and a moderate or intense physiotherapy program for treatment of lameness in overweight dogs with osteoarthritis. J Am Vet Med Assoc 2006;229(11):1756–60.
10. Chauvet A, Laclair J, Elliott DA, et al. Incorporation of exercise, using an underwater treadmill, and active client education into a weight management program for obese dogs. Can Vet J 2011;52(5):491–6.
11. Kathmann I, Cizinauskas S, Doherr MG, et al. Daily controlled physiotherapy increases survival time in dogs with suspected degenerative myelopathy. J Vet Intern Med 2006;20(4):927–32.
12. Gallucci A, Dragone L, Menchetti M, et al. Acquisition of involuntary spinal locomotion (spinal walking) in dogs with irreversible thoracolumbar spinal cord lesion: 81 dogs. J Vet Intern Med 2017;31(2):492–7.
13. Hodgson MM, Bevan JM, Evans RB, et al. Influence of in-house rehabilitation on the postoperative outcome of dogs with intervertebral disk herniation. Vet Surg 2017;46(4):566–73.
14. Zidan N, Fenn J, Griffith E, et al. The effect of electromagnetic fields on postoperative pain and locomotor recovery in dogs with acute, severe thoracolumbar intervertebral disc extrusion: a randomized placebo-controlled, prospective clinical trial. J Neurotrauma 2018;35(15):1726–36.
15. Bruno E, Canal S, Antonucci M, et al. Perilesional photobiomodulation therapy and physical rehabilitation in post-operative recovery of dogs surgically treated for thoracolumbar disk extrusion. BMC Vet Res 2020;16(1):120.
16. Martins Â, Gouveia D, Cardoso A, et al. A comparison between body weight-supported treadmill training and conventional over-ground training in dogs with incomplete spinal cord injury. Front Vet Sci 2021;8:597949.
17. Martins Â, Gouveia D, Cardoso A, et al. Functional neurorehabilitation in dogs with an incomplete recovery 3 months following intervertebral disc surgery: a case series. Animals (Basel) 2021;11(8):2442.
18. Gallucci A, Dragone L, Al Kafaji T, et al. Outcome in cats with acute onset of severe thoracolumbar spinal cord injury following physical rehabilitation. Vet Sci 2021;8(2):22.
19. Millis D, Levine D. Canine rehabilitation and physical therapy. 2nd edition. Saunders Elsevier; 2014.
20. Zink C, Van Dyke JB. Canine sports medicine and rehabilitation. 2nd edition. Wiley-Blackwell; 2018. https://doi.org/10.1002/9781119380627.
21. Baltzer WI. Rehabilitation of companion animals following orthopaedic surgery. N Z Vet J 2020;68(3):157–67.
22. Kirkby Shaw K, Alvarez L, Foster SA, et al. Fundamental principles of rehabilitation and musculoskeletal tissue healing. Vet Surg 2020;49(1):22–32.
23. Holler PJ, Brazda V, Dal-Bianco B, et al. Kinematic motion analysis of the joints of the forelimbs and hind limbs of dogs during walking exercise regimens. Am J Vet Res 2010;71(7):734–40.
24. Breitfuss K, Franz M, Peham C, et al. Surface electromyography of the vastus lateralis, biceps femoris, and gluteus medius muscle in sound dogs during walking and specific physiotherapeutic exercises. Vet Surg 2015;44(5):588–95.

25. McLean H, Millis D, Levine D. Surface electromyography of the vastus lateralis, biceps femoris, and gluteus medius in dogs during stance, walking, trotting, and selected therapeutic exercises. Front Vet Sci 2019;6:211.
26. Carr JG, Millis DL, Weng HY. Exercises in canine physical rehabilitation: range of motion of the forelimb during stair and ramp ascent. J Small Anim Pract 2013; 54(8):409–13.
27. Lauer SK, Hillman RB, Li L, et al. Effects of treadmill inclination on electromyographic activity and hind limb kinematics in healthy hounds at a walk. Am J Vet Res 2009;70(5):658–64.
28. Millard RP, Headrick JF, Millis DL. Kinematic analysis of the pelvic limbs of healthy dogs during stair and decline slope walking. J Small Anim Pract 2010;51(8): 419–22.
29. Durant AM, Millis DL, Headrick JF. Kinematics of stair ascent in healthy dogs. Vet Comp Orthop Traumatol 2011;24(2):99–105.
30. Kopec NL, Williams JM, Tabor GF. Kinematic analysis of the thoracic limb of healthy dogs during descending stair and ramp exercises. Am J Vet Res 2018; 79(1):33–41.
31. McCormick W, Oxley JA, Spencer N. Details of canine hydrotherapy pools and treadmills in 22 hydrotherapy centres in the United Kingdom. Vet Rec 2018; 183(4):128.
32. Nganvongpanit K, Boonchai T, Taothong O, et al. Physiological effects of water temperatures in swimming toy breed dogs. Kafkas Univ Vet Fak Derg 2014; 20(2):177–83.
33. Levine D, Marcellin-Little DJ, Millis DL, et al. Effects of partial immersion in water on vertical ground reaction forces and weight distribution in dogs. Am J Vet Res 2010;71(12):1413–6.
34. Bertocci G, Smalley C, Brown N, et al. Aquatic treadmill water level influence on pelvic limb kinematics in cranial cruciate ligament-deficient dogs with surgically stabilised stifles. J Small Anim Pract 2018;59(2):121–7.
35. Barnicoat F, Wills AP. Effect of water depth on limb kinematics of the domestic dog (Canis lupus familiaris) during underwater treadmill exercise. Comp Exerc Physio 2016;12(4):199–207.
36. Parkinson S, Wills A, Tabor G, et al. Effect of water depth on muscle activity of dogs when walking on a water treadmill. Comp Exerc Physiol 2018;14(2):79–89.
37. Preston T, Wills AP. A single hydrotherapy session increases range of motion and stride length in Labrador retrievers diagnosed with elbow dysplasia. Vet J 2018; 234:105–10.
38. Fish FE, DiNenno NK, Trail J. The "dog paddle": stereotypic swimming gait pattern in different dog breeds. Anat Rec (Hoboken) 2021;304(1):90–100.
39. Marsolais GS, McLean S, Derrick T, et al. Kinematic analysis of the hind limb during swimming and walking in healthy dogs and dogs with surgically corrected cranial cruciate ligament rupture. J Am Vet Med Assoc 2003;222(6):739–43.
40. Fisher CJ, Scott KC, Reiter HK, et al. Effects of a flotation vest and water flow rate on limb kinematics of Siberian Huskies swimming against a current [published online ahead of print, 2021 Dec 1]. Am J Vet Res 2021;1–8. https://doi.org/10.2460/ajvr.21.02.0021.
41. Nganvongpanit K, Kongsawasdi S, Chuatrakoon B, et al. Heart rate change during aquatic exercise in small, medium and large healthy dogs. Thai J Vet Med 2011;41(4):455–61.
42. Nganvongpanit K, Yano T. Side effects in 412 Dogs from swimming in a chlorinated swimming pool. Thai J Vet Med 2012;42:281–6.

43. Chanou K, Gerodimos V, Karatrantou K, et al. Whole-body vibration and rehabilitation of chronic diseases: a review of the literature. J Sports Sci Med 2012;11(2):187–200.
44. Stania M, Juras G, Słomka K, et al. The application of whole-body vibration in physiotherapy - a narrative review. Physiol Int 2016;103(2):133–45.
45. Williams S, Whatman C, Hume PA, et al. Kinesio taping in treatment and prevention of sports injuries: a meta-analysis of the evidence for its effectiveness. Sports Med 2012;42(2):153–64.
46. Kalron A, Bar-Sela S. A systematic review of the effectiveness of Kinesio Taping–fact or fashion? Eur J Phys Rehabil Med 2013;49(5):699–709.
47. Molle S. Kinesio Taping Fundamentals for the Equine Athlete. Vet Clin North Am Equine Pract 2016;32(1):103–13.
48. Corti L. Massage therapy for dogs and cats. Top Companion Anim Med 2014;29(2):54–7.
49. Riley LM, Satchell L, Stilwell LM, et al. Effect of massage therapy on pain and quality of life in dogs: a cross sectional study. Vet Rec 2021;e586. https://doi.org/10.1002/vetr.586.
50. Lane DM, Hill SA. Effectiveness of combined acupuncture and manual therapy relative to no treatment for canine musculoskeletal pain. Can Vet J 2016;57(4):407–14.
51. Crook T, McGowan C, Pead M. Effect of passive stretching on the range of motion of osteoarthritic joints in 10 labrador retrievers. Vet Rec 2007;160(16):545–7.
52. Kieves NR, Bergh MS, Zellner E, et al. Pilot study measuring the effects of bandaging and cold compression therapy following tibial plateau levelling osteotomy. J Small Anim Pract 2016;57(10):543–7.
53. Szabo SD, Levine D, Marcellin-Little DJ, et al. Cryotherapy improves limb use but delays normothermia early after stifle joint surgery in dogs. Front Vet Sci 2020;7:381.
54. Millard RP, Towle-Millard HA, Rankin DC, et al. Effect of cold compress application on tissue temperature in healthy dogs. Am J Vet Res 2013;74(3):443–7.
55. Akgun K, Korpinar MA, Kalkan MT, et al. Temperature changes in superficial and deep tissue layers with respect to time of cold gel pack application in dogs. Yonsei Med J 2004;45(4):711–8.
56. Scialoia D, Swartzendruber AJ. The R.I.C.E protocol is a myth: a review and recommendations. Sport J 2020. thesportjournal.org/article/the-r-i-c-e-protocol-is-a-myth-a-review-and-recommendations.
57. Draper DO, Harris ST, Schulthies S, et al. Hot-Pack and 1-MHz ultrasound treatments have an additive effect on muscle temperature increase. J Athl Train 1998;33(1):21–4.
58. Millard RP, Towle-Millard HA, Rankin DC, et al. Effect of warm compress application on tissue temperature in healthy dogs. Am J Vet Res 2013;74(3):448–51.
59. Levine D, Millis DL, Mynatt T. Effects of 3.3-MHz ultrasound on caudal thigh muscle temperature in dogs. Vet Surg 2001;30(2):170–4.
60. Steiss JE, Adams CC. Effect of coat on rate of temperature increase in muscle during ultrasound treatment of dogs. Am J Vet Res 1999;60(1):76–80.
61. Acevedo B, Millis DL, Levine D, et al. Effect of therapeutic ultrasound on calcaneal tendon heating and extensibility in dogs. Front Vet Sci 2019;6:185.
62. Johnson KD, Levine D, Price MN, et al. The effect of TENS on osteoarthritic pain in the stifle of dogs. Proceedings of the 2nd international symposium on rehabilitation and physical therapy in veterinary medicine, Knoxville, TN; 2002, p.199.

63. Currier DP, Ray JM, Nyland J, et al. Effects of electrical and electromagnetic stimulation after anterior cruciate ligament reconstruction. J Orthop Sports Phys Ther 1993;17(4):177–84.
64. Knaflitz M, Merletti R, De Luca CJ. Inference of motor unit recruitment order in voluntary and electrically elicited contractions. J Appl Physiol (1985) 1990; 68(4):1657–67.
65. Sawaya SG, Combet D, Chanoit G, et al. Assessment of impulse duration thresholds for electrical stimulation of muscles (chronaxy) in dogs. Am J Vet Res 2008; 69(10):1305–9.
66. Hady LL, Schwarz PD. Recovery times for dogs undergoing thoracolumbar hemilaminectomy with fenestration and physical rehabilitation: a review of 113 cases. J Vet Med Ani Heal 2015;7(8):278–89.
67. Inês Rodrigues Gonçalves F, Neves Rocha Martins AP, Ferreira Alves MM. Functional neurorehabilitation in dogs with cervical neurologic lesion. J. Vet Sci Tech 2016;7:1–6.
68. Frank LR, Roynard PFP. Veterinary neurologic rehabilitation: the rationale for a comprehensive approach. Top Companion Anim Med 2018;33(2):49–57.
69. Martins Â, Gouveia D, Cardoso A, et al. Nervous system modulation through electrical stimulation in companion animals. Acta Vet Scand 2021;63(1):22.
70. Johnson JM, Johnson AL, Pijanowski GJ, et al. Rehabilitation of dogs with surgically treated cranial cruciate ligament-deficient stifles by use of electrical stimulation of muscles. Am J Vet Res 1997;58(12):1473–8.
71. Gaynor JS, Hagberg S, Gurfein BT. Veterinary applications of pulsed electromagnetic field therapy. Res Vet Sci 2018;119:1–8.
72. Gwechenberger M, Rauscha F, Stix G, et al. Interference of programmed electromagnetic stimulation with pacemakers and automatic implantable cardioverter defibrillators. Bioelectromagnetics 2006;27(5):365–77.
73. Inoue N, Ohnishi I, Chen D, et al. Effect of pulsed electromagnetic fields (PEMF) on late-phase osteotomy gap healing in a canine tibial model. J Orthop Res 2002; 20(5):1106–14.
74. Stefani RM, Barbosa S, Tan AR, et al. Pulsed electromagnetic fields promote repair of focal articular cartilage defects with engineered osteochondral constructs. Biotechnol Bioeng 2020;117(5):1584–96. https://doi.org/10.1002/bit.27287.
75. Sullivan MO, Gordon-Evans WJ, Knap KE, et al. Randomized, controlled clinical trial evaluating the efficacy of pulsed signal therapy in dogs with osteoarthritis. Vet Surg 2013;42(3):250–4.
76. Pinna S, Landucci F, Tribuiani A, et al. The effects of pulsed electromagnetic field in the treatment of osteoarthritis in dogs: clinical study. Pak Vet J 2013;33(1): 96–100.
77. Alvarez LX, McCue J, Lam NK, et al. Effect of targeted pulsed electromagnetic field therapy on canine postoperative hemilaminectomy: a double-blind, randomized, placebo-controlled clinical trial. J Am Anim Hosp Assoc 2019;55(2):83–91.
78. Pryor B, Millis DL. Therapeutic laser in veterinary medicine. Vet Clin North Am Small Anim Pract 2015;45(1):45–56.
79. Barger BK, Bisges AM, Fox DB, et al. Low-level laser therapy for osteoarthritis treatment in dogs at Missouri veterinary practices. J Am Anim Hosp Assoc 2020;56(3):139–45.
80. Anders JJ, Lanzafame RJ, Arany PR. Low-level light/laser therapy versus photobiomodulation therapy. Photomed Laser Surg 2015;33(4):183–4.

81. Chung H, Dai T, Sharma SK, et al. The nuts and bolts of low-level laser (light) therapy. Ann Biomed Eng 2012;40(2):516–33.
82. Hochman-Elam LN, Heidel RE, Shmalberg JW. Effects of laser power, wavelength, coat length, and coat color on tissue penetration using photobiomodulation in healthy dogs. Can J Vet Res 2020;84(2):131–7.
83. Ryan T, Smith R. An investigation into the depth of penetration of low level laser therapy through the equine tendon in vivo. Ir Vet J 2007;60(5):295–9.
84. Rogatko CP, Baltzer WI, Tennant R. Preoperative low level laser therapy in dogs undergoing tibial plateau levelling osteotomy: a blinded, prospective, randomized clinical trial. Vet Comp Orthop Traumatol 2017;30(1):46–53.
85. Renwick SM, Renwick AI, Brodbelt DC, et al. Influence of class IV laser therapy on the outcomes of tibial plateau leveling osteotomy in dogs. Vet Surg 2018;47(4):507–15.
86. Kennedy KC, Martinez SA, Martinez SE, et al. Effects of low-level laser therapy on bone healing and signs of pain in dogs following tibial plateau leveling osteotomy. Am J Vet Res 2018;79(8):893–904.
87. Looney AL, Huntingford JL, Blaeser LL, et al. A randomized blind placebo-controlled trial investigating the effects of photobiomodulation therapy (PBMT) on canine elbow osteoarthritis. Can Vet J 2018;59(9):959–66.
88. Shmalberg J, Memon MA. A retrospective analysis of 5,195 patient treatment sessions in an integrative veterinary medicine service: patient characteristics, presenting complaints, and therapeutic interventions. Vet Med Int 2015;2015:983621.
89. Alvarez LX, Repac JA, Kirkby Shaw K, et al. Systematic review of postoperative rehabilitation interventions after cranial cruciate ligament surgery in dogs. Vet Surg 2022;51(2):233–43.

Guidelines to Home Exercises and Lifestyle Modifications for Common Small Animal Orthopedic Conditions

Carolina Medina, DVM, DACVSMR, CVA, CVPP

KEYWORDS

• Home exercises • Range of motion • Orthopedic • Osteoarthritis • Assistive devices

KEY POINTS

- Home exercises should be selected according to tissue healing principles, the patient's ability and orthopedic condition, and the projected treatment goals.
- Progression of exercises or plan modification should be implemented according to the patient's individual goals and clinical status.
- Lifestyle modifications using assistive devices, such as a support harness, can be recommended to assist the patient in performing their daily tasks.

 **Video content accompanies this article at http://www.vetsmall.theclinics.com.**

Patients with orthopedic conditions are likely to benefit from a home exercise program to improve their range of motion, weight-bearing, strength, and overall mobility. The first thing to consider is the patient's current mobility status. Assessing a pet's mobility is imperative to treatment planning (please refer to Christina Montalbano's article, "Comprehensive Mobility Assessment," in this issue for details on assessing a patient's mobility). Based on their current mobility evaluation and clinical diagnosis, specific exercises should be chosen that would improve their overall status. For example, if an osteoarthritic patient has decreased range of motion in one or more joints, range of motion exercises should be incorporated into the treatment plan. The second factor to consider is the projected goal of therapy. For example, a pet that is non–weight-bearing in the acute postoperative phase should perform exercises that promote weight-bearing. The final consideration is the owner's time and ability. In order for the owner to be actively involved in their pet's care, choosing a home exercise program that will be feasible for the owner to perform will allow better owner compliance.

Coral Springs Animal Hospital, 2160 North University Drive, Coral Springs, FL 33071, USA
E-mail address: cmedina@coralspringsanimalhosp.com

Vet Clin Small Anim 52 (2022) 1021–1032
https://doi.org/10.1016/j.cvsm.2022.03.006

GUIDELINES FOR HOME EXERCISES

Exercises should be selected according to tissue healing principles, the patient's ability and orthopedic condition, and the projected treatment goals. Progression of exercises should be applied according to the patient's individual goals and clinical status. It is important not to push a patient beyond their current level of tissue healing, as it could delay healing and be a source of chronic pain for the patient.

Common Therapeutic Exercises

When structuring a home exercise program, the owner's accessibility and compliance should be considered. It is the author's opinion that most clients will be more compliant if the exercises are easy to perform and can be completed in a short time period. Asking the owner during your history taking about their time commitment and what tricks their pet knows can help the veterinarian develop a successful home exercise program. The exercises chosen for home use are typically easy to perform and differ from what is conducted professionally in a hospital setting in both complexity and advancement. When instructing pet owners on home exercises, perform an in-person demonstration with the owner and ask the owner to video the demonstration for their reference. Giving clients handouts with diagrams and written instruction can also improve their compliance. You might also create your own library of exercise videos and give clients access as you are treating their pets.

Deciding on how many repetitions and sets to perform and how often to perform the home exercises should be based on the individual pet's condition and any comorbidities, the pet's current mobility status, and the phase of tissue healing. It is common to start with less repetitions (ie, 4–6 repetitions) and usually 1 set, then gradually advance the pet to higher repetitions (ie, 8–12 repetitions) and more sets (ie, 2–3 sets), as the pet builds strength. The frequency of when the exercises should be performed is also individualized to the patient. Typically for patients with osteoarthritis, in which their condition is progressive and lifelong, exercises are usually recommended a few times a week (ie, 2–3 times a week), and modified over the course of the pet's life as their mobility changes. In cases that are more acute in nature, such as a post-operative femoral head ostectomy, home exercises should be performed daily, and initially with exercises that promote weight-bearing and progressing to exercises that build strength.

Passive range of motion decreases pain, lubricates joints, and improves joint range of motion. To perform a passive range of motion, the patient should be comfortable and either in lateral recumbency or standing. The bones proximal and distal to the joint should be supported, and hands should be placed close to the joint. Hands should move slow, and with steady motion move the distal limb segment while holding the proximal limb segment in a fixed position. Place the joint in its most tolerable flexion position, hold for 10 to 30 seconds, release, perform 3 to 10 repetitions, and then perform joint extension in a similar manner (**Fig. 1**, Video 1). A study was conducted on Labrador retrievers with osteoarthritis in the elbows, carpi, and stifles. Owners were instructed on how to perform passive a range of motion: holding flexion and extension for 10 seconds each for 10 repetitions, twice a day for 3 weeks. Goniometric measurements demonstrated a significant increase in range of motion measured as a mean angular increase in joint flexion of 14.6°, and an average of 7% to 23% increase in overall joint range of motion.[1]

Walking is an excellent exercise as it is low impact and helps maintain range of motion. Walking induces range of motion in the following manner: approximately 30° in the shoulders, 45° in the elbows, 90° in the carpi, 35° in the hips, 40° in the stifles,

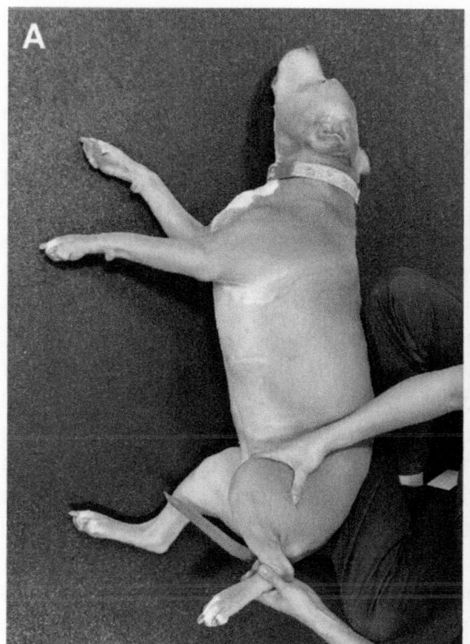

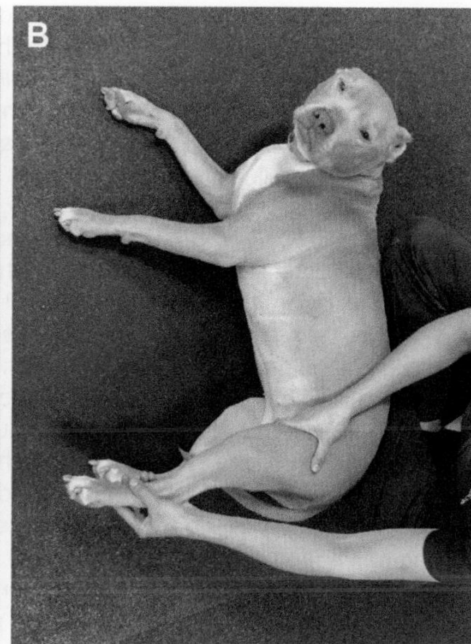

Fig. 1. Passive range of motion of the stifle joint. (*A*) Stifle flexion. (*B*) Stifle extension.

and 35° in the tarsi.[2] To make proper recommendations for walks, one should ask the owner if their pet is used to going on walks, how long their typical walks are, if they notice any lameness or fatigue during the walk and if so, when on the walk does the lameness or fatigue occur. Walk recommendations are different for patients with osteoarthritis compared with postoperative patients. Patients with osteoarthritis should be encouraged to go on daily walks. If walking is not routine for an osteoarthritic patient, inform the owner to start with short walks, that is, 5 to 10 minutes, and monitor for lameness or signs of fatigue. If that length of time is tolerated, a 5-min increase per walk per week can be added to get the pet to comfortably walk for about 30 to 45 minutes if the pet is able. If the pet is not able to walk that long, then walks should be curbed to the time just before lameness or fatigue occurs. If a patient is postoperative, walking instructions are given based on tissue healing principles, that is, a postoperative TPLO case could start 5-min leash walks 2 to 3 times a day starting 2 weeks postoperative if the patient has started to bear weight.

Uneven surface walking, such as walking on an air mattress or uneven terrain, enhances proprioception, promotes weight-bearing, and strengthens the stabilizer muscles. This can be incorporated into part of the routine walk for about 3 to 5 minutes pending patient strength, balance, and tolerance. Incline ramp walking promotes increased flexion, extension, and range of motion of the hip, shoulder extension and range of motion, elbow flexion and extension, and carpal flexion.[3,4] Incline ramp walking also increases strength in the pelvic limb muscles especially the quadriceps, semitendinosus, semimembranosus, and gluteal muscles. Decline ramp walking results in decreased range of motion of the hips with increased range of motion of the stifles and tarsi, as well as increased strength of the thoracic limb muscles especially the triceps.[5] The addition of ramp walking can be added after the walks for 4 to 12 repetitions, starting with lower repetitions and gradually increasing them as the pet develops strength.

Cavaletti pole exercise improves proprioception and weight-bearing, strengthens the flexors, and elongates the stride length.[6] Walking over cavaletti poles increases the range of motion compared with walking on a flat surface. The elbows, stifles, and tarsi have increased range of motion, especially flexion, during cavaletti pole walking.[4] Cavalettis are constructed by placing either PVC pipes, broomsticks, pool noodles, or similar linear obstacles on the ground or at various heights, and the pet is instructed to walk over the poles ideally not touching or moving the poles (**Fig. 2**, Video 2). Typically, 4 to 6 objects are used, and 3 to 12 repetitions should be performed based on the pet's ability. The height of the cavaletti poles impacts the degree of range of motion. Walking over cavaletti poles at the level of the carpi, increases flexion in the carpi, elbows, stifles, and tarsi compared with ground walking.[7] Initially, pole height should be just slightly above the pet's carpus. Increasing the pole height over time should be encouraged once the lower height has been mastered, keeping in mind that too high may make the pet try to jump over the poles which would defeat the purpose of the exercise. Cavaletti poles should be spaced at appropriate distances apart, determined by the dog's natural stride length. The distance between the poles should be just wide enough to allow for a single step between the poles at a normal walking gait speed.[8]

There are a variety of weight-shifting exercises that promote weight-bearing. One is with the patient standing stationary, gently pushing their body on one side to create a rebound weight shift so the pet catches their balance and engages their muscles to stay standing (Video 3). When performing this exercise, you can do 3 to 12 repetitions quickly, or slowly holding the gentle push for 10 to 30 seconds for 3 to 12 repetitions. Another weight-bearing exercise is the cookie stretch, in which you show a treat to the pet and then lure it to follow the treat as you move the treat from its nose to its hip. As the pet moves its body to follow the treat, they will increase weight distribution to the limbs on the same side as the treat lure, in addition to pushing off the opposite limbs, and stretching the paraspinal muscles on the opposite side (**Fig. 3**, Video 4). To perform this exercise, have the patient hold the side crunch for 10 to 30 seconds for 3 to 12 repetitions.

The sit-to-stand exercise increases flexion of the tarsi, stifles and hips.[9] This exercise also strengthens the quadriceps, biceps femoris, semitendinosus, semimembranosus, gastrocnemius, and gluteal muscles. Sit-to-stands are performed by asking the patient to sit, immediately stand, and then repeat for 3 to 12 repetitions.

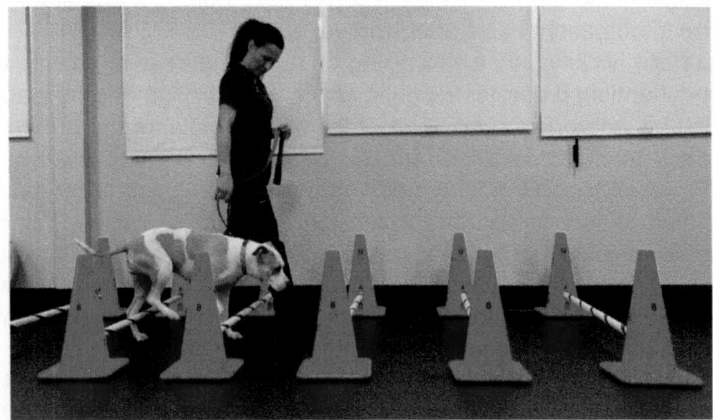

Fig. 2. Cavalettis.

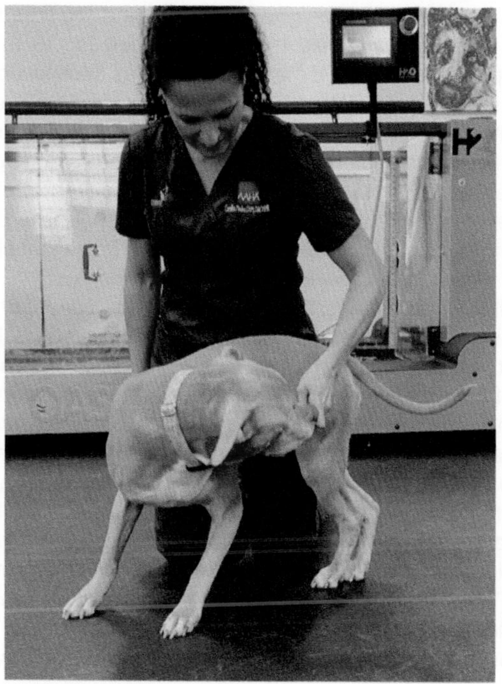

Fig. 3. Cookie stretch.

The three-leg stand exercise strengthens the limbs that maintain contact with the ground when performing this exercise. To strengthen the thoracic limbs, with the patient standing square, lift the unaffected thoracic limb off the ground and extend the limb forward in front of the patient (**Fig. 4**, Video 5). To strengthen the pelvic limbs,

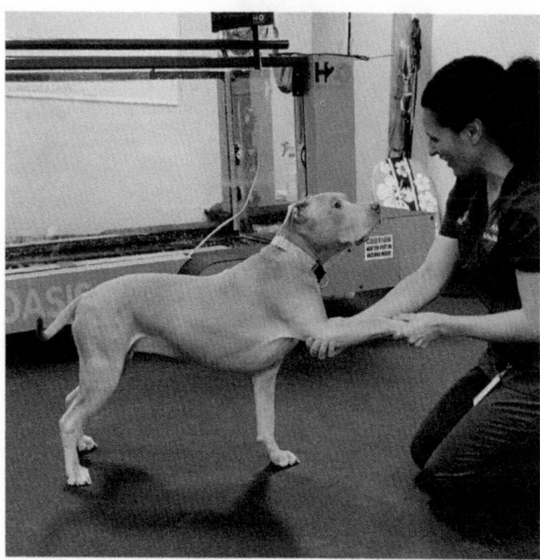

Fig. 4. Three-leg stand of the thoracic limb.

lift the unaffected pelvic limb off the ground and extend the limb behind the patient (**Fig. 5**, Video 6). The patient should hold this position for 10 to 30 seconds, and perform 3 to 12 repetitions as able. If the patient buckles or sinks down, this is an indication that it is possibly painful, fatigued, or is not strong enough yet for the exercise. Once the patient has mastered the three-leg stand, you can advance them to a two-leg stand. A two-leg stand is performed with the patient standing square, simultaneously lifting one thoracic limb and the diagonal pelvic limb off the ground (**Fig. 6**; Video 7). This movement should be repeated with the opposite diagonal limb pair. This exercise strengthens all limbs as well as the core. The patient should hold this position for 10 to 30 seconds, and perform 3 to 12 repetitions.

Backwards walking strengthens the semitendinosus, semimembranosus, gluteal muscles, and triceps. It is performed by asking the pet to step backwards which creates extension of the hips, stifles, tarsi, and elbows. You can encourage the patient by standing in front of them with a treat or toy and moving forward so the dog steps backwards to focus on the reward (Video 8). This can also be performed standing next to the patient, using a reward in front and the leash to help gently guide them backwards. Instruct the pet to take 10 steps backwards for 3 to 12 repetitions.

Side stepping strengthens the abductors and adductors of all limbs in particular the pectoralis, pectineus, and gluteal muscles. This exercise is performed by standing on the side of the patient facing them, then you take a step forward gently nudging the pet to step sideways (Video 9). Instruct the pet to take 10 steps sideways in each direction for 3 to 12 repetitions.

Examples of home exercises for common orthopedic conditions.

- Osteoarthritis
  - Passive range of motion can maintain and improve joint health, particularly when the active range of motion is limited. It can be performed daily by the pet owner, and it is best to perform before walks and exercises.
  - Walks are essential for all patients with osteoarthritis.

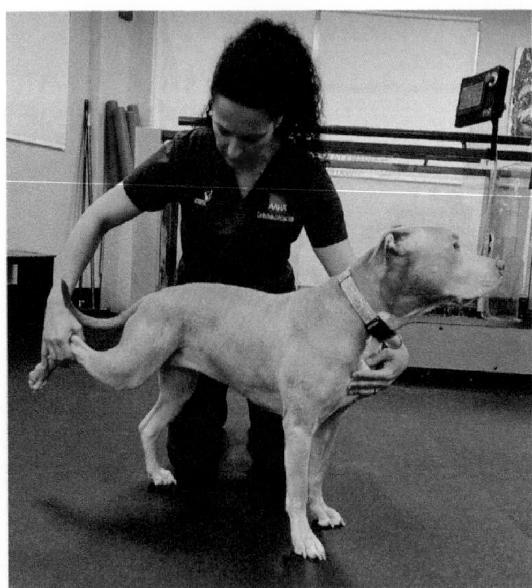

Fig. 5. Three-leg stand of the pelvic limb.

  - Cavalettis can be performed to increase the range of motion of the elbows, stifles, and tarsi.
  - Sit-to-stands can be conducted with patients with osteoarthritis in the pelvic limbs, as they improve the range of motion in the tarsi, stifles, and hips, and strengthen the quadriceps, semitendinosus, semimembranosus, gastrocnemius, and gluteal muscles.
  - Three-leg stands can be used to strengthen the limbs.
  - Backwards walking is used to increase the range of motion in the hips, stifles, tarsi, and elbows, as well as strengthen the semitendinosus, semimembranosus, gluteal muscles, and triceps.
  - Side stepping strengthens the pectorals, pectineus, and gluteal muscles.
- Elbow dysplasia
  - Passive range of motion, particularly elbow extension, should be conducted as the sequela of elbow dysplasia is osteoarthritis.
  - Walks are essential for all patients with osteoarthritis.
  - Rebounding and cookie stretches can be incorporated in the early postoperative phase or when there is less weight-bearing.
  - Cavalettis can be performed to increase the range of motion in the elbows.
  - Three-leg stands on the thoracic limbs strengthen the thoracic limbs.
  - Backwards walking is used to increase the range of motion in the elbows and strengthen the triceps.
- Hip dysplasia
  - Passive range of motion, especially hip extension, should be conducted as hip dysplasia leads to osteoarthritis.
  - Walks are essential for all patients with osteoarthritis.
  - Rebounding and cookie stretches can be incorporated in the early postoperative phase or when there is less weight-bearing.
  - Three-leg stands on the pelvic limbs strengthen the pelvic limbs.
  - Backwards walking is used to increase the range of motion in the hips, and strengthen the semitendinosus, semimembranosus, and gluteal muscles.
  - Side stepping strengthens the pectineus and gluteal muscles.
- Cranial cruciate ligament disease
  - Care must be taken if there is stifle instability as it is painful, and exercises that do not cause increased pain should be selected.
  - Gentle passive range of motion and leash walks can help improve or maintain joint range of motion.
  - Rebounding and cookie stretches can be incorporated in the early postoperative phase when there is less weight-bearing.
  - Cavalettis can be performed to increase the active range of motion in the stifles.
  - Three-leg stands on the pelvic limbs are used to strengthen the pelvic limbs.
  - Backwards walking is used to increase the stifle range of motion and strengthen the semitendinosus, semimembranosus, and gluteal muscles.
  - Side stepping strengthens the pectineus and gluteal muscles.
- Biceps brachii tendinopathy
  - Passive range of motion of both the shoulder and elbow should be performed. Care should be taken not to stretch the bicep in the acute phase.
  - Three-leg stands on the thoracic limbs strengthen the thoracic limbs.
  - Backwards walking is used to increase the range of motion in the elbows and strengthen the triceps.
  - Side stepping strengthens the pectoral muscles.

- Calcaneal tendinopathy
  - Care must be taken if there is tarsal instability as it is painful, and exercises that do not cause increased pain should be selected.
  - Gentle passive range of motion and leash walks can help improve tarsal range of motion. Care should be taken not to hyper-flex the tarsus as this elongates the calcaneal tendon risking further injury.
  - Rebounding and cookie stretches can be incorporated in the early postoperative phase or when there is less weight-bearing.
  - Cavalettis can be performed to increase the range of motion in the tarsus.
  - Backwards walking is used to increase the tarsal range of motion and strengthen the semitendinosus, semimembranosus, and gluteal muscles.
- Iliopsoas strain or tendinopathy
  - Rebounding and cookie stretches can be incorporated to promote weight-bearing.
  - Three-leg stands on the pelvic limbs strengthen the pelvic limbs.
  - Backwards walking is used to increase the range of motion of the hips, and strengthen the semitendinosus, semimembranosus, and gluteal muscles.
  - Side stepping strengthens the pectineus and gluteal muscles.

LIFESTYLE MODIFICATIONS

Recommendations for modifying the pet's home and/or certain activities in the home are important as patients recover from an orthopedic condition or suffer from progressive lifelong osteoarthritis. A thorough history including details of the home environment is important to know prior to making recommendations for lifestyle modifications. An understanding of the patient's ability, limitations, and comorbidities is also essential prior to making recommendations.

Lifestyle Modification Recommendations

- Slings and harnesses can be used to support the body during weak ambulation or in the early postoperative phase when weight-bearing is limited. Slings are

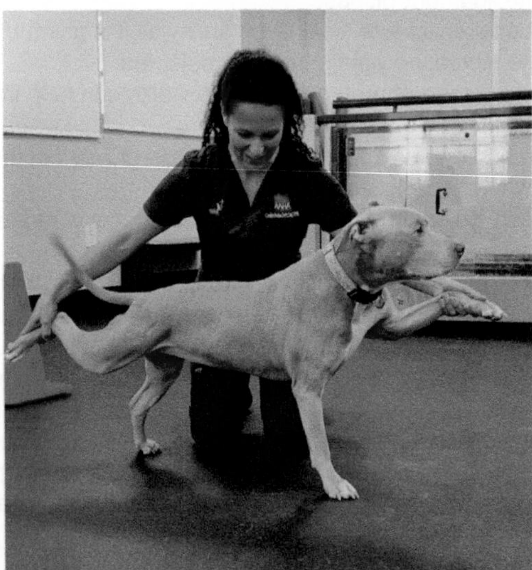

Fig. 6. Two-leg stand.

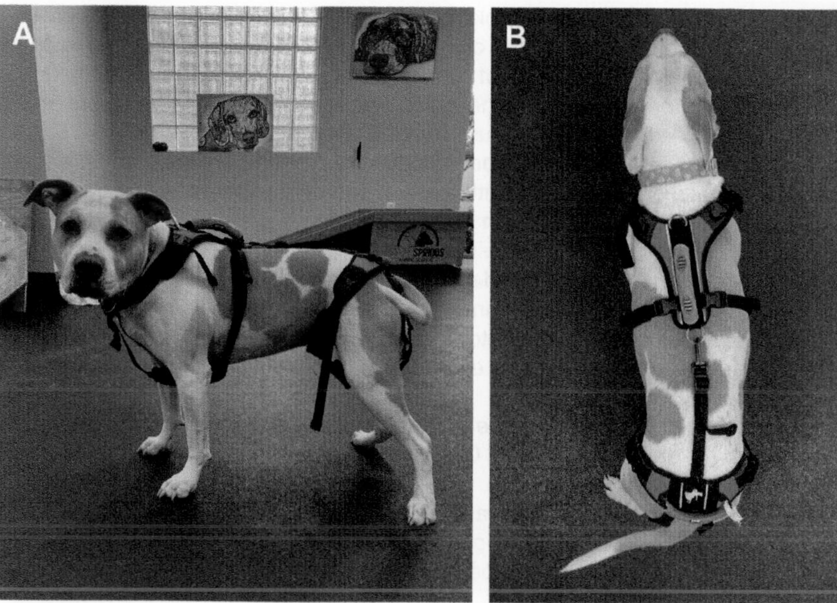

Fig. 7. Assistive device - harness. (*A*) Harness (side view). (*B*) Harness (top view).

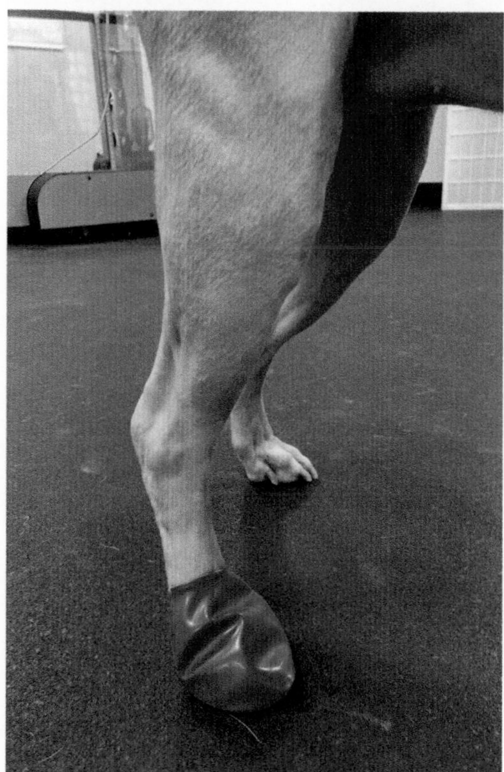

Fig. 8. Assistive device - Bootie.

typically made of soft comfortable material that goes under the pet's abdomen or chest, and it has straps for the owner to hold on to and provide support to the pet's body. There are a variety of support harnesses, including ones that support only the thoracic limbs or only the pelvic limbs or all four limbs. Some are able to be worn by the pet for ease of use (**Figs. 6** and **7**).

- Footing: skid resistance dog socks, foot applications such as traction pads or traction material, and footing with traction can help enable ambulation (**Fig. 8**).
- Placing mats and/or runners on slippery flooring in the home provides traction and ease of mobility around the house.
- Ramps and stairs can be placed next to the owner's bed/sofa to facilitate the pet getting on and off the furniture in a gradual and lower impact manner.
- Soft bedding provides comfort to arthritic joints.
- An elevated food bowl makes it easier for pets to eat without falling or overusing their neck and shoulders.
- Wheelchairs or carts can provide mobility for those pets who have very limited or have lost the ability to ambulate. Carts are available for the pelvic limbs (hind cart) and for all limbs (quad cart).
- Tarsal devices assist with increasing tarsal flexion and keep the hind paw in an anatomically correct standing position limiting knuckling. It is used as a mobility aid for unstable or weak distal pelvic limbs especially when knuckling is present (**Fig. 9**).

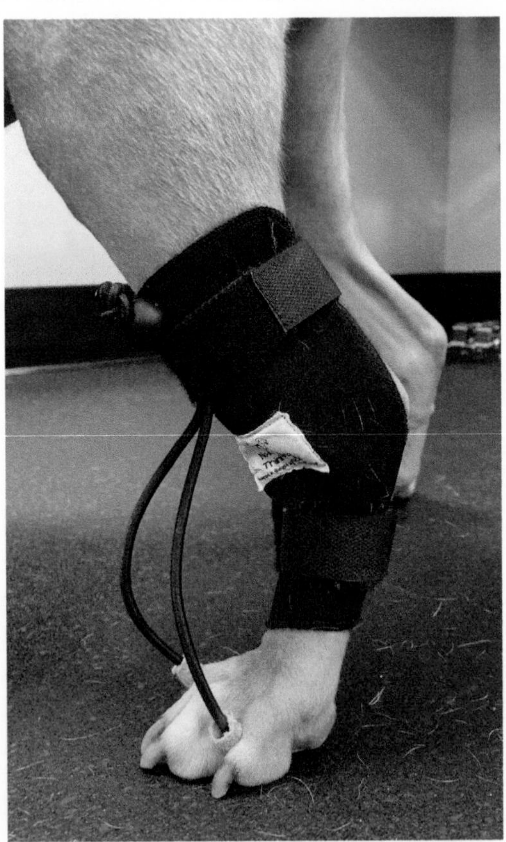

Fig. 9. Assistive Device – Toe up.

Pets with osteoarthritis and other orthopedic conditions benefit from a home exercise program, as well as lifestyle modifications based on their condition. Home exercises can be performed to improve a pet's range of motion, weight-bearing, strength, and overall mobility. A home exercise program should be designed to improve the patient's impairments, and progression of exercises should occur depending on the patient's response and ability to master each exercise. Considerations for the patient's current mobility status, clinical diagnosis, comorbidities, treatment goals, and the owner's availability should be adhered to.

CLINICS CARE POINTS

- Passive range of motion and stretching decreases pain, lubricates joints, and improves joint range of motion and muscle flexibility.
- Cavaletti pole exercises improve proprioception and weight-bearing, strengthen the flexor muscles, and elongate the stride length.
- Sit-to-stand exercise increases flexion of the tarsi, stifles and hips, and strengthens the quadriceps, biceps femoris, semitendinosus, semimembranosus, gastrocnemius, and gluteal muscles.
- Backwards walking strengthens the semitendinosus, semimembranosus, gluteal muscles, and triceps.
- Side stepping strengthens the pectoralis, pectineus, and gluteal muscles.

DISCLOSURE

The author has no conflicts of interest associated with this publication.

SUPPLEMENTARY DATA

Supplementary data related to this article can be found online at doi:10.1016/j.cvsm.2022.03.006.

REFERENCES

1. Crook T, McGowan C, Pead M. Effect of passive stretching on the range of motion of osteoarthritic joints in 10 Labrador retrievers. Vet Rec 2007;160(16):545–7.
2. Hottinger HA, DeCamp CE, Olivier NB, et al. Noninvasive kinematic analysis of the walk in healthy large-breed dogs. Am J Vet Res 1996;57:381–8.
3. Carr J, Millis DL, Weng HY. Exercises in Canine Physical Rehabilitation: range of motion of the forelimb during stair and ramp ascent. J Sm Anim Pract 2013;54(8):409–13.
4. Holler PJ, Brazda V, Dal-Bianco B, et al. Kinematic motion analysis of the joints of the forelimbs and hindlimbs of dogs during walking exercise regimens. Am J Vet Res 2010;71:734–40.
5. Millard RP, Headrick JF, Millis DL. Kinematic analysis of the pelvic limbs of healthy dogs during stair and decline slope walking. J Small Anim Pract 2010;51(8):419–22.
6. McCauley L, Van Dyke J. Therapeutic Exercise. In: Zink C, Van Dyke J, editors. Canine Sports Medicine and Rehabilitation. 2nd Edition. Hoboken, NJ: John Wiley & Sons, Inc; 2018. p. 177–207.
7. Weigel JP, Millis D. Biomechanics of Physical Rehabilitation and Kinematics of Exercise. In: Millis D, Levine D, Taylor R, editors. Canine Rehabilitation and Physical Therapy. 2nd edition. Philadelphia, (PA): Elsevier Saunders; 2014. p. 401–30.

8. Drum MG, Marcellin-Little DJ, Davis MS. Principles and Applications of Therapeutic Exercises for Small Animals. Vet Clin North Am Small Anim Pract 2015;45(1): 73–90.
9. Feeney LC, Lin CF, Marcellin-Little DJ, et al. Validation of two-dimensional kinematic analysis of walk and sit-to-stand motion in dogs. Am J Vet Res 2007;68: 277–82.

Extracorporeal Shockwave Therapy for Musculoskeletal Pathologies

Leilani Alvarez, DVM, CCRT, CVA

KEYWORDS

- Extracorporeal Shockwave Therapy • Shockwave therapy • Shockwave • ESWT
- ECSW

KEY POINTS

- Extracorporeal shockwave therapy (ESWT) offers a safe, noninvasive treatment of multiple musculoskeletal conditions
- ESWT machines are not comparable in treatment protocols
- The greatest evidence for electrohydraulic units is improved bone healing
- Radial pressure wave therapy seems beneficial for the treatment of osteoarthritis

INTRODUCTION

Extracorporeal shockwave therapy (ESWT) offers a noninvasive treatment option for many musculoskeletal conditions. Advances in both the human and veterinary fields have demonstrated benefits in the treatment of chronic repetitive injuries that typically do not respond well to surgical intervention. The use of ESWT became widely accepted in equine sports medicine before it was adopted in canine patients. Musculoskeletal conditions that can benefit from EWST are wide ranging from improved bone healing to tendinopathies and osteoarthritis. As evidence continues to build, more small animal patients with musculoskeletal disorders may benefit from ESWT.

HISTORY/BACKGROUND

ESWT has been in use for several decades. ESWT initially gained medical acceptance in the 1970s as a lithotripsy treatment of urinary, salivary, and renal calculi.[1–3] More recent advances show evidence in human clinical trials for use of nonunion fractures, tendinopathies, plantar fasciopathy, epicondylitis, and other uses.[1]

Shockwaves are nonlinear, high-pressure, and high-velocity acoustic waves characterized by low tensile amplitude, short rise time to peak pressure, and a short

Integrative and Rehabilitative Medicine, Schwarzman Animal Medical Center, 510 East 62nd Street, New York, NY 10065, USA
E-mail address: Leilani.Alvarez@amcny.org

Vet Clin Small Anim 52 (2022) 1033–1042
https://doi.org/10.1016/j.cvsm.2022.03.007 vetsmall.theclinics.com

duration (less than 10 milliseconds).[1] Examples of natural shockwaves include thunder, bangs from explosions, and airplanes as they break the sound barrier. A shockwave generates a single pulse with a wide frequency range (16–20 MHz), high-pressure amplitude (up to 100 MPa), and short rise time (5–10 nanoseconds) **Fig. 1**.[2] Shockwave therapy differs from therapeutic ultrasonography in that it has no thermal effect, has minimal tissue absorption, and is low frequency.[2,3] Shockwaves transmit mechanical energy into tissues according to their acoustic impedance. Water and gel have the lowest impedance allowing for best transmission of shockwaves. The sharp, rapid increase in pressure waves is followed by a negative pressure drop (**Fig. 1**) that leads to generation of cavitation bubbles with subsequent collapse; this leads to increased cellular permeability and production of free radicals followed by generation of anti-inflammatory cytokines and growth factors. The ultimate effect is purported to reduce pain and inflammation and remodel soft tissues.[3]

TYPES OF DEVICES

Shockwave therapy devices can be generally divided into 2 groups: focused and unfocused.[4] There are 3 types of focused shockwave generators: electrohydraulic, electromagnetic, and piezoelectric. Unfocused generators create radial (also known as pneumatic/ballistic/dispersive) pressure waves with much lower energy compared with focused ones. Radial waves may be more accurately described as pressure waves because they are longer, slower, less intense, and do not generate true shockwaves[4,5] (see **Fig. 1**). Radial waves are also shallower in penetration (~3.5 cm) compared with focused shockwaves (10–12 cm).[4,5] Focused shockwaves and unfocused radial waves are similar in that they both generate mechanical sound waves, both require a medium to transmit energy, and both can be clinically effective.[5,6] Treatment methods also vary in amount of energy delivered, generally categorized as high (>0.6 mJ/mm^2), medium (0.08–0.28 mJ/mm^2), or low (<0.08 mJ/mm^2) energy.[1]

Electrohydraulic units have a spark plug in the trode (ie, the handheld device that is used to administer the treatment) that fires within a fluid medium releasing focused energy waves (**Figs. 2** and **3B**). Piezoelectric units have crystals that expand and deform

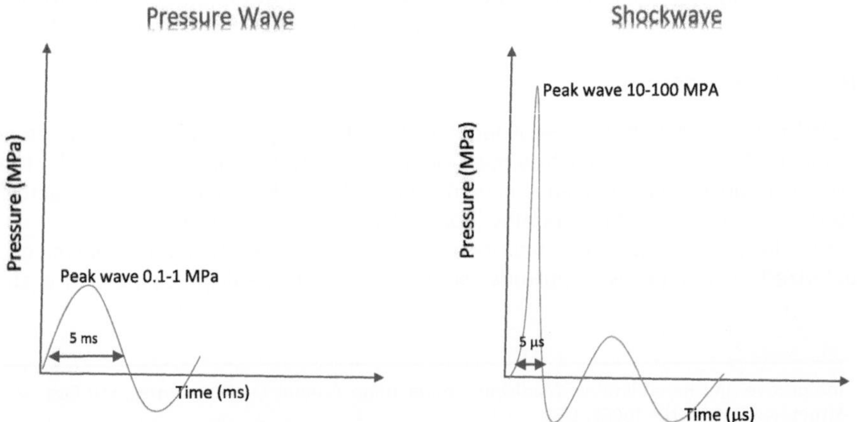

Fig. 1. Radial pressure waves are low energy density and not focused compared with focused shock waves with high energy density that have a rapid increase and decrease in energy. The duration to reach a peak wave is also much longer for a radial pressure wave (~5000 μs) compared with focused shockwave (~5 μs).

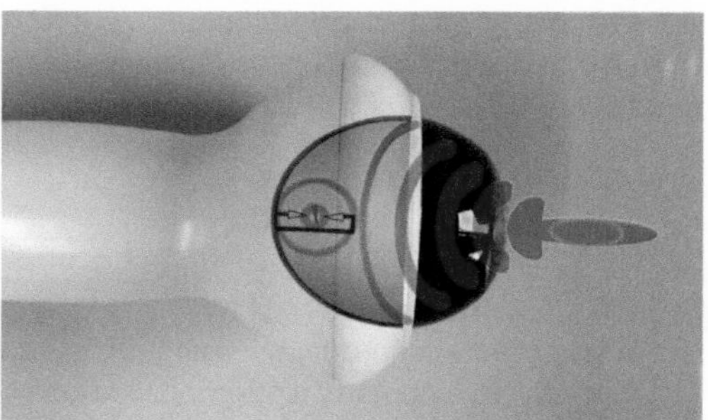

Fig. 2. Electrohydraulic trode with spark plug generating a focused shockwave. Depth of penetration is determined by the thickness of the bulb trode head. (Photo courtesy of PulseVet ®, a Zomedica ® Company, with written permission.)

when stimulated by high-voltage electricity delivering a focused, low-energy ultrasonic wave (**Fig. 3**A). Electromagnetic units have induction coils that generate opposing magnetic fields that are focused on an acoustic lens to generate low-pressure acoustic waves. It is important to note that although all focused devices deliver shockwaves, energy settings are not comparable, because the amplitude and focal depth vary considerably between machines yielding acoustic field properties with very different values.[7] Although it may be possible to find settings on 2 machines that are the same in 1 property, the other properties will differ significantly. For example, to yield the same pressure (mPA), the energy (Joules) measurement would need to drop by a factor of almost 10 in an electromagnetic unit when compared with an electrohydraulic generator.[7] In addition, the depth of penetration is generally deeper for focused shockwave units (up to 12 cm) compared with radial pressure waves (3–4 cm).[5–7] Another consideration between various machines is the difference

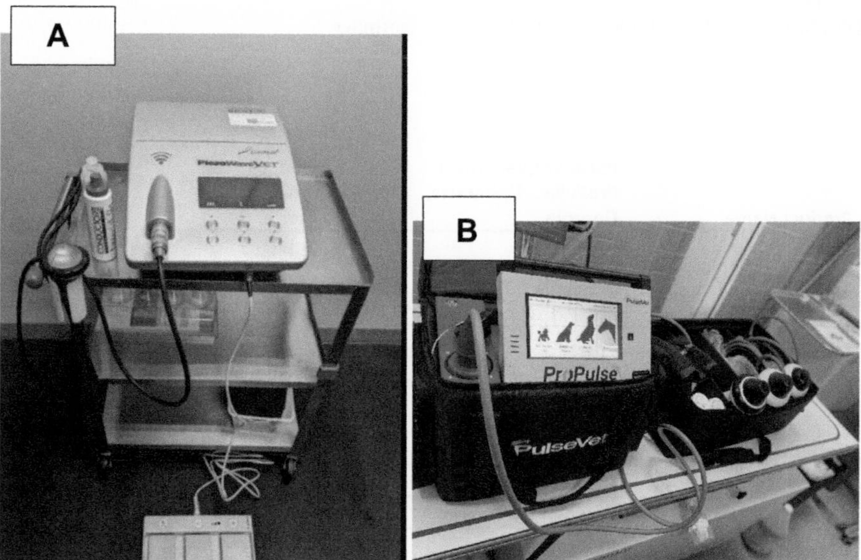

Fig. 3. (*A*) Piezoelectric generator. (*B*) Electrohydraulic generator. ([*A*] Photo courtesy of Dr. Missy Webber with written permission.)

in cost. There is the initial cost of acquisition of the device, which is variable among companies, and electrohydraulic generators have additional costs to replenish the pulses after approximately 20,000 to 50,000 pulses (**Table 1**).

INDICATIONS AND TREATMENT PROTOCOLS

The Food and Drug Administration has approved ESWT as a treatment for plantar fasciopathy.[4,8] There are also multiple high-quality clinical trials supporting the use of ESWT for treating tendinopathies in humans throughout the body, especially calcific shoulder tendinopathy.[1,4–6,8]

Indications in veterinary literature point to wide-ranging uses for musculoskeletal conditions including fracture healing, tendinopathies, chronic myofascial and lumbosacral pain, osteoarthritis, and wound healing.

Treatments generally range from 500 to 1500 pulses per location per treatment. Published literature and the author's preference is to administer a total of 2 to 3 treatments 2 to 3 weeks apart (**Table 2**).[1,3,4] Radial pressure wave devices may require more treatments (3–5 sessions) when compared with electrohydraulic units (1–3 treatments).[4–6] There are no randomized controlled clinical trials in animals demonstrating superiority between various machines or treatment protocols.

In general, it is recommended to clip the hair to allow better contact with the patient skin and use gel to improve transmission of the shockwaves and thereby reduce acoustic impedance. It may also be helpful to keep the trode perpendicular to the tissues and to move the trode during treatment to ensure the focused waves penetrate the tissue of interest. Finally, due to relatively high acoustic waves, ear plugs can be beneficial for both the human personnel administering treatment and the patients.

Table 1
Product comparisons for veterinary shockwave machines

Product Name	Pulse Vet,VersaTron ProPulse, Alpharetta, Georgia	PiezoWave2 Vet, Alpharetta, Georgia	Swiss DolorClast, Nyon, Switzerland MasterPuls, Tägerwilen, Switzerland
Type of wave	Focused	Focused	Unfocused
Type of generator	Electrohydraulic	Piezoelectric	Radial
Peak pressure (MPa)	70	15	0.4
Penetration depth	Trodes: 5 mm (0–25 mm) 20 mm (0–40 mm) X-trode (0–93 mm)	F7G3 gel[b] pads range in 5-mm increments (30–40 mm)	5 mm 15 mm 20 mm
Sedation	Yes, except for X-trode[a]	No (**Fig. 5**)	Yes
Must replenish Pulses	Yes	No	No
Easily portable	Yes	Yes	Yes
Lifetime cost	$$$	$	$

[a] Manufacturer suggests that sedation may not be needed in all patients.
[b] Gel pads are removable on the treatment trode allowing for various depths of penetration.

Table 2
General treatment protocols used by author[a]

Condition	# Pulses	Trode	Energy[c]	Sedation	Number of Treatments	Frequency
Shoulder tendinopathy (dogs ≥ 20 kg)	1000 (Divided 500/500 cranial/lateral)	20 mm	E6	Yes	2–3	2 wk
Hip osteoarthritis	1000[b]	X-trode	E5-6	No	1-3	2-3 wk
Elbow osteoarthritis	500–800[b]	X-trode	E3-5	No	1-3	2-3 wk
Lumbosacral pain (dogs ≥ 20 kg)	1000	X-trode	E6	No	1–3	2–3 wk
Acute/subacute myopathies	500 (Focused on muscle)	5 mm 20 mm	E5-6	Yes	2–3	2 wk

[a] Note these treatments protocols are for PulseVet electrohydraulic generator and are used by the author based on personal experience and should not be misinterpreted as evidence or superiority over other published protocols.
[b] For patients smaller than 20 kg, fewer pulses are delivered- 500 for 5 to 10 kg, 600 for 11 to 15 kg, 750 for 16 to 20 kg, 800 for 20 kg+.
[c] Higher energy levels (E7-8) are available, but not personally used by this author. These settings may be useful for promoting bone healing/malunions.

REVIEW OF CURRENT EVIDENCE

Bone Healing

Cancellous bone is most susceptible to shockwaves due to its multiple tissue interfaces (bone, fat, and connective tissue) resulting in greater reflection and energy transmission compared with compact bone.[2] Because most of the energy is deposited into cancellous bone, it stimulates osteoblasts to promote bone healing. Shockwaves have a low relative risk of adverse effects on healthy, intact bone.

Kieves and colleagues[9] prospectively studied the effects of ESWT on 42 dogs (50 stifles) recovering from tibial plateau leveling osteotomy (TPLO). Treatment consisted of 1000 pulses using electrohydraulic ESWT (PulseVet, VersaTron, Alpharetta, Georgia, USA) or sham treatment to the osteotomy site immediately and 2 weeks post-TPLO. Radiographs were evaluated 8 weeks postoperatively by 3 blinded, board-certified radiologists and found to have superior osteotomy healing in the ESWT group. This is considered a high-quality level 2 evidence study with low risk of bias.

Barnes and colleagues[10] also evaluated the effect of electrohydraulic ESWT (PulseVet, VersaTron, Alpharetta, Georgia, USA) on osteotomy healing in 39 dogs following tibial tuberosity advancement (TTA); this was an unblinded randomized controlled study. Dogs were divided into groups evaluating autologous bone graft with ESWT, autologous bone graft without ESWT, ESWT without autologous bone graft, and neither therapy. ESWT consisted of 1000 pulses delivered to the stifle with a 5-mm electrohydraulic trode. Radiographic densitometry demonstrated higher osteotomy gap density at 4 weeks postoperatively compared with no treatment and ESWT-only groups at 4 weeks postoperatively. No significant difference was found between any of the groups at 8 weeks. This is also a high-quality level 2 study with moderate risk of bias due to unblinding.

More recently, Barnes and colleagues[11] evaluated the effects of electrohydraulic ESWT (PulseVet, VersaTron, Alpharetta, Georgia, USA) post-TPLO in 16 dogs. ESWT consisted of 1000 pulses administered at 0 and 2 weeks postoperatively.

ESWT dogs had improved weight-bearing (higher peak vertical force [PVF] and vertical impulse [VI]) than control dogs. As in the Barnes TTA study, no difference in osteotomy healing was found between ESWT and control groups at 8 weeks. Additional outcome measures (thigh girth, pain scores, and goniometry) were also not different between study groups. This was also a level 2 evidence study.

Tendinopathy

Low-level evidence exists from 2 retrospective studies in dogs with shoulder tendinopathy demonstrating improvement in lameness following treatment with electrohydraulic ESWT.

Becker and colleagues[12] conducted a retrospective study with 15 client-owned dogs diagnosed with shoulder lameness (biceps tendinopathy, medial shoulder instability or supraspinatus tendinopathy) that had failed conservative management. ESWT (PulseVet, VersaTron, Alpharetta, Georgia, USA) was administered 3 times at 750 pulses, 3 to 4 weeks apart. Nine dogs were examined 3 to 4 weeks after the last treatment, and all had improved or resolved lameness. Long-term follow-up via telephone interview in 11 dogs (844 $\pm$ 543 days mean time after treatment) noted improvement or resolution by their owners in 7 of 11 dogs (64%). This study is considered level 4 evidence due to retrospective nature with a high risk of bias due to lack of objective outcome measures, lack of control group, recall bias, and lack of blinding of investigators and owners.

Another retrospective study with 29 client-owned dogs with confirmed biceps or supraspinatus tendinopathy demonstrated 85% success as determined by owner assessment 11 to 220 weeks following therapy.[13] Treatment consisted of 3 treatments 3 weeks apart with an electrohydraulic generator (PulseVet, VersaTron, Alpharetta, Georgia, USA) as well as therapeutic exercise. This is also deemed a level 4 study with high risk of bias.

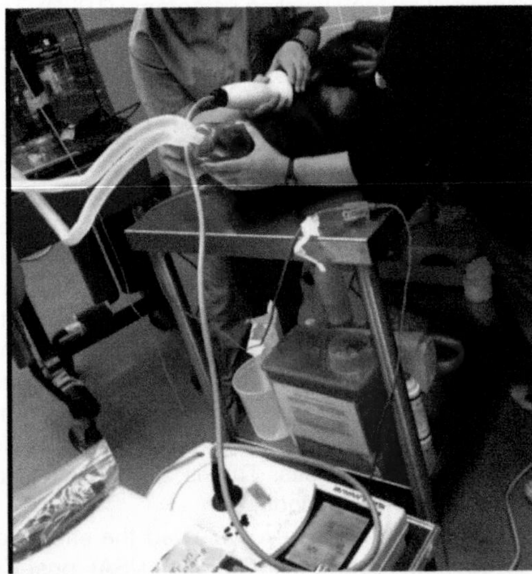

Fig. 4. Use of a focused shockwave electrohydraulic generator to treat a dog with shoulder tendinopathy under sedation.

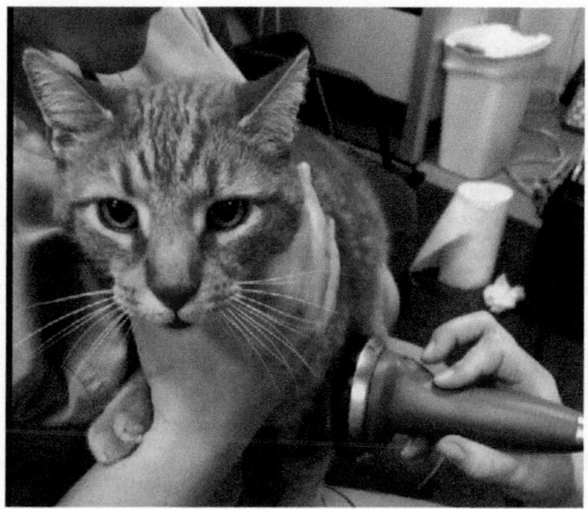

Fig. 5. Feline patient receiving piezoelectric extracorporeal shockwave therapy for elbow osteoarthritis unsedated. (Photo courtesy of ELvation USA Vet, Alpharetta, Georgiawith written permission.)

Treatment of shoulder tendinopathy in these studies was administered under sedation and was well tolerated (**Fig. 4**). Sedation was used for all published studies using EWST for the treatment of canine shoulder tendinopathy.

Desmopathy

Gallagher and colleagues[14] evaluated the effects of ESWT on patellar ligament desmitis in 19 dogs recovering from TPLO. Dogs were treated with electrohydraulic ESWT (PulseVet, VersaTron, Alpharetta, Georgia, USA) 600 pulses at energy level 6 with a 5-mm trode focused on the patellar ligament at 4 and 6 weeks postoperatively. Mean patellar ligament thickness was significantly lower in the ESWT treatment group at 6 and 8 weeks compared with the control group. This constitutes a high-quality level 2 study with low risk of bias.

Osteoarthritis

There are studies showing benefits of radial pressure wave therapy (RPWT) for the treatment of osteoarthritis in dogs.

In a randomized clinical trial, 30 dogs with hip dysplasia received RPWT to 1 limb and the contralateral limb served as a no treatment control.[15] Patients received a total of 3 treatments spaced 1 week apart delivering 2000 pulses at 0.1 to 0.3 mJ/mm^2 (MasterPuls, Tägerwilen, Switzerland) to the coxofemoral joint. Outcomes were measured at day 0, 30, 60, and 90 and included subjective visual analog pain scale by a blinded veterinarian and owner as well as objective gait analysis (PVF, VI, and symmetry index [SI]). PVF improved in the treated limb compared with the contralateral limb. Pain and lameness improved in both groups and did not differ between treated and control limbs during the treatment period. Owners reported improvements in quality of life and level of activity; however, given the contralateral limb served as a control in the same dogs, it is difficult to qualify the meaning of these data. Petechiation was noted in 20% of treated dogs, but the therapy was otherwise well tolerated. This was a level 2 study with moderate risk of bias due to allocation of controls.

Mueller and colleagues[16] prospectively studied the effects of RPWT on 18 dogs with naturally occurring hip osteoarthritis compared with 6 untreated dogs. A total of 3 treatments spaced 1 week apart delivered 2000 pulses (Swiss DolorClast Vet, Electro

Medical Systems, Nyon, Switzerland) to the affected coxofemoral joints. Force plate analysis demonstrated significant improvements in PVF, VI, and SI in treated dogs at 3 and 6 months posttreatment. No adverse effects were reported. This constitutes a level 2 study with low risk of bias.

In a small, randomized controlled study with 7 dogs suffering from naturally occurring stifle osteoarthritis, electrohydraulic shockwave was administered 3 times at 3 week intervals consisting of 1500 pulses (divided into 4 areas around the stifle) at 0.14 mJ/mm^2 (product name not provided).[17] Although improvements were noted during the 98-day study period, none reached statistical significance between treatment and sham control dogs for PVF, VI, stifle range of motion, or owner subjective outcome measures. Mild discomfort and petechiation were noted as minor side effects of treatment. This is considered a level 2 study with moderate risk of bias due to low subject numbers.

In a study by Millis and colleagues, dogs with hip and elbow osteoarthritis received a single electrohydraulic (PulseVet, VersaTron, Alpharetta, Georgia, USA) shockwave treatment.[18] Steady improvement was shown from day 0 to day 28 when compared with baseline in peak vertical force, comfortable range of motion, and lameness at both a walk and trot. Dogs in the control group showed a continuous decline in these measurements when compared with baseline, highlighting the value of shockwave treatment in osteoarthritis. However, these data were presented in abstract form only and the study remains unpublished.[18]

Future Research

A large, prospective study is currently being conducted at The Ohio State University to evaluate the effects of electrohydraulic ESWT (PulseVet, ProPulse, Alpharetta, Georgia, USA) on chronic low back pain in dogs. Systematic review and meta-analysis has demonstrated efficacy of ESWT in humans with chronic back pain.[19] This study may add to the objective data demonstrating additional benefits of ESWT for musculoskeletal conditions in dogs.

USE OF EXTRACORPOREAL SHOCKWAVE THERAPY SHOULD BE AVOIDED NEAR:

- Malignant masses. Note, however, that if the neoplasm is removed, recent research points to beneficial effects of ESWT in patients with cancer.[20]
- Gravid uterus due to concern for damage to the fetus.[21]
- Lung parenchyma due to the presence of gas and where formation of gas bubbles could lead to pneumothorax.[21]
- Growth plates due to concern for altering growth rate (either dampening or accelerating); however, this has recently been questioned.[22]
- Brain and spinal cord for risk of nerve damage; however, some report it can improve nerve regeneration.[23,24]
- Large vessels and patients with coagulopathies, due to risk of bleeding/petechiation.[21]

SIDE EFFECTS

ESWT is generally very well tolerated and safe for most patients. Side effects can include pain during treatment, local bruising, ecchymosis and/or petechiae, hematoma, and local swelling at the site of treatment.[5,8]These are typically short-lasting and expected to resolve within 48 to 72 hours after treatment.[25] In addition, some patients may experience aversion to the loud noise during treatment and may induce patient anxiety.

CLINICS CARE POINTS

- Aim for a minimum of 2 shockwave treatments spaced 2 to 3 weeks apart
- Keep the shockwave trode perpendicular to the tissue of interest for maximal effect
- Clip hair and use ultrasound gel to improve shockwave penetration
- Avoid using shockwave over areas of the lungs or large vessels

DISCLOSURE

The author has nothing to disclose. No funding or grants were received in the research for this manuscript.

REFERENCES

1. Chung B, Wiley JP. Extracorporeal shockwave therapy: A review. Sport Med 2002;32(13):851–65.
2. McClure SR, Van Sickle D, White R. Effects of extracorporeal shockwave therapy on bone. Vet Surg 2004;33:40–8.
3. Durant A, Millis D. Applications of extracorporeal shockwave in small animal rehabilitation. In: Millis DL, Levine DL, editors. Canine Rehabilitation and Physical therapy, 2w. St. Louis: Elsevier; 2014. p. 381–92.
4. Speed C. A systematic review of shockwave therapies in soft tissue conditions: focusing on the evidence. Br J Sport Med 2014;48(21):1538–42.
5. Elia Martinez JM, Schmitt J, Tenias Burillo JM, et al. Comparison between extracorporeal shockwave therapy and radial pressure wave therapy in plantar fasciitis. Rehabilitacion (Madr) 2020;54(1):11–8.
6. DeLuca S, Robinson DM, Yun PH, et al. Similar functional gains using radial versus combined shockwave therapy in management of plantar fasciitis. J Foot Ankle Surg 2021;60(6):1098–102.
7. Cleveland RO, McAteer JA. The physics of shockwave lithotripsy. ed 2. Smith's Textbook of Endourology. Hamilton, Ontario: BC Decker Inc; 2007.
8. Roerdink RL, Dietvorst M, van der Zwaard B, et al. Complications of extracorporeal shockwave therapy in plantar fasciitis: Systematic review. Int J Surg 2017;46:133–45.
9. Kieves NR, MacKay CS, Adducci K, et al. High energy focused shock wave therapy accelerates bone healing. A blinded, prospective, randomized canine clinical trial. Vet Comp Orthop Traumatol 2015;28(6):425–32.
10. Barnes K, Lanz O, Werre S, et al. Comparison of autogenous cancellous bone grafting and extracorporeal shock wave therapy on osteotomy healing in the tibial tuberosity advancement procedure in dogs: Radiographic densitometric evaluation. Vet Comp Orthop Traumatol 2015;28(3):207–14. https://doi.org/10.3415/VCOT-14-10-0156.
11. Barnes K, Faludi A, Takawira C, et al. Extracorporeal shock wave therapy improves short-term limb use after canine tibial plateau leveling osteotomy. Vet Surg 2019;48(8):1382–90. https://doi.org/10.1111/vsu.13320.
12. Becker W, Kowaleski M, McCarthy RJ, et al. Extracorporeal shockwave therapy for shoulder lameness in dogs. J Am Anim Hosp Assoc 2015;51:15–9. https://doi.org/10.5326/JAAHA-MS-6175.

13. Leeman JJ, Shaw KK, Mison MB, et al. Extracorporeal shockwave therapy and therapeutic exercise for supraspinatus and biceps tendinopathies in 29 dogs. Vet Rec 2016;179(5):385. https://doi.org/10.1136/vr.103487.
14. Gallagher A, Cross AR, Sepulveda G. The effect of shock wave therapy on patellar ligament desmitis after tibial plateau leveling osteotomy. Vet Surg 2012; 41(4):482–5. https://doi.org/10.1111/j.1532-950X.2012.0095.
15. Souza AN, Ferreira MP, Hagen SC, et al. Radial shock wave therapy in dogs with hip osteoarthritis. Vet Comp Orthop Traumatol 2016;29(2):108–14.
16. Mueller M, Bockstahler B, Skalicky M, et al. Effects of radial shockwave therapy on limb function of dogs with hip osteoarthritis. Vet Rec 2007;160(22):762–5.
17. Dahlberg J, Fitch G, McClure SR, et al. The evaluation of extracorporeal shockwave therapy in naturally occurring osteoarthritis of the stifle joint in dogs. Vet Comp Orthop Traumatol 2005;18(3):147–52.
18. Francis, DA, Millis, DL, Evans, M, Moyers, T. Clinical Evaluation of Extracorporeal shock wave therapy for management of canine osteoarthritis of the elbow and hip joint. Proceedings of the 31st Annual Conference of the Veterinary Orthopedics Society, Big Sky Montana, USA. 2004; Feb 22 to 27: p13.
19. Yue L, Sun MS, Chen H, et al. Extracorporeal shockwave therapy for treating chronic low back pain: A systematic review and meta-analysis of randomized controlled trials. Biomed Res Int 2021;2021:5937250. https://doi.org/10.1155/2021/5937250.
20. Crevenna R, Mickel M, Keilani M. Extracorporeal shock wave therapy in the supportive care and rehabilitation of cancer patients. Support Care Cancer 2019; 27(11):4039–41.
21. Desai M, Sun Y, Buchholz N, et al. Treatment selection for urolithiasis: percutaneous nephrolithomy, ureteroscopy, shock wave lithotripsy, and active monitoring. World J Urol 2017;35(9):1395–9.
22. Lohrer H, Nauck T, Korakakis V, et al. Historical ESWT Paradigms Are Overcome: A Narrative Review. Biomed Res Int 2016;2016:3850461.
23. Wu YH, Lun JJ, Chen WS, et al. The electrophysiological and functional effect of shock wave on peripheral nerves. Conf Proc IEEE Eng Med Biol Soc 2007;2007: 2369–72.
24. Mense S, Hoheisel U. Shock wave treatment improves nerve regeneration in the rat. Muscle Nerve 2013;47(5):702–10.
25. Schmitz C, Császár NB, Milz S, et al. Efficacy and safety of extracorporeal shock wave therapy for orthopedic conditions: a systematic review on studies listed in the PEDro database. Br Med Bull 2015;116(1):115–38.

Conditioning Dogs for an Active Lifestyle

Julia Tomlinson, BVsc, MS, PhD*, Megan Nelson, BS, CVT

KEYWORDS

• Canine fitness • Canine exercise • Canine training • Sports-specific training

KEY POINTS

- Conditioning prepares the body for the demands of physical activity so that the activity can be performed with relative ease and enjoyment and with the goal of injury prevention.
- The foundation of conditioning for an activity is sports or activity-specific training, and this training needs to be more than once a week.
- A certain amount of fatigue is needed to gain fitness in an individual, but that should be balanced with adequate recovery time.

GENERAL PRINCIPLES OF CONDITIONING

When training to maximize function and to prevent injury in sports, experts in equine sports medicine agree the best approach is to train for the sport that the athlete competes in.[1,2] The same is true for a leisure activity. Although this seems as an obvious statement, the body needs to train for the speed needed (appropriate muscle fiber selection) and hone the specific movements needed for the sport or leisure activity (fine motor control and balance). Dogs training agility less than one hour a week needed to use more triceps muscle fibers to complete a simple trotting task after a warm-up as compared to dogs who trained more often.[3] Fatigue has a detrimental effect on accuracy of movement[4] and so likely increases injury risk. During activity, metabolism needs to increase and waste products need to be removed, conditioning upregulates this process.[5,6] Stamina also needs to be trained for both mind and body; a field trial dog needs to maintain concentration over long periods of time while continuing to run. Stamina alone is not enough. Consider a dog who has spent the summer swimming and retrieving in the water, then abruptly switches to hunting in dense cover as the weather cools. This dog may have excellent stamina but extensor muscles of the rear limbs will not be conditioned enough. Swimming produces 20° less stifle extension than at a fast walk,[7] and joints will not be adequately conditioned for the long periods of impact during land-based retrieving.

Twin Cities Animal Rehabilitation and Sports Medicine Clinic, 12010 Riverwood Drive, Burnsville, MN 55337, USA
* Corresponding author.
E-mail address: Drjulia@tcrehab.com

Vet Clin Small Anim 52 (2022) 1043–1058
https://doi.org/10.1016/j.cvsm.2022.03.008
vetsmall.theclinics.com

Conditioning has 2 main components:

1. Sports or activity specific: this is practicing the exact movements required for a particular sport or activity, either in short sequences or at full level.
2. "Cross training" or combined training: in human sports medicine this training is often doing sports-related movements with a different load to improve strength and reduce injury risk.[8] For example, a baseball pitcher practicing the motions of a throw holding a 3 lb weight or a sprinter running in water.

Conditioning programs should focus on activity-specific practice (eg, speed, distance, jump height) along with strengthening. In the veterinary field, with the plethora of individuals giving advice on training canine athletes, there is a lot of emphasis on body awareness and strength and balance via other non–sport-specific exercises that have value but should not predominate. Spending enough time on activity-specific training is important to ensure the body is building the right type of tissue strength and exercise capacity. In an experiment using young dogs on a treadmill trotting for 55 weeks, their triceps muscle fibers became predominantly slow twitch type I muscle; this was a change from the faster twitch type II fibers needed for sprinting.[9]

"Cross" training (combination training) is often mentioned in the world of canine conditioning. The main sports training principle is that "power athletes should train power and endurance athletes should train endurance."[10] True cross-training can achieve sport-specific goals. A study of netball (similar to basketball) players doing the chest pass movement at lower speed when compared with a group doing close to sport-specific speed showed no significant difference between groups in improvement of throw velocity. Part of the effect of this training was the repeated *intent* to move the load as rapidly as possible, a difficult challenge in our patients. It is difficult to use true cross-training for some canine athletes and relatively easy in others. Hunting/field dogs can just carry a weighted dummy in their mouth on walks. We can mimic sport-related movements and provide resistance during work at lower than sport-specific speeds—resisted swims are the most appropriate training modality for improving stroke rate in swimmers.[11]

A sample cross-training program from human medicine is in the sport of netball:

- Single leg landing after a jump holding the ball
- Single leg squat holding the ball
- Balance one leg back, bend, and straighten while holding the ball
- Core work

In veterinary sports medicine, we can use sports-specific motions as a conditioning exercise by isolating a movement or activity normally performed during sport. Often the moments will be performed more slowly than when competing, and this will still strengthen tissues because the animal is moving the same load (the body) and making the same movements that happen at higher speed during the actual sport.

For example, jump works as combined training for an agility dog:

- Single jump from standstill (no advantage of momentum to aid in propulsion)
- Practice tight turns (wraps) from standstill over a single jump
- Single or combination jumping at speed using varying distances as lead out (to keep tissues trained for impact)

It is particularly important for both the juvenile and elderly dog to regularly practice an activity at lower loads/slower speed in order to train accuracy of movement (eg, slow turns, catching a simple throw of the ball or frisbee from a standstill). Exercise causes the creation of new nerves in the hippocampus of people, which is the center of learning and memory in the brain.[12] The trainer should challenge balance and coordination with varied movements that mimic the skills needed for the sport or leisure activity. Train for focus and drive using short periods, then building up to the requisite concentration time needed for the activity.

CLINICS CARE POINTS

There are several different types of training that focus on speed and strength and on endurance. The methods used depend on the sport but include the following:

- Interval training—high-intensity workouts interspersed with rest or relief periods
- Circuit training—moving from one specific exercise to another every few minutes can repeat the circuit
- Fartlek training—periods of intense effort alternate with periods of less strenuous effort in a continuous workout
- Plyometric training—rapid movements that need fast stretch or contraction of muscles, for example, rapid, targeted jumps (**Fig. 1**)

Basic principles of increasing workload depend mostly on the dog's performance and ability to endure the current workload. Usually increases are weekly. It is best to work on staging up only one parameter at a time, distance, speed, or number of repetitions, focusing on what is most useful for the sport or leisure activity. For example, a technique used in sled dogs is as follows: if dogs are maintaining within 10% of the maximum allowed speed while pulling the sled during the last 30 minutes of the workout, then the distance of the next workout is increased by 25%.[13]

Exercise is advised to be at lower speeds in order to build endurance, rather than at close to maximum effort—in practice this means exercise at a trot is appropriate when starting out. High-intensity intervals help exercise tolerance even if the sport or leisure activity itself is at a slower speed and intensity. This training pushes the cardiovascular system, increases plasma volume by driving water intake after submaximal exercise, and pushes the respiratory and other systems to increase metabolism.[14]

One challenge for practitioners is designing an appropriate fitness stress test. Return to resting pulse rate has been used as a gauge of baseline fitness; however, in dogs it has the added challenge of anticipatory response. Pulse rate can be markedly

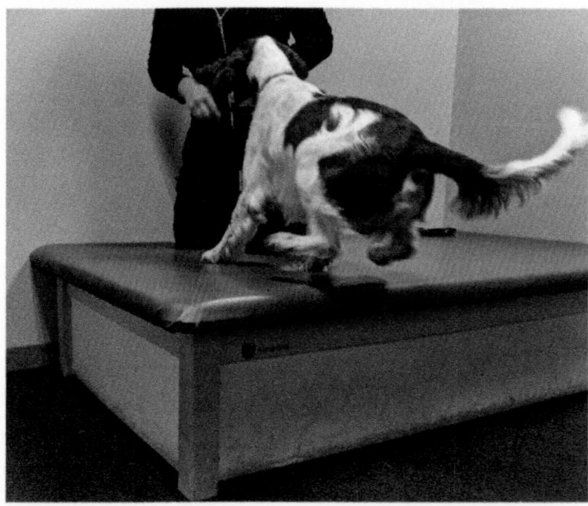

Fig. 1. A plyometric exercise, jumping rapidly on and off a target surface from a standing position with the goal of increasing muscle power.

elevated in anticipation of activity; respiratory rate can also increase in some dogs.[15] Studies in sporting dogs show when pulse rate is taken as much as 5 minutes after training or competing, heart rates remain high, which may be due to the measuring method causing stress. An example protocol would be using a simple validated heart rate monitor[16] when working a dog until a heart rate of 150 to 160 bpm is achieved, then measuring heart rate every 1 minute during rest to determine how quickly it falls to baseline. The remote method of measuring may remove some of the stressors that keep heart rate high. At this time, only intra-dog comparison will have value in interpreting response to conditioning and that depends on many environmental factors.

Core strength training is part of most human athletic programs. The center of gravity is a lot lower in quadrupeds, although the epaxial and hypaxial muscles still act to stabilize the trunk in motion and absorb torque. The spine moves differently in dogs as compared with humans, with lateral bending of the spine in dogs during protractions.[17] As in humans, a weak core possibly leads to excessive trunk motion. Training the core (**Fig. 2**) requires modeling a sustained muscle contraction; challenges to maintain core stability while moving can be added once this has been achieved. A hand placed on the ventral abdomen can check for muscle engagement during the exercise.

Trainers should watch the posture of the athlete; the spine should be in neutral unless specific targeting of flexors or extensors is needed. For example, jumping dogs use spinal flexors a lot, and the muscle group may become predominant with dogs lacking reach over jumps; in that case extensors may need to be targeted.

SPECIFIC CONSIDERATIONS FOR JUVENILE DOGS

Training of the young athlete should be well-rounded. Early specialization causes fewer muscle groups to be worked, resulting in imbalance. In human athletic medicine, recovery stress consensus is that before puberty, focus should be on agility, balance, and coordination.[18] The juvenile canine athlete also has a period of maximal neuroplasticity where foundations of sport should be taught via general proprioceptive challenges, working on confidence and familiarization with equipment in short, frequent sessions. Building strength is focused on after musculoskeletal maturity is reached.

Exercise will remodel tissue in the young[19] as it does in mature athletes, and some light strength work is warranted. A study on young Retrievers aged 11 to 24 months showed that treadmill running for 25 minutes 3 times a week adequately stimulated bone formation with no resorption.[20] Strenuous work can be detrimental to joints of

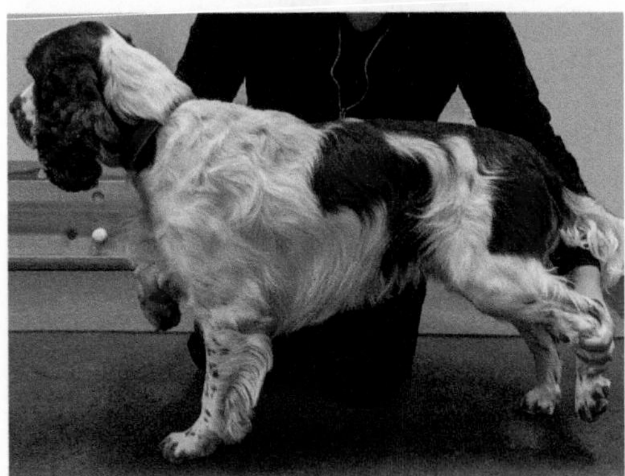

Fig. 2. Simple exercise aimed at recruitment of abdominal and epaxial muscles to maintain balance while the 2 opposite limbs are lifted.

immature dogs.[21] Therefore, one reasonable approach may be to allow the immature dog to free run and play but avoid repetitive actions at high speed (eg, keep ball play to very short sessions of a few reps at a time). Similarly, avoiding long (particularly forced, eg, jogging with a puppy) durations of activity seems reasonable. There is no consensus on exercising young dogs at this time, but the Authors' rule of thumb is to start with very short training walks, then build to a continuous walk of 20 to 30 minutes once midgrowth is achieved. After that, lengthen walks by 10 minutes a week, maximum distance 5 miles until musculoskeletal maturity. It is best to avoid going on a run or biking with a dog until they have reached musculoskeletal maturity.

Sports-specific training is started once closer to maturity. Thoroughbred racehorses used to be working at a trotting gait for a large percentage of each training week; however, they work at a gallop when they race. A study found that the risk of dorsometacarpal disease (shin splints) at 1.5 years decreased with accumulation of distance that those horses were exercised at the canter and galloping speeds.[6,22] Analysis of daily training information and health reports of 2-year-old Thoroughbreds in 5 commercial stables showed that survival during 1 year of racing was significantly greater when exercised at a hard gallop versus breezing (moderate gallop).

CONDITIONING THE INEXPERIENCED ADULT

If conditioning for a specific activity starts when the dog is already an adult, the foundations of the activity need to be worked on. The trainer can and should train for activity-specific proprioception in the inexperienced adult.

Training age is a term used to describe ability based on a combination of chronologic age and experience. There are 3 different factors in estimating training age:

1. Sport specific—the duration the athlete has been performing the sport
2. General training—the duration the athlete has done any training (strength, conditioning)
3. Lifestyle—a general measure of how active the athlete is (do they go on walks, run in the yard, or do they only train agility 1 day a week and do nothing else?)

Training age should always be considered when prescribing exercises for conditioning, as a dog with a relatively inactive lifestyle will struggle to be an athlete. Agility dogs with less than 4 years of experience are more prone to injury, and this is not an effect of chronologic age.[23]

Chronologic age does have some effect on conditioning, as dogs and humans age their muscle size decreases (sarcopenia),[24] and this can only be partially offset by training and nutrition. Exercise progression should be slower in older athletes, with longer recovery time between bouts of exercise, as aged dogs show less adaptability to a treadmill exercise.[25] A rule of thumb for interval training would be to double rest time (eg, from 3 to 6 minutes between sessions of high intensity) but it is very dog dependent and training age should be considered. A fit, older dog can usually tolerate an exercise progression similar to a younger adult. Depending on the baseline level of fitness of an older dog, conditioning sessions may be more appropriately spaced every third day as opposed to every other day, with increases in duration every 4 sessions instead of every 3. The clinician should observe the dog exercising and make appropriate decisions based on the individual.

PROVIDING ADEQUATE REST

There is a certain amount of fatigue needed to push conditioning in an individual, but that should be balanced with recovery time. Time is needed for tissue building and repair. The term "under-recovery" is used in human sports medicine, and this under-recovery can accumulate, resulting in overtraining syndrome. Symptoms of overtraining syndrome include continuous muscle soreness and even endocrinological disturbances. Much longer rest periods are needed to resolve this.[26] As our dogs cannot self-advocate and will keep exercising due to drive and willingness to please, we need to err on the side of caution. The trainer should be aware of signs of fatigue, watching for lack of full recovery of respirations in interval training, and/or loss of form (body position during training), and cut the session short if needed. The American Sports Medicine College recommends strength training 2 to 3x a week for novice individuals and 4 to 5 days a week for more experienced athletes.[27] Training for endurance at low speeds (trot, scaling up to canter) can be done up to 6 days a week although it is advised to only increase distance once weekly. In older dogs, if there are signs of excess fatigue when increasing weekly, then every 2 weeks is warranted.

CONSIDERATIONS BEFORE EXERCISE

Warm up: the goal of warm up is to improve performance and reduce the risk of muscle injury. Warm up increases muscle temperature and metabolism as well as muscle fiber function.[28] It also increases soft tissue flexibility.[29] There are no scientific research studies on the effect of stretching on performance of exercising dogs. In human medicine stretching before exercise is not recommended, as it may reduce muscle performance.[30] The benefit of stretching immediately after exercise is controversial; a metanalysis found that muscle stretching before, after, or both before and after exercise did not reduce delayed-onset muscle soreness.[31]

Excitement can contribute to warm up but works against focus. Just 5 minutes of warm up exercise (1 minute of brisk walk and of trot, 0.5 minute of canter, 2.5 minutes of tight turns around the owner, and stepping over low obstacles) improved the efficiency of muscle activity in the triceps at trot in healthy dogs.[1] Warm up should be repeated if there is more than 20 minutes of inactivity between runs.

Climate: working dogs' body temperature has been shown to reach as high as 42°C (107 F) when undergoing strenuous exercise outside in temperatures around 22°C (72 F).[32] Brachycephalic dogs are far less heat tolerant.[33] Heat dissipation in temperate to warm conditions is usually more problematic than exercising at low temperatures. Cold conditions do decrease air moisture, and so fluid losses from the respiratory tract can be higher than expected. Very low temperatures (−12 C/10 F) can damage airway lining, and intense exercise at less cold temperatures can cause airway damage, known as "ski asthma."[34]

SPECIFIC ACTIVITIES

Following are a few examples of particular canine sport or leisure activities with guidelines on how to condition for the activity. Specific conditioning for activities is important, even if the activity is for leisure and not a formal sport (eg, going snowshoeing or cross-country skiing with the owner on weekends). The guidelines in this article can be used for any activity performed as part of an active lifestyle. In some of the following examples, sample protocols are given.

Field Trial

Field trial competitors are elite athletes who need to train for speed, strength, and stamina. In the case of the dog used as an example here, the individual was already a fit athlete but was facing some challenges in performance. As practitioners treating sporting dogs, it is rare for us to have to design a training program and more usual for us to have to alter a program to improve fitness while avoiding changes in sports-specific behavioral training.

A 4-year-old male Labrador presented to our clinic in Minnesota for a baseline sporting examination. The dog spends time in Texas with his trainer from January to April and then goes back and forth between Texas and home in the Midwest over the summer. He has shown some issues with heat intolerance and has a negative test for exercise-induced collapse. He has worked with a field veterinarian on some cooling strategies (rubbing alcohol on legs, belly, getting him wet, fan in the vehicle, pushing water intake). The owner reported that the dog "tends to get pretty high" (meaning excited) when he works and is full on sprinting out; however, he runs out of steam on the way back from a long retrieve.

Current activity level: 30-minute walks twice a day. Training schedule Monday through Friday, 50:50 land work to swimming. Land work is generally in the morning and water in the afternoon.

Land work is marks (object a dog sees thrown for it to retrieve, usually a game bird or a training bumper) 3 to 4 x 100 yards along with blinds (placed unseen by the dog) 3 × 300 yards, not necessarily on the same day.

He takes Mondays off if he has a weekend trial.

He does go trail running 4 to 5 miles with his owner on some of his days off or goes out in the kayak/swims.

Current warm up consists of some down to stand transitions, brisk walking to get him to a light pant, and cool down is walking.

Examination findings: good muscle and joint symmetry, lean to moderate muscle bulk. Minor lack of extensibility in shoulder supporting muscles.

Assessment: his lack of stamina is likely due to several factors: heat intolerance, excitement/drive using up energy reserves before he works, and having more type I endurance style muscles than type II speed muscles, as he does a lot of lower intensity endurance work at home with his owner (walks, running with owner).

The dog and owner need to work using high-intensity interval training; this has the goal of improving metabolite disposal, which in turn slows muscle fatigue and also helps adaptation to heat loss. Progression should be applied cautiously, to apply enough pressure to elicit change but to avoid overheating. If he does this interval training after he swims, he will be wet and therefore cooler for the exercise. Intervals allow recovery during the session. It should ideally take only 2 minutes to recharge but he may need to start with 5-minute breaks, and with time the rest period can be reduced.

Goals: improve exercise tolerance/sprinting stamina by training him to metabolize waste products more quickly and to cool better. Build strength without excess muscle bulk as that would be detrimental to cooling. Maintain joint health.

Plan:

Cooling:

- White sheet for when he is aired out at events, to reflect sun.
- Reduce warm up when greater than 60°F outside, concentrate on walk time only.
- Wet legs, belly before land work.
- Cooling fan placed as a crosswind in the vehicle, not head on.
- Use flavoring to push water intake.
- Use width of tongue, frantic head movements and panting rate as indicators of heat, and when to implement active cooling or see a veterinarian, but take rectal temperature if concerned.
- Cooling plan in emergency—best plan is to immerse in the training pond for 10 minutes.

Training schedule

Rest is as important as sport-specific conditioning. Implement 1 day off (excluding walks, light play) midweek if no trial that weekend. If trialing at the weekend, then give him Friday and Monday off.

1. Strength training—target shoulder muscles and knee extensors. Latter is important for jumping/leaping and will not get exercised when swimming.

   Two of his training days a week after swim work do "push-ups"

   A. For his front legs do push-ups. Start with 10 reps 4 on the floor, in 2 weeks change to doing them on a decline (**Fig. 3**) and 4 weeks from onset, increase reps to 15x

   B. For his rear do sit to stands with front on platform (training tip, works best if start in a sit, put his front feet on a pedestal and lure him to stand, **Fig. 4**). Eventual goal is he lowers himself into a sit and then pushes into a stand all with front feet on the bucket. Start with 5 reps, add 2 reps a week until he can do 15 reps with good form, quality over quantity. Do not progress in number until he can do the current assignment without difficulty for at least 4 days.

2. High-intensity interval training

   Two other training days a week after swimming perform high intensity interval training (HIIT)—short fast bumper retrieves using 2 bumpers to keep him moving.

   Week 1: 2 minutes retrieves, 2 minutes rest, 2 minutes retrieves 2 minutes rest, 1 minute retrieves.

   Week 2: 2 minutes retrieves, 2 minutes rest, 2 minutes retrieves 2 minutes rest, 2 minutes retrieves.

   Week 3: 3 minutes retrieves, 2 minutes rest, 2 minutes retrieves 2 minutes rest, 2 minutes retrieves.

   Week 4: 3 minutes retrieves, 2 minutes rest, 3 minutes retrieves 2 minutes rest, 2 minutes retrieves.

   Week 5: 3 minutes retrieves, 2 minutes rest, 3 minutes retrieves 2 minutes rest, 3 minutes retrieves.

   Week 6 onward: 3 minutes retrieves, 2 minutes rest, 3 minutes retrieves 2 minutes rest, 3 minutes retrieves 2 minutes rest 3 minutes retrieves

   If he does not return to baseline respiration rate after 2 minutes of rest then lengthen rest time to 5 minutes; this may be dependent on ambient

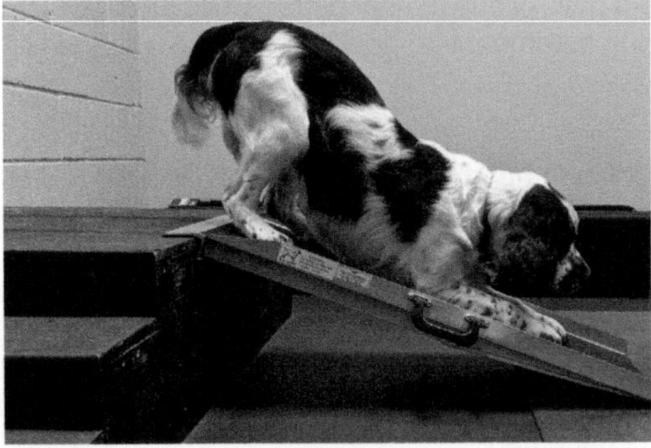

Fig. 3. A push up involves the dog flexing elbows and shoulders to touch the lower limb to the floor while keeping the rear standing. In this case the dog is standing on a ramp so more weight is shifted forward (decline push up).

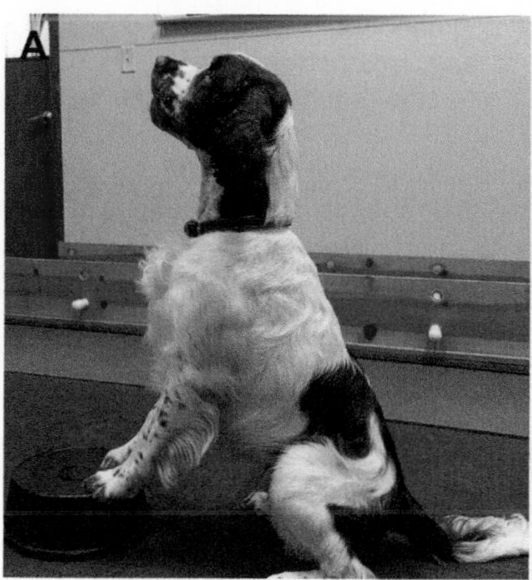

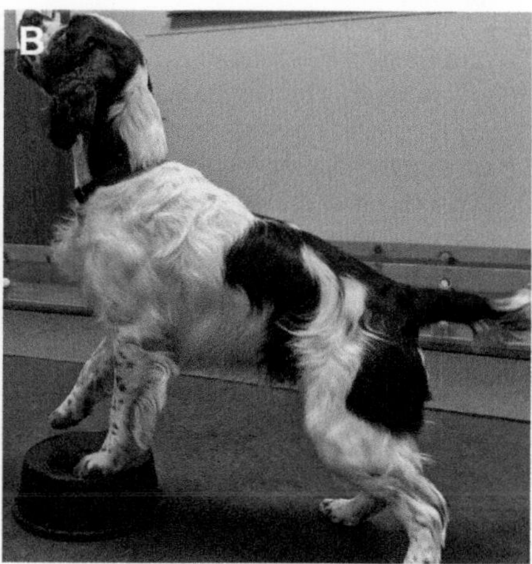

Fig. 4. (*A, B*) Sit to stands with front on a platform; the goal is to have the dog push with his rear and make little use of his front limbs during the exercise.

temperature. Being wet from swimming should prevent overheating but if ambient temperature greater than 70 F then monitor carefully, reduce rate of progression, and skip one interval if needed.

3. Flexibility

Manual therapies (light massage, demonstrated in clinic) on shoulders in the evening of every working day for 1 to 2 minutes. Follow with stretch into play bow position and then stretch front feet up on the second step of the stairs, rear on the floor, and reach for a treat to elongate spine.

Winter conditioning:

- Find a pole barn or agility arena available for rent to do indoor HIIT work, aim for 3 days a week of speed work
- Keep up the walks
- Strength work frequency increases to every other day instead of 2 days a week
- One of the three HIIT sessions a week can be replaced with rapid jumping on and off a stable ottoman if more feasible. 25x in a row after warm up

Outcome: "We had a very memorable experience at a field trial this weekend. We won a tough qualifying stake down in St. Louis. The conditioning program designed for us has been extremely beneficial physically and also mentally. It has provided an additional venue for us to learn to be a team in a very positive way, while at the same time building physique. Injuries are my biggest concern with the sport. But by working with you I feel as though we are doing everything we can to proactively address that issue."

Running with a Human

For a dog running with most people, they will be at a rapid trot; this is a relatively energy efficient gait (greater than 70% of the energy of propulsion being from elastic recoil).[35] Concerns are mostly related to impact and cooling; steadily increasing distance is advised. Start with measuring time trotting, then once intervals are combined and the goal distance of 2 to 3 miles of continuous speed is reached; distance can be added. Lengthen distance only once weekly, adding a mile to one of the runs. The running surface is often concrete; it is better to advise trail running.

Sample protocol: running a 5 km with your dog handout for owners.

Avoid training on consecutive days—take at least 1 day off between sessions.

(Clinician may start an individual at week 1 or a later week depending on baseline activity level and strength.)

Puppies and skeletally immature dogs should not follow this program.

Advise owners, if their dog shows any signs of heat exhaustion or lameness while following this program, seek veterinary attention immediately.

Warm up: before every training session, be sure to spend at least 5 minutes warming up; this will help warm up muscles, lubricate joints, and will help to prevent injury such as sprains and strains.

- Walk at a brisk pace for 5 minutes
- Then have your dog weave in a figure-eight around your legs (if small) or around 2 objects placed $^{3}/_{4}$ of their body length apart for 30 seconds.

Cool down: after every training session, spend a few minutes cooling down to allow heart rate and respiratory rate to return to normal and allow muscles to relax.

- Walk at a brisk pace for 5 minutes, then at a more leisurely pace for 3 more minutes.
- Then have your dog stand up onto their hind legs and put their front feet up on the stairs, hold this position for 10 seconds.
- Provide clean, cool water for your dog (**Table 1**).

Agility

Agility is usually a speed sport; the average dog runs a course in 45 to 60 seconds. The goal of conditioning is to ensure the dog can comfortably run for 60 seconds at a time and will practice obstacles for sports-specific training and conditioning of joints for impact. Experimental models show that load, repetition, and loading rate all affect how much stress cartilage can take without damage.[36] What we do not know in dogs (or people) is the load rate, force, and rest required to build joint strength and avoid damage. It is recommended in training that tissues are exposed regularly to force for adequate strength, generally 2 to 3 x per week.

Experience has an effect on injury rate in agility.[23,37] Practice on a full course is needed every week and is usually done in a formal class. In addition to once weekly practice on a full course, further at home practice is recommended on 2 other days. Short sequences (eg, jump-tunnel-weaves-jump) are often more feasible at home than full courses. Inclement weather can affect practice, and often the trainer has to compromise with single jump work indoors.

Work on jump forces has shown that take off in horses and dogs is mostly rear limb muscle work plus some elastic recoil from distal joints. Lift and reach are forelimb muscle work. As jump height increases, muscle work at the shoulder and stifle increases.[38] Jumping at speed versus from a standstill significantly increases the force of impact when landing. This force is as high as 4.5x body weight in the forelimbs when landing from a hurdle jump at high speed.[39]

Some agility competitors choose to train and trial at a lower jump height to preventatively decrease risk of injury; however, there is no proof that lower height is preventative; this becomes particularly a question in experienced athletes as they age. A lowering of jump height will result in pacing changes and changes in the parabolic arc of jumps, enabling dogs to speed up, translating to a faster motion with less experience at this pace and potentially greater risk of injury. It is harder to correct a movement error and correct course at higher speeds.

Table 1
Example of conditioning a dog to run 5 km/3 miles with a person

Week	Session 1	Session 2	Session 3
1	Warm up • Jog 60 s • Walk 90 s *Repeat 8 times* (20 min) Cool down	Warm up • Jog 60 s • Walk 90 s *Repeat 8 times* (20 min) Cool down	Warm up • Jog 60 s • Walk 90 s *Repeat 8 times* (20 min) Cool down
2	Warm up • Jog 90 s • Walk 1 min *Repeat 8 times* (18 min) Cool down	Warm up • Jog 90 s • Walk 1 min *Repeat 8 times* (18 min) Cool down	Warm up • Jog 90 s • Walk 1 min *Repeat 8 times* (18 min) Cool down
3	Warm up • Jog 90 s • Walk 1 min • Jog 3 min • Walk 2 min • Jog 90 s • Walk 1 min • Jog 3 min • Walk 2 min • Jog 90 s • Walk 1 min • Jog 3 min • Walk (20.5 min) Cool down	Warm up • Jog 90 s • Walk 1 min • Jog 3 min • Walk 2 min • Jog 90 s • Walk 1 min • Jog 3 min • Walk 2 min • Jog 90 s • Walk 1 min • Jog 3 min • Walk (20.5 min) Cool down	Warm up • Jog 3 min • Walk 2 min • Jog 3 min • Walk 2 min • Jog 3 min • Walk 2 min • Jog 3 min (18 min) Cool down
4	Warm up • Jog 3 min • Walk 2 min • Jog 5 min • Walk 2 min • Jog 3 min • Walk 2 min • Jog 3 min • Walk 2 min (22 min) Cool down	Warm up • Jog 5 min • Walk 2 min • Jog 5 min • Walk 2 min • Jog 5 min • Walk 1 min • Jog 2 min (22 min) Cool down	Warm up • Jog 5 min • Walk 2 min • Jog 5 min • Walk 2 min • Jog 5 min • Walk 1 min • Jog 2 min (22 min) Cool down
5	Warm up • Jog 7 min • Walk 2 min • Jog 5 min • Walk 1 min • Jog 5 min • Walk 2 min • Jog 2 min (24 min) Cool down	Warm up • Jog 7 min • Walk 2 min • Jog 5 min • Walk 1 min • Jog 5 min • Walk 2 min • Jog 2 min (24 min) Cool down	Warm up • Jog 7 min • Walk 1 min • Jog 7 min • Walk 2 min • Jog 6 min (23 min) Cool down
6	Warm up • Jog 7 min • Walk 1 min • Jog 7 min • Walk 2 min • Jog 6 min (24 min) Cool down	Warm up • Jog 9 min • Walk 2 min • Jog 7 min • Walk 1 min • Jog 5 min (24 min) Cool down	Warm up • Jog 9 min • Walk 2 min • Jog 7 min • Walk 1 min • Jog 5 min (24 min) Cool down

(*continued on next page*)

Table 1
(continued)

Week	Session 1	Session 2	Session 3
7	Warm up • Jog 13 min • Walk 3 min • Jog 8 min (24 min) Cool down	Warm up • Jog 13 min • Walk 3 min • Jog 8 min (24 min) Cool down	Warm up • Jog 13 min • Walk 3 min • Jog 8 min (24 min) Cool down
8	Warm up • Jog 16 min • Walk 2 min • Jog 6 min (24 min) Cool down	Warm up • Jog 16 min • Walk 2 min • Jog 6 min (24 min) Cool down	Warm up • Jog 16 min • Walk 2 min • Jog 6 min (24 min) Cool down
9	Warm up • Jog 20 min Cool down	Warm up • Jog 20 min Cool down	Warm up • Jog 20 min Cool down
10	Warm up • Jog 25 min Cool down	Warm up • Jog 25 min Cool down	Warm up Jog 25 min Cool down
11	Warm up Jog 30 min Cool down	Warm up • Jog 30 min Cool down	Warm up • Jog 30 min Cool down
12	Warm up • Jog 35 min Cool down	Warm up • Jog 35 min Cool down	Warm up • Jog 35 min Cool down Add 5 min a week until you complete 5k!

The training days are 3 nonconsecutive days a week. Running time is listed as opposed to distance.

Straight Line Racing

Racing Greyhounds undergo high-intensity workouts, including galloping, trials, and racing, on average 2 times per week.[40] Any dog who will be racing following a lure line should practice close to maximum speed 2 days a week. The problem for any trainer is simulating the intense prey drive if they do not have access to a lure. For this reason, there are generally groups or organizations that provide a once weekly practice. In addition to that, the dog should chase an object (frisbee, ball, even a remote-control car) at high speed for multiple repetitions to mimic close to the distance ran with the lure. Straight line racing is usually over a distance of 150 to 200 yards.

Conditioning involves steadily lengthening sprint distance or, failing that, the time sprinted in rapidly repeating intervals.

Sample protocol:

This is for an unconditioned but generally fit dog, with the goal of running 150 to 200 yards. Owner has a lure at home.

(Rest days are numbered but not listed)

- Day 1 and day 3: 10 min walk out for warm up. Run him with the frisbee 5 x 30 feet. Cool down 5-minute walk then do active stretches.
- Day 5 and day 7: same regimen but 10 × 30 feet with the frisbee
- Day 9: run him with the straight line 50 yards x 2
- Day 11: 50 yards x 4 (this is broken down to 50 yards to ensure some rest between repetitions)

- Day 13: 100 yards x 3
- Day 16: 150 yards x 3
- Day 19: 150 yards x 4

Sledding/Skijoring and Bikejoring

Training for sledding, skijoring, and bikejoring is very similar, the latter being "a type of dryland mushing requiring high-intensity effort, with speed peaks close to 42 km/h."[41] Dogs should be medium to large size and generally fit (daily walks off leash so the dog is moving freely and at a brisk pace) before starting formal conditioning.

Goals of conditioning are to work on strength and endurance. In order to achieve the speed (ranging from slow canter to full gallop) and distance while pulling, many owners start conditioning with their dog running next to a bicycle or golf cart. Adding 25% of previous distance when the dog is performing without maximal effort. Once the target distance is achieved, then the load of pulling can be added. Rollerblades can be used for skijoring and an all-terrain vehicle for a sled team. Training should be at least 3 days a week or more frequent for professional mushers.

Protection Dog Sports

This sport is more complex than other canine sports as multiple disciplines including obedience, jumping, tracking, and protection work are practiced. It is most similar to 3-day eventing in the horse world except that when competing in this sport, all of the disciplines are often completed on the same day. Ring sports, in particular, require that the dog is on the field for the longest duration, often as long as 45 minutes at the highest levels. The dogs perform obedience, jumping (Palisade, Long Jump, Hurdle) and protection (biting a decoy-person wearing bite protection). At level 3, the highest level in Mondioring, there are a total of 17 exercises. These exercises are completed without interruption. Goals of conditioning are concentration, stamina, and strength. Obedience work requires a long duration of heeling with head lifted to watch the handler; retrieves can involve a 3 lb dumbbell. Long periods of concentration are required.

Lower height jumps are used to build foundational skills and strength with the goal of honing jumping mechanics. Subsequently, height is built incrementally by 2 to 4″ a week to get to 1.2 m (~47 inches), which is level 3 maximum points. Exposure to jumps at a greater than 0.75 m (30 inches) height is minimized for injury prevention; the dog should jump the greater heights only once or twice during a practice session and do more repetitions of lower jumps. The long jump is similarly practiced at incremental distance until the level 3 maximum points goal of 4 m (~13 feet) is reached. Forelimb and rear targeted strengthening apply for the Palisade jump (scaling a wall height from 1.8–2.3 m). Working with a decoy for protection training is often only feasible once weekly, and so tug replaces some of the work. Jaw and neck strength for bite work is achieved from tug exercises and balance work. Introducing dogs to decoy work starts with a short lead out distance, then incrementally building up distance and speed. The decoy can help guide the height of the bite and the resistance provided.

Flyball

Flyball is short sprints over relatively low jumps. The challenge is conditioning for impact on the box as the dog retrieves the ball and turns. Starting with the jump sequence and retrieving a ball on the ground will pattern turning at speed. Introducing the box is generally started at short distances, which should translate to slower speed; this in turn should be lower impact than the full flyball relay set up and should be slower, giving the dog time to learn the motions. Once the dog is conditioned to perform the 2 separate tasks of jumps and box turns, they are combined: first with a single jump and box combination and then adding jumps until the full set up is practiced.

WORKING DOGS

Conditioning for work should be specific to the job. Mental and physical stamina are important as well as strength. The Penn Vet Working Dog Center Fit to Work Program has been developed[42] and provides a step-by-step assessment and conditioning program.

SUMMARY

Sports- or activity-specific training should take up the bulk of training time. Combined or cross-training should focus on actions needed for the sport as well as general strength.

DISCLOSURE

No commercial or financial conflicts of interest.

REFERENCES

1. Rivero JL. A scientific background for skeletal muscle conditioning in equine practice. J Vet Med A Physiol Pathol Clin Med 2007;54(6):321–32.
2. Boston RC, Nunamaker DM. Gait and speed as exercise components of risk factors associated with onset of fatigue injury of the third metacarpal bone in 2-year-old Thoroughbred racehorses. Am J Vet Res 2000;61(6):602–8.
3. L.H. Fuglsang-Damgaard, A.P. Harrison, A.D. Vitger. Altered muscle activation in agility dogs performing warm-up exercises: an acoustic myography study. Comp Exerc Physiol, v. 17 ,.3 pp. 251-262.
4. Rampinini E, Impellizzeri FM, Castagna C, et al. Effect of match-related fatigue on short-passing ability in young soccer players. Med Sci Sports Exerc 2008;40(5):934–42.
5. Miller B, Hamilton K, Boushel R, et al. Mitochondrial respiration in highly aerobic canines in the non-raced state and after a 1600-km sled dog race. PLoS One 2017;12:e0174874.
6. Davis MS, Bonen A, Snook LA, et al. Conditioning increases the gain of contraction-induced sarcolemmal substrate transport in ultra-endurance racing sled dogs. PLoS One 2014;9(7):e103087.
7. Marsolais GS, McLean S, Derrick T, et al. Kinematic analysis of the hind limb during swimming and walking in healthy dogs and dogs with surgically corrected cranial cruciate ligament rupture. J Am Vet Med Assoc 2003;222(6):739–43.
8. Cronin J, McNair PJ, Marshall RN. Velocity specificity, combination training and sport specific tasks. J Sci Med Sport 2001;4(2):168–78.
9. Parsons D, Musch TI, Moore RL, et al. Dynamic exercise training in foxhounds. II. Analysis of skeletal muscle. J Appl Physiol 1985;59(1):190–7.
10. Kasper K. Sports training principles. Curr Sports Med Rep 2019;18(4):95–6.
11. Crowley E, Harrison AJ, Lyons M. The impact of resistance training on swimming performance: a systematic review. Sports Med 2017;47(11):2285–307.

12. Erickson KI, Voss MW, Prakash RS, et al. Exercise training increases size of hippocampus and improves memory. Proc Natl Acad Sci U S A 2011;108(7):3017–22.
13. Davis MS, Barrett MR. Effect of conditioning and physiological hyperthermia on canine skeletal muscle mitochondrial oxygen consumption. J Appl Physiol (1985) 2021;130(5):1317–25.
14. Ready AE, Morgan G. The physiological response of siberian husky dogs to exercise: effect of interval training. Can Vet J 1984;25(2):86–91.
15. Lopedote M, Valentini S, Musella V, et al. Changes in pulse rate, respiratory rate and rectal temperature in working dogs before and after three different field trials. Animals (Basel) 2020;10(4):733.
16. Shull SA, Rich SK, Gillette RL, et al. Heart rate changes before, during, and after treadmill walking exercise in normal dogs. Front Vet Sci 2021;8:641871.
17. Reitmaier S, Schmidt H. Review article on spine kinematics of quadrupeds and bipeds during walking. J Biomech 2020;102:109631.
18. Jayanthi NA, Post EG, Laury TC. Fabricant PD. Health Consequences of Youth Sport Specialization. J Athl Train 2019;54(10):1040–9.
19. Kiviranta I, Tammi M, Jurvelin J, et al. Moderate running exercise augments glycosaminoglycans and thickness of articular cartilage in the knee joint of young beagle dogs. J Orthop Res 1988;6(2):188–95.
20. Vrbanac Z, Brkljaca Bottegaro N, Skrlin B, et al. The effect of a moderate exercise program on serum markers of bone metabolism in dogs. Animals (Basel) 2020; 10(9):1481.
21. Kiviranta I, Tammi M, Jurvelin J, et al. Articular cartilage thickness and glycosaminoglycan distribution in the canine knee joint after strenuous running exercise. Clin Orthop Relat Res 1992;283:302–8.
22. Verheyen KL, Henley WE, Price JS, et al. Training-related factors associated with dorsometacarpal disease in young Thoroughbred racehorses in the UK. Equine Vet J 2005;37(5):442–8.
23. Cullen KL, Dickey JP, Bent LR, et al. Survey-based analysis of risk factors for injury among dogs participating in agility training and competition events. J Am Vet Med Assoc 2013;243(7):1019–24.
24. Pagano TB, Wojcik S, Costagliola A, et al. Age related skeletal muscle atrophy and upregulation of autophagy in dogs. Vet J 2015;206(1):54–60.
25. Strasser A, Simunek M, Seiser M, et al. Age-dependent changes in cardiovascular and metabolic responses to exercise in beagle dogs. Zentralbl Veterinarmed A 1997;44(8):449–60.
26. Kellmann M, Bertollo M, Bosquet L, et al. Recovery and Performance in Sport: Consensus Statement. Int J Sports Physiol Perform 2018;13(2):240–5.
27. Kraemer WJ, Adams K, Cafarelli E, et al. American College of Sports Medicine. American College of Sports Medicine position stand. Progression models in resistance training for healthy adults. Med Sci Sports Exerc 2002;34(2):364–80.
28. McGowan CJ, Pyne DB, Thompson KG, et al. Warm-up strategies for sport and exercise: mechanisms and applications. Sports Med 2015;45:1523–46.
29. Tsolakis C, Bogdanis GC. Acute effects of two different warm-up protocols on flexibility and lower limb explosive performance in male and female high level athletes. J Sports Sci Med 2012;11(4):669–75.
30. Shrier I. Does stretching improve performance? A systematic and critical review of the literature. Clin J Sport Med 2004;14(5):267–73.
31. Herbert RD, de Noronha M, Kamper SJ. Stretching to prevent or reduce muscle soreness after exercise. Cochrane Database Syst Rev 2011;(7):CD004577.

32. Osinchuk S, Taylor SM, Shmon CL, et al. Comparison between core temperatures measured telemetrically using the CorTemp® ingestible temperature sensor and rectal temperature in healthy Labrador retrievers. Can Vet J 2014;55(10):939–45.
33. Davis MS, Cummings SL, Payton ME. Effect of brachycephaly and body condition score on respiratory thermoregulation of healthy dogs. J Am Vet Med Assoc 2017;251(10):1160–5.
34. Davis MS, McKiernan B, McCullough S, et al. Racing Alaskan sled dogs as a model of "ski asthma. Am J Respir Crit Care Med 2002;166(6):878–82.
35. Gregersen CS, Silverton NA, Carrier DR. External work and potential for elastic storage at the limb joints of running dogs. J Exp Biol 1998;201(Pt 23):3197–210.
36. Vincent TL, Wann AKT. Mechanoadaptation: articular cartilage through thick and thin. J Physiol 2019;597(5):1271–81.
37. Sellon DC, Martucci K, Wenz JR, et al. A survey of risk factors for digit injuries among dogs training and competing in agility events. J Am Vet Med Assoc 2018;252(1):75–83.
38. Cullen KL, Dickey JP, Brown SH, et al. The magnitude of muscular activation of four canine forelimb muscles in dogs performing two agility-specific tasks. BMC Vet Res 2017;13(1):68.
39. Pfau T, Garland de Rivaz A, Brighton S, et al. Kinetics of jump landing in agility dogs. Vet J 2011;190(2):278–83.
40. Palmer AL, Rogers CW, Stafford KJ, et al. Cross-Sectional Survey of the Training Practices of Racing Greyhounds in New Zealand. Animals (Basel) 2020;10(11): 2032.
41. Benito M, Boutigny L. Cardiovascular clinical assessment in greyster dogs in bikejöring training. Animals (Basel) 2020;10(9):1635.
42. Farr BD, Ramos MT, Otto CM. The Penn vet working dog center fit to work program: a formalized method for assessing and developing foundational canine physical fitness. Front Vet Sci 2020;7:470.

Economic and Clinical Benefits of Orthopedic/ Sports Medicine and Rehabilitation

Juliette Hart, DVM, MS, CCRT, CVA, DACVSMR[a,b,c,d,*]

KEYWORDS

• Sports medicine and rehabilitation • Orthopedic medicine • Pain management
• Recovery • Orthopedics

KEY POINTS

- Orthopedic/Sports Medicine and Rehabilitation can be a vital and valuable addition to not only specialty and Emergency (ER) practices, but general practices as well
- Key strategies to successfully incorporate Orthopedic/Sports Medicine and Rehabilitation into your practice include:
  - Identify Orthopedic/Sports Medicine and Rehabilitation equipment needs early on to build and successfully run the service.
  - Fulfill staffing needs and requirements to ensure excellent patient care during treatments.
  - Schedule and design the optimum workflow early on to maximize space and hospital options, build on staff efficiency, and support hospital financial goals.
- Orthopedic/Sports Medicine and Rehabilitation communication are vital to partnership within general practice, specialty services and Critical Care/Emergency, quickly building caseload internally in order to build external capacity and referrals from the larger referral community.

INTRODUCTION

Sports medicine is frequently defined as medicine that focuses on the prevention, diagnosis and treatment of conditions that impact the function of athletes. Given the high number of equine athletes and their use for sporting activities, this definition

[a] Diplomate, Veterinary Sports Medicine and Rehabilitation – Small Animal; [b] Specialty Advisory Board, Sports Medicine and Rehabilitation – NVA Compassion First Hospitals; [c] Medical Director and Sports Medicine and Rehabilitation Department Head, Animal Emergency and Specialty Center, 17701 Cottonwood Drive, Parker, CO 80134, USA; [d] Certified in Veterinary Acupuncture (Large and Small Animal) and Rehabilitation

* Animal Emergency and Specialty Center, 17701 Cottonwood Drive, Parker, CO 80134,
E-mail address: juliettehart@gmail.com

Vet Clin Small Anim 52 (2022) 1059–1067
https://doi.org/10.1016/j.cvsm.2022.03.011

is quite applicable and accepted in equine veterinary medicine. However, it causes some confusion when applied to small animals since many owners do not consider their dog a canine athlete. Although many owners may believe that 'canine sports medicine' also applies to their companion animal, to avoid this confusion completely, the term orthopedic medicine may be more appropriate. This term conveys the goal of providing focused, nonsurgical care for musculoskeletal conditions, potentially appealing to a larger audience.

Previous articles in this issue covered many of the diagnostic and treatment modalities available for an Orthopedic/Sports Medicine and Rehabilitation service. The implementation of orthopedic/sports medicine and rehabilitation therapy continues to vary widely in the different types of practices. Yet, this implementation benefits the patient and can also result in economic benefits to the practice. But how does a hospital (whether general practice or specialty/Emergency) put it all together and incorporate Orthopedic Sports Medicine and Rehabilitation into practice? It can seem like a daunting project to embark upon. However, with careful planning and early determination of service goals and needs of the hospital, this incredible patient care resource can be built in a way that is not only financially advantageous but will contribute to the larger goal of excellent patient care within the hospital.

When a hospital is considering adding a Orthopedic/Sports Medicine and Rehabilitation service or offering some Orthopedic Medicine services, it is important to look at the overarching goals of the department, both independently and within the larger hospital. Consider the objectives of the American College of Veterinary Sports Medicine and Rehabilitation early on in hospital discovery:

- State-of-the-art veterinary care
- Research advancing scientific knowledge and the practice of evidence-based medicine
- Continuing education for veterinarians, students, and owners/handlers of pets, animal athletes, and working animals
- Public awareness of the benefits of working with certified specialists in veterinary sports medicine and rehabilitation.[1]

Whether the service is housed in academia, private practice (general practice or specialty private practice), these shared goals can be achieved in a variety of settings. Regardless of location, there are some simple starting goals in a practice offering Orthopedic/Sports Medicine and Rehabilitation.

- The primary care veterinarian, veterinary specialists, and the Orthopedic/Sports Medicine and Rehabilitation specialist (if applicable) are partners in case management and responsible for the medical diagnosis and decisions regarding appropriate rehabilitative care of a veterinary patient.
- Depending on the injury and repair, specific recommendations are made.[2]
- Communication and documentation between the Orthopedic/Sports Medicine and Rehabilitation team members and within all other services are critical.
- The Orthopedic/Sports Medicine and Rehabilitation team approach involves an evaluation or an assessment of the patient, the team documents their findings, meets, and decides together the most effective plan for intervention.[2]
- The rehabilitation plan and any home therapy and therapeutic exercises must be also communicated clearly to the owner and be successfully accomplished by the owner and the patient.
- An effective Orthopedic/Sports Medicine and Rehabilitation team contributes to the execution of the home program and can improve compliance if the team is

also supportive of the owner's process at home. If the owner is confident and an active member of the rehabilitation team, the team expects to see better compliance and communication. When things at home go well, that can be fantastic feedback; however, just as important is client communication of setbacks, struggles at home, and everything in between.
- Ultimately, the Orthopedic/Sports Medicine and Rehabilitation team becomes a supportive resource at home for the patient and client.

Although many Orthopedic/Sports Medicine and Rehabilitation practices have been successfully set up in academia and veterinary teaching hospitals, there are often additional unique challenges regarding integration into private practice (both specialty only, stand-alone, general practice, and Specialty and Emergency practices). If considering Orthopedic/Sports Medicine and Rehabilitation integration into private practice (general practice or Specialty/ER), a key question can be asked before a team begins: Is your practice considering integration of a new Orthopedic/Sports Medicine and Rehabilitation service into your existing general practice or Specialty and Emergency practice?

Consider partnering with a nearby Specialty and Emergency practice if you are a stand-alone practice or general practice. This not only builds a good relationship with the partner hospital but also provides that service to the Orthopedic/Sports Medicine and Rehabilitation patient appointments that may need more urgent care during their rehabilitation appointment (ie, the diabetic patient in crisis, patient with an elevated temperature, owner expressing concerns with lethargy, the doctor appreciates neurologic decline, acute vomiting, diarrhea, etc.).

For practices with an established orthopedic surgery group, consider the benefits of having a service that partners with the surgery team. Separation of the medical and surgical management of mobility disorders (ie, Orthopedic Medicine and Orthopedic Surgery as practiced at Colorado State University Veterinary Teaching Hospital) facilitates improved patient care, which in turn will result in economic benefits to the practice. For example, a geriatric, obese Labrador with chronic hip dysplasia would be seen by the Orthopedic/Sports Medicine and Rehabilitation team, freeing up appointment slots for the next surgical case. More specifically, both services receive consultations that fit within their specialty. This separation of care is beneficial for the client and the hospital; this integration allows the surgery team to spend more time in the OR, and the large number of chronic nonsurgical cases that require long-term osteoarthritis, pain and nutrition management is well taken care of within the Orthopedic/Sports Medicine and Rehabilitation service.

Physical Space

When considering a stand-alone private practice or integration into an existing Specialty and Emergency practice, one needs to carefully evaluate the needs for a dedicated rehabilitation space. Underwater treadmills, room for gait analysis, pressure-sensitive walkways, mobility gym (with therapeutic exercise equipment), and sporting equipment (agility) all will consume significant space in any building.

Diagnostic Capabilities

Does your hospital have dedicated diagnostics available (eg, radiology, anesthesia monitoring equipment, musculoskeletal ultrasound, bloodwork/diagnostic lab submission equipment/technology) and the capability to perform sedated and/or anesthetized procedures? If yes to the latter, is there dedicated recovery space? Although this physical footprint can be challenging, it is an important process to consider in terms of increasing value to the practice, as well as supporting Orthopedic/Sports Medicine and Rehabilitation needs in your area.

Staffing

When considering additional patient diagnostics and treatment options, it is important to also consider staffing. The following questions should be considered:

- Do you have dedicated team members responsible for patient intake, scheduling, phone calls?
- Do you have dedicated support staff to perform treatments, diagnostics, recovery, and therapeutic exercise training with the owner?
- Consider your rehabilitation team will most likely be with the patient ("hands-on") for the majority of the appointment—if your treatment appointments are only 30 to 45 minutes, a staff member will likely be with that patient the full 30 to 45 minutes, and unable to fill medications, answer phones, check patients out, etc.

One can consider the efficiency and effectiveness of one to two support staff per Orthopedic/Sports Medicine and Rehabilitation specialist, rehabilitation certified veterinarian or rehabilitation certified therapist. That designation affords one support member working with the patient at all times, and a "float" person to help when there are multiple patients, aid in restraint, assist in getting any modality equipment to the team members working with the patients, etc. If the practice has a diplomate in Orthopedic/Sports Medicine and Rehabilitation, then a dedicated technician (comfortable with sedation/anesthesia) and an assistant are essential to the process to maintain efficiency.

Incorporating into an existing Specialty and Emergency practice grants the Orthopedic/Sports Medicine and Rehabilitation service faster integration by using a centralized pharmacy, centralized Radiology (for radiographs, MSK, computed tomography, magnetic resonance imaging) with dedicated Radiology technicians and staff to facilitate procedures and also allocates the Orthopedic/Sports Medicine and Rehabilitation team more effectively to perform treatments and work through their day without decreasing efficiency, and minimizing appointment delay impact. Consultations can come through the Orthopedic/Sports Medicine and Rehabilitation team and then can be scheduled for any additional procedures, medications can be filled, patients can be recovered in the centralized anesthesia and recovery services, scheduling can occur, and then during discharge exercises can be reviewed with the owner in detail, similar to existing services in the hospital (Orthopedic Surgery, Neurology/Neurosurgery, etc.).

A Typical Day in Orthopedic/Sports Medicine and Rehabilitation

Within a Specialty and Emergency practice, morning cage-side rounds are an important integration piece in this scenario, as having a Sports Medicine and Rehabilitation diplomate present at morning rounds allows the emergency team to use rehabilitation support for any down/geriatric patient, surgeons/Neurology can discuss the orthopedic and neurologic cases undergoing surgery that day, and any painful cases in hospital (regardless of specialty) can be discussed so that ultimately patient care is at the forefront. In Orthopedic/Sports Medicine and Rehabilitation, you often have the opportunity to take primary case responsibility (neurologic dogs, geriatric dogs, stable postoperative neurology/orthopedic cases). After cage-side rounds, consider a 15- to 20-minute Orthopedic/Sports Medicine and Rehabilitation rounds so everyone on the team is aware of cases, reasons for visit, special owner or patient needs, and the team can review case selection, roles for the day, and any administrative duties (client callbacks, emails, scheduling, insurance paperwork, etc.)

Morning rounds are a vital part of the communication and efficiency of any veterinary service within a hospital, whether specialty or general practice. Although there are many experiences that make clinical training successful, clinic "rounds," where the veterinary team meets to discuss patients or topics, are still regarded as a central learning opportunity.[3] Whether the practice has an electronic "whiteboard" or a physical whiteboard, an external visual tool allows the team to communicate throughout the day. As with any specialty within veterinary medicine, the scheduled day can often change based on the needs of the patients, and as the Orthopedic/Sports Medicine and Rehabilitation teams go about their day, notes on the whiteboard help communicate changes, where people are located, additional needs and procedures, and any concerns. In Specialty and Emergency practices, an assigned "floater" Orthopedic/Sports Medicine and Rehabilitation team member is often used to help refill medications, process insurance, run bloodwork, submit samples, perform postoperative rehabilitation treatments, and facilitate any pickups/transfers in the hospital although the assigned schedule for the day is running efficiently.

Schedule

In human healthcare, the contribution margin has already been used to assess the profitability of a given service or department.[4] Although veterinary medicine continues to evolve with regard to balancing patient care and financial goals—specifically with regards to Orthopedic/Sports Medicine and Rehabilitation:

- How does the service set up a schedule that allows maximum patient care, efficient staffing, and financial goals?
- How many people are necessary in the Orthopedic/Sports Medicine and Rehabilitation team?
- How many patients are the team members safely able to see in a day?
- What are the chain-limiting modalities that need alternative solutions to maximize efficiency?
  - An underwater treadmill is a frequently used treatment modality in Orthopedic/Sports Medicine and Rehabilitation, and if the practice has 1 or 2 units, this important tool often determines the minimum and maximum efficiency within a scheduled day
  - The number of physical modality machines is also important to consider when planning the schedule.
  - Once the modalities have been identified, a schedule can be built around each modality used, staff member(s) needed, and any additional equipment needed.

It is common practice in Orthopedic/Sports Medicine and Rehabilitation to run concurrent "schedule tracks"—each rehabilitation veterinarian or therapist has a track of scheduled appointments, and depending on staffing, there can be one to four concurrent tracks of patients being seen on a typical day within a Orthopedic/Sports Medicine and Rehabilitation department. When scheduling, it is vital to consider the needs of every patient (temperament, ambulation status, systemic/health status, etc.) so the team has visibility into how many staff members are needed for each patient, and how best to allocate modalities (ie, if you have multiple underwater treadmills, but only one Class IV laser, etc.)

General Practice Integration

Are you considering adding in Orthopedic/Sports Medicine and Rehabilitation into your existing general practice? In these cases, implementation can often be streamlined. General practitioners are seeing cases every day that can benefit from rehabilitation.

- Routine wellness ("I noticed she doesn't jump into her cat tree as much anymore.")
- Geriatric evaluation ("He seems to be slowing down, and can't walk as far.")
- Primary lameness ("I noticed he's had a limp after the dog park.")
- Postsurgery ("She just seems weaker in that leg.")
- Weight ("I know she needs to lose weight, but she loves her food.")

All of the above examples are common, and with your physical examination, you may find that many of your patients would benefit from a structured rehabilitation program focusing on weight loss, muscle strengthening, pain control, and improving mobility long term. As with many patients, conversations about diet, nutrition, and supplements can often be helpful in maintaining their pet's lifelong mobility and function.

For the cases that require additional diagnostics or specialty referral may be recommended, consider partnering with your local Orthopedic/Sports Medicine and Rehabilitation Specialist. With a team approach, your patients will benefit, and your clients will look to you as a resource for their pets.

Postoperative Cases

In addition to the regular caseload, an excellent value add with low-time commitment to consider is Orthopedic/Sports Medicine and Rehabilitation integration into both postoperative orthopedic surgeries and neurologic cases. Consider assigning your "float" Orthopedic/Sports Medicine and Rehabilitation assistant to this role as a service cannot specifically predict when a surgery will depart the operating room—it is feasible to predict a 2-h window, but a surgery may run shorter or longer depending on the specifics of the surgery and patient, so it often less disruptive to the day if the "float" team member can tackle the postoperative treatments.

Additionally, having that "float" team member support the discharge process gives the surgery teams time to discharge their patient, while the Orthopedic/Sports Medicine and Rehabilitation support team member can then review and reinforce the Surgery discharges, importance of wearing an e-collar, review icing if appropriate, and all home exercises and stretching for that particular patient—also setting up the relationship early with the owner regarding the importance of rehabilitation and recovery at home.

Many hospitals will integrate a "Orthopedic/Sports Medicine and Rehabilitation postoperative rehabilitation package" and associated fee folded into all orthopedic and neurologic surgery case estimates for the owner, which can include one to two treatments although the patient is hospitalized. Additionally, at discharge, the first consultation can be set up in conjunction with the 2-week incision check (or suture removal) with both the Surgery and Orthopedic/Sports Medicine and Rehabilitation teams (scheduling for both appointments can be done at the time of initial discharge). At that 2 week appointment, the Orthopedic/Sports Medicine and Rehabilitation team evaluates the patient and determines if continued treatments are recommended, or full recovery can be augmented with a home exercise program. It is often at this time the Orthopedic/Sports Medicine and Rehabilitation team can evaluate the incision, identify concerns, and provide another resource for the client to support recovery at home.

Treatments

Determining treatment times and modalities is important to maximize staffing efficiencies as well. Do you allow clients in with the patients for your appointments? If yes, consider the additional time needed for communication, and also ensure that privacy is maintained with any other patients and clients in your rehabilitation/therapy space.

If you do not allow clients in the rehabilitation spaces, it often creates better efficiency of the day (both planned and unplanned). This is very important especially in a Specialty and Emergency hospital as there may be very sick, immune compromised, and painful patients in the treatment area, and both safety and care need to be considered with each patient in the Orthopedic/Sports Medicine and Rehabilitation space. The decision to allow clients in your space is a personal one, and it is important to consider the risks, pros, and cons of each opportunity and make the choice that is best for your business model.

When deciding how to set up your schedule:

- How much time is needed for each treatment?
- How much time does it take to check in and check out a patient?
- Many practices use treatment windows from 30 to 90 minutes depending on the services provided.

Choosing a time commitment for treatments naturally determines the flow of how many patients a Orthopedic/Sports Medicine and Rehabilitation service can see in a day, what efficiencies the practice has, and the financial goals of the practice.

Whether the Orthopedic/Sports Medicine and Rehabilitation service runs 4 to 5 days a week or 7 days a week, consider staffing options, as well as evening/weekend appointments. These options are often very attractive to owners, with evening and weekend appointments being chosen by clients. Potential downside is staffing needs after hours and weekends. Also consider the potential of charging for late cancels and missed (no show) appointments.

Additional Diagnostic Options: Pressure Sensitive Walkway

The use of objective gait analysis in clinical practice has steadily increased in recent years. As systems also become more affordable, equipment has become more readily available in both academia and private practice. Although frequently used in an academic setting, pressure-sensitive walkways can be both a value add for the Orthopedic/Sports Medicine and Rehabilitation Service and for critical research needs within the Specialty.

With research available on both force plate and pressure-sensitive walkway systems, for ease of discussion (and feasibility in private practice) pressure-sensitive walkways will be discussed in this section. Systems can vary in the overall physical dimension, measurement capabilities, as well as the degree of computerized automation[5,6]

Many pressure-sensitive walkways have a much smaller footprint, so if the hospital has a dedicated quiet and open space (roughly 8–10 dog-body lengths), a pressure-sensitive walkway may be used. In a hospital setting, the pressure-sensitive walkway can be used not only for objective gait analysis within Orthopedic/Sports Medicine and Rehabilitation but can also support Orthopedic Surgery, and Neurology Services by providing a resource to objectively measure and track lameness (and improvements) over time.

Additionally, if there is interest within the hospital, research opportunities based on objective gait analysis can be a valuable asset that contributes to the Orthopedic/Sports Medicine and Rehabilitation peer-reviewed literature library. You can also consider eliciting interest from local agility groups, and the hospital can offer objective gait analysis for the "team"—it not only opens the practice up to sporting dogs but also allows active canine (and feline) athletes the opportunity for an objective evaluation and potential treatment options to maintain their athletic ability over time.

Acupuncture/Integrative Medicine

Integrative medicine can also provide benefits not only for patients of Orthopedic/Sports Medicine and Rehabilitation but for every additional service in the hospital. A 2015 study solicited survey responses from general practices in Florida to evaluate the profitability of acupuncture and clients' perception of the service. A total of 68% of surveyed acupuncture clients and 65% of primary care clients responded that they would be more likely to use a veterinarian who offered acupuncture.[7]

Putting It all Together

With all the possibilities available with regard to treatment options and patients with Orthopedic/Sports Medicine and Rehabilitation, how does a hospital set up a service during launch, during initial growth, and then into maturity?

- Map out the space (what is the clinic footprint?)
- What equipment is necessary?
    - What is needed for day 1 start?
    - What is ideal for the long term?
- Identify staffing needs for startup and long term
- Finetune schedule efficiencies

With regard to equipment, possibly the largest single piece of equipment is an underwater treadmill. This particular equipment uses a very large footprint in the hospital—if you have one installed, will you reach a point in the future where a hospital can consider a second underwater treadmill or potentially a large pool. Does your floor plan support future additions?

Start Small and Build from Within

Orthopedic/Sports Medicine and Rehabilitation is an exciting and dynamic service. When a new service starts, a common pitfall is trying to be "too busy" from the start to maximize equipment use and staff time. A good guideline is to consider spending your ramp-up time training your team to maximize efficiency for the long term.

Consider adding in-house consultations and postoperative cases when starting to build out the Orthopedic/Sports Medicine and Rehabilitation service. Once the team is confident in the care, schedule, and flow, the service can start to see referrals from the larger referral community.

Orthopedic/Sports Medicine and Rehabilitation is a supportive and exciting part of many hospitals. With careful planning, staff training, and continuing education, your Orthopedic/Sports Medicine and Rehabilitation service will quickly grow and thrive.

CLINICS CARE POINTS

- Availability is critical early on in establishing an efficient and vital Orthopedic/Sports Medicine and Rehabilitation service. Injuries are happening in real time, and owners do not want to wait 4 weeks to be seen before starting a comprehensive recovery plan
- Use your resources: start small (internal hospital referrals) to build up caseload
- Efficiency is key: the number of cases a Orthopedic/Sports Medicine and Rehabilitation service can see is one key to productivity.

- Orthopedic/Sports Medicine and Rehabilitation cases require hands-on staffing the entire visit and that is a chain limiting step and should be factored into all models

DISCLOSURE

The author of this article has no commercial or financial conflicts of interest.

REFERENCES

1. American College of Veterinary Sports Medicine and Rehabilitation, vsmr.org
2. Millis DL, Levine D. Canine rehabilitation and physical therapy. 2nd edition. Elsevier; 2014. p. 30.
3. Lane IF, Cornell KK. Teaching tip: making the most of hospital rounds. J Vet Med Educ 2013;40(2):145–51.
4. Macario A, Dexter F, Traub RD. Hospital profitability per hour of operating room time can vary among surgeons. Anesth Analg 2001;93:669–75.
5. Duerr FM. Canine lameness. Wiley Blackwell; 2020.
6. Lascelles BD, Roe SC, Smith E, et al. Evaluation of a pressure sensitive walkway system for measurement of vertical limb forces in clinically normal dogs. Am J Vet Res 2006;67(2):277–82.
7. Shmalberg J, Marks D. Profitability and financial benefits of acupuncture in small animal private practice. Am J Traditional Chin Vet Med 2015;10(1):p43–8, 6p.

Printed and bound by CPI Group (UK) Ltd, Croydon, CR0 4YY

03/10/2024

01040474-0007